Social Phobia

SOCIAL PHOBIA
Diagnosis, Assessment, and Treatment

Edited by

RICHARD G. HEIMBERG
MICHAEL R. LIEBOWITZ
DEBRA A. HOPE
FRANKLIN R. SCHNEIER

THE GUILFORD PRESS
New York London

© 1995 The Guilford Press
A Division of Guilford Publications, Inc.
72 Spring Street, New York, NY 10012

Printed in the United States of America

This book is printed on acid-free paper.

Last digit is print number: 9   8   7   6   5   4   3   2   1

Library of Congress Cataloging-in-Publication Data

Social phobia: diagnosis, assessment, and treatment / edited by
    Richard G. Heimberg . . . [et al.].
        p.   cm.
    Includes bibliographical references and index.
    ISBN 1-57230-012-4
    1. Social phobia.   I. Heimberg, Richard G.
    [DNLM: 1. Phobic Disorders.   WM 178 S6778 1995]
RC552.S62S653   1995
616.85′225—dc20
DNLM/DLC
for Library of Congress   95-34091
                                                                    CIP

Contributors

Anne Marie Albano, PhD, Child and Adolescent Anxiety Disorders Program, Center for Stress and Anxiety Disorders, Department of Psychology, University at Albany, State University of New York, Albany, NY

David H. Barlow, PhD, Center for Stress and Anxiety Disorders, Department of Psychology, University at Albany, State University of New York, Albany, NY

Monroe A. Bruch, PhD, Department of Counseling Psychology, University at Albany, State University of New York, Albany, NY

Gillian Butler, PhD, Department of Psychiatry, Oxford University, Oxford, England

Tim F. Chapman, PhD, Institute for Health, Health Policy and Aging Research, Rutgers University, New Brunswick, NJ; New York State Psychiatric Institute, New York, NY

Jonathan M. Cheek, PhD, Department of Psychology, Wellesley College, Wellesley, MA

Robin L. Chene, MD, Dean Foundation for Health, Research and Education, Madison, WI

David M. Clark, DPhil, Department of Psychiatry, Warneford Hospital, Oxford University, Oxford, England

Jonathan R. T. Davidson, MD, Department of Psychiatry and Behavioral Sciences, Duke University Medical Center, Durham, NC

Patricia Marten DiBartolo, MA, Child and Adolescent Anxiety Disorders Program, Center for Stress and Anxiety Disorders, Department of Psychology, University at Albany, State University of New York, Albany, NY

Dirk Taylor Elting, MA, Department of Psychology, University of Nebraska–Lincoln, Lincoln, NE

Abby J. Fyer, MD, Department of Psychiatry, College of Physicians and Surgeons, Columbia University, New York, NY; New York State Psychiatric Institute, New York, NY

John H. Greist, MD, Dean Foundation for Health, Research and Education, Madison, WI

Leora R. Heckelman, PhD, Department of Psychiatry, College of Physicians and Surgeons, Columbia University, New York, NY; St. Luke's–Roosevelt Hospital, New York, NY

Richard G. Heimberg, PhD, Social Phobia Program, Center for Stress and Anxiety Disorders, Department of Psychology, University at Albany, State University of New York, Albany, NY

Debra A. Hope, PhD, Department of Psychology, University of Nebraska–Lincoln, Lincoln, NE

James W. Jefferson, MD, Dean Foundation for Health, Research and Education, Madison, WI

Harlan R. Juster, PhD, Social Phobia Program, Center for Stress and Anxiety Disorders, Department of Psychology, University at Albany, State University of New York, Albany, NY

David J. Katzelnick, MD, Dean Foundation for Health, Research and Education, Madison, WI

Kenneth A. Kobak, MSSW, Dean Foundation for Health, Research and Education, Madison, WI

Robin M. Kowalski, PhD, Department of Psychology, Western Carolina University, Cullowhee, NC

Mark R. Leary, PhD, Department of Psychology, Wake Forest University, Winston-Salem, NC

Michael R. Liebowitz, MD, Department of Psychiatry, College of Physicians and Surgeons, Columbia University, New York, NY; New York State Psychiatric Institute, New York, NY

Salvatore Mannuzza, PhD, Department of Psychiatry, College of Physicians and Surgeons, Columbia University, New York, NY; New York State Psychiatric Institute, New York, NY

Randall D. Marshall, MD, Department of Psychiatry, College of Physicians and Surgeons, Columbia University, New York, NY; New York State Psychiatric Institute, New York, NY

Daniel W. McNeil, PhD, Department of Psychology, West Virginia University, Morgantown, WV

Susan Mineka, PhD, Department of Psychology, Northwestern University, Evanston, IL

P. V. Nickell, MD, Department of Psychiatry, Medical College of Pennsylvania, Allegheny General Hospital, Pittsburgh, PA

Nicholas L. S. Potts, MD, Department of Psychiatry and Behavioral Sciences, Duke University Medical Center, Durham, NC

Ronald M. Rapee, PhD, School of Behavioural Sciences, Macquarie University, Sydney, New South Wales, Australia

Barry J. Ries, MS, Department of Psychology, Oklahoma State University, Stillwater, OK

Franklin R. Schneier, MD, Department of Psychiatry, College of Physicians and Surgeons, Columbia University, New York, NY; New York State Psychiatric Institute, New York, NY

Cynthia L. Turk, MS, Department of Psychology, Oklahoma State University, Stillwater, OK

Thomas W. Uhde, MD, Department of Psychiatry and Behavioral Neurosciences, School of Medicine, Wayne State University, Detroit, MI

Adrian Wells, PhD, Department of Psychiatry, Oxford University, Oxford, England

Richard Zinbarg, PhD, Department of Psychology, University of Oregon, Eugene, OR

Preface

Social phobia is the least well known of the anxiety disorders, and it is also the least well understood. Although it was discussed by Marks and Gelder as early as 1966, it did not become an official part of the diagnostic nomenclature until the publication of the third edition of the *Diagnostic and Statistical Manual of Mental Disorders* (DSM-III; American Psychiatric Association, 1980). As a result, research on social phobia lagged behind research on other anxiety disorders, and social phobia was referred to as "the neglected anxiety disorder" (Liebowitz, Gorman, Fyer, & Klein, 1985, p. 729).

While the inclusion of social phobia in DSM-III marked the beginning of serious efforts to understand this debilitating disorder, DSM-III described social phobia as something akin to a specific phobia of a social situation. Social phobia was believed to be a relatively rare disorder. It was further stated that social phobia was rarely incapacitating and that a patient was unlikely to have more than one social phobia. However, time and increased attention to social phobia have proven these ideas to be fallacious. Most individuals with social phobia experience fear of multiple situations (Holt, Heimberg, Hope, & Liebowitz, 1992; Liebowitz et al., 1985; Turner, Beidel, Dancu, & Keys, 1986), and the functional impairment associated with social phobia can be extreme, ranging from increased alcohol and substance abuse, depression, and suicidal ideation to unemployment and financial dependence (Schneier, Johnston, Hornig, Liebowitz, & Weissman, 1992). The seriousness and breadth of impairment associated with social phobia is reflected in the revised third edition and the fourth edition of the *Diagnostic and Statistical Manual of the Mental Disorders* (DSM-III-R and DSM-IV; American Psychiatric Association, 1987, 1994). As defined in DSM-III-R, social phobia is the third most common psychiatric disorder, behind major depression and alcohol dependence. Its lifetime prevalence rate of 13.3% (Kessler et al., 1994) clearly asserts that social phobia is a serious mental health problem, worthy of the attention of clinicians and researchers alike.

Since 1980, research on social phobia has increased exponentially. We have learned much more about it, and there is much to be happy about. Although there is still a distance to go, we have seen the development of increasingly sophisticated theoretical models. Several treatments, both pharmacological and cognitive-behavioral, have been developed and have shown to be effective at reducing the anxiety, avoidance, and impairment associated with social phobia. The next few years should produce further advancements in the diagnosis, assessment, and treatment of social phobia.

We are very excited about this book and what it represents. We have gathered together many of the world's leaders in the diagnosis, assessment, and treatment of social phobia. In the book's several chapters, the contributors present state-of-the-art reviews and analyses, providing the reader with a thorough and comprehensive resource on almost every aspect of social phobia. We believe that these works will prove useful to both the novice and the expert and to both the clinician and the researcher interested in social phobia.

The book is organized into five sections. In Part I, chapters on diagnostic issues by Heckelman and Schneier, epidemiology and family studies by Chapman, Mannuzza, and Fyer, and descriptive psychopathology by Rapee provide the reader with a thorough knowledge of the history and clinical presentation of individuals with social phobia.

In Part II, chapters are presented on several different theoretical and empirical approaches to the conceptualization of social phobia. Clark and Wells present a new and sophisticated cognitive model of social phobia. Leary and Kowalski present an application of their self-presentational model of social anxiety, representative of the best work on shyness and social anxiety from a social psychological perspective. Nickell and Uhde provide us with the most current thinking about the neurobiological underpinnings of social phobia. Mineka and Zinbarg present a thorough and comprehensive review of conditioning and ethological studies of several species, which suggests that social phobia may not be the specific province of human beings and which helps us to think about social phobia in broader perspective. Finally, Bruch and Cheek examine the developmental and temperamental underpinnings of social phobia.

Part III is devoted to the assessment of social phobia. Greist, Kobak, Jefferson, Katzelnick, and Chene provide us with an invaluable guide to the clinical interview with social phobics and to the use of structured interviews and clinician-administered assessment devices. McNeil, Ries, and Turk provide a thorough review and analysis of self-report, behavioral, and physiological assessment approaches. Elting and Hope discuss the area of cognitive assessment, that is, the assessment of information-processing styles and biases, which may be so important to the understanding of social phobia.

Part IV concerns treatment and has a little bit of something for everyone involved in the treatment of adults with social phobia. Heimberg and Juster provide a comprehensive review of the literature on the outcome of cognitive-behavioral treatments for social phobia, and this is followed by a thorough discussion by Butler and Wells of the application of cognitive-behavioral techniques. Similarly, in the realm of pharmacological treatment approaches, Potts and Davidson review the empirical literature on treatment, and Liebowitz and Marshall examine the many issues involved in the clinical application of these treatments to individuals with social phobia.

In Part V, Albano, DiBartolo, Heimberg, and Barlow extend the effort to the diagnosis, assessment, and treatment of children and adolescents with social phobia. This is an area of research that desperately requires our attention, and Albano et al. set us on the right track.

Social Phobia: Diagnosis, Assessment, and Treatment does not provide everything one needs to know about social phobia. We do not yet know everything we need to know, so research continues. However, the book is a comprehensive resource, and we hope it will stimulate you to think about social phobia in new ways.

As always, in efforts of this magnitude, there are many people to thank, and we can never adequately express our gratitude to all of them. One person in particular deserves our deepest thanks. Karen Law, administrative coordinator of the Social Phobia Program of the Center for Stress and Anxiety Disorders at the University at Albany and administrative assistant to Richard Heimberg, was responsible for so many aspects of this project. Thanks, Karen.

RICHARD. G. HEIMBERG, PhD
MICHAEL R. LIEBOWITZ, MD
DEBRA A. HOPE, PhD
FRANKLIN R. SCHNEIER, MD

REFERENCES

American Psychiatric Association. (1980). *Diagnostic and statistical manual of mental disorders* (3rd ed.). Washington, DC: Author.

American Psychiatric Association. (1987). *Diagnostic and statistical manual of mental disorders* (3rd ed., rev.). Washington, DC: Author.

American Psychiatric Association. (1994). *Diagnostic and statistical manual of mental disorders* (4th ed.). Washington, DC: Author.

Holt, C. S., Heimberg, R. G., Hope, D. A., & Liebowitz, M. R. (1992). Situational domains of social phobia. *Journal of Anxiety Disorders, 6,* 63–77.

Kessler, R. C., McGonagle, K. A., Zhao, S., Nelson, C. B., Hughes, M., Eshleman, S., Wittchen, H.-U., & Kendler, K. S. (1994). Lifetime and 12-month prevalence of

DSM-III-R psychiatric disorders in the United States. *Archives of General Psychiatry, 51,* 8–19.

Liebowitz, M. R., Gorman, J. M., Fyer, A. J., & Klein, D. F. (1985). Social phobia: Review of a neglected anxiety disorder. *Archives of General Psychiatry, 42,* 729–736.

Marks, I. M. & Gelder, M. G. (1966). Different ages of onset in varieties of phobias. *American Journal of Psychiatry, 123,* 218–221.

Schneier, F. R., Johnson, J., Hornig, C. D., Liebowitz, M. R., & Weissman, M. M. (1992). Social phobia: Comorbidity and morbidity in an epidemiologic sample. *Archives of General Psychiatry, 49,* 282–288.

Turner, S. M., Beidel, D. C., Dancu, C. V., & Keys, D. J. (1986). Psychopathology of social phobia and comparison to avoidant personality disorder. *Journal of Abnormal Psychology, 95,* 389–394.

Contents

Part I. History and Clinical Presentation

1. Diagnostic Issues   3
   Leora R. Heckelman and Franklin R. Schneier

2. Epidemiology and Family Studies of Social Phobia   21
   Tim F. Chapman, Salvatore Mannuzza, and Abby J. Fyer

3. Descriptive Psychopathology of Social Phobia   41
   Ronald M. Rapee

Part II. Theoretical and Empirical Approaches

4. A Cognitive Model of Social Phobia   69
   David M. Clark and Adrian Wells

5. The Self-Presentation Model of Social Phobia   94
   Mark R. Leary and Robin M. Kowalski

6. Neurobiology of Social Phobia   113
   P. V. Nickell and Thomas W. Uhde

7. Conditioning and Ethological Models of Social Phobia   134
   Susan Mineka and Richard Zinbarg

8. Developmental Factors in Childhood
   and Adolescent Shyness   163
   Monroe A. Bruch and Jonathan M. Cheek

Part III. Assessment

9. The Clinical Interview   185
   *John H. Greist, Kenneth A. Kobak, James W. Jefferson,
   David J. Katzelnick, and Robin L. Chene*

10. Behavioral Assessment: Self-Report, Physiology, and
    Overt Behavior   202
    Daniel W. McNeil, Barry J. Ries, and Cynthia L. Turk

11. Cognitive Assessment   232
    Dirk Taylor Elting and Debra A. Hope

Part IV. Treatment

12. Cognitive-Behavioral Treatments: Literature Review   261
    Richard G. Heimberg and Harlan R. Juster

13. Cognitive-Behavioral Treatments: Clinical Applications   310
    Gillian Butler and Adrian Wells

14. Pharmacological Treatments: Literature Review   334
    Nicholas L. S. Potts and Jonathan R. T. Davidson

15. Pharmacological Treatments: Clinical Applications   366
    Michael R. Liebowitz and Randall D. Marshall

Part V. Special Populations

16. Children and Adolescents: Assessment and Treatment   387
    *Anne Marie Albano, Patricia Marten DiBartolo,
    Richard G. Heimberg, and David H. Barlow*

Index   427

PART I

History and
Clinical Presentation

CHAPTER ONE

Diagnostic Issues

LEORA R. HECKELMAN
FRANKLIN R. SCHNEIER

The term "social phobia" (*phobie des situations sociales*) was first coined by Janet (1903) to describe patients who feared being observed while speaking, playing the piano, or writing. Syndromes of shyness, social anxiety, and social avoidance had been described as early as the time of Hippocrates (as quoted in Marks, 1969), who reported this case: "through bashfulness, suspicion, and timorousness, will not be seen abroad; . . . He dare not come in company, for fear he should be misused, disgraced, overshoot himself in gestures of speeches. . . . He thinks every man observed him . . ." (p. 362).

Persons with social phobia experience excessive fear of being humiliated or judged negatively in social or performance situations. In feared situations, they tend to be self-conscious and self-critical, and they often experience physical symptoms of anxiety, such as blushing, palpitations, sweating, and trembling. The extent of situations feared by persons with social phobia ranges from fear of a single discrete setting, such as performing on stage, to fear of virtually all interpersonal contacts. The anxiety in social situations often is part of a vicious cycle in which anticipatory anxiety at the prospect of entering feared settings leads to avoidance, which in turn increases both anticipatory anxiety and anxiety in social situations.

While persons with social phobia generally fear embarrassment or negative evaluation, the perceived causes of embarrassment vary widely. Some individuals are concerned that people will notice a symptom of anxiety, such as blushing, trembling hand or voice, or sweating. Others fear that they will speak an awkward phrase, make a mistake, or act in some other way that will embarrass or humiliate them. Some fear that they will be embarrassed by fleeing a feared situation without explanation.

The feared cause of embarrassment is often unlikely, as in the experienced actor who begins to fear that he will flee the stage, or it may be so excessive as to become catastrophic, as in the young woman who fears that her date will despise her if she stammers once. Low self-esteem is common. Persons with social phobia have at least some awareness that their fears are irrational or excessive.

Some physical manifestations of the disorder, such as blushing or averting the gaze, are relatively specific to social anxiety. Other anxiety symptoms, such as sweating, palpitations, trembling hand or speech, or urge to defecate, are common to many anxiety states. Typical panic disorder symptoms of dizziness and dyspnea seem to be less common in social phobic anxiety episodes. The person with social phobia is also generally aware from the start of an anxiety reaction that it is related to social or performance fear and rarely fears dying during an episode, unlike persons with panic disorder.

Some persons with social phobia report no physical symptoms of anxiety, but only self-consciousness and fear. The apprehension and worrying may begin minutes, days, or even months before an anticipated difficult social or performance situation. This anticipatory anxiety may include worrying and physical symptoms of anxiety and may in itself be impairing. The greatest source of impairment, however, is often phobic avoidance. It may be subtle, as in avoiding consistent eye contact or avoiding initiating social conversation, or extreme, as in avoiding all interpersonal contacts outside his or her immediate family. Some people may build their lives around the limitations of social phobia: choosing a "back room" job over a better position for which they are otherwise well qualified or settling for an unhappy relationship rather than facing the anxiety of meeting new people.

HISTORY OF THE DIAGNOSIS

The emergence of social phobia as a specific diagnostic entity is relatively recent. Early classifications of the first and second editions of the *Diagnostic and Statistical Manual of Mental Disorders* (DSM-I and DSM-II; American Psychiatric Association, 1952, 1968) grouped all phobias together, consonant with a psychoanalytic perspective that considered phobic symptoms to be the product of unacceptable instinctual urges (Freud, 1926/1961). Following the findings of Marks and Gelder (1966) that particular phobias could be distinguished by characteristic ages of onset, specific criteria for social phobia were established in the third edition of the DSM (DSM-III; American Psychiatric Association, 1980), a diagnostic system that attempted to be neutral with respect to theories of etiology. The central feature of social phobia was excessive fear of observation or scrutiny in discrete, performance-oriented situations. These situations included public speaking or specific acts such as writing or using a urinal in front of other people. Persons who met the criteria for avoidant personality disorder, in which many social situations were typically avoided, were excluded from the diagnosis of social phobia. The DSM-III definition also required that the disturbance must cause "significant distress" and that fears must be recognized by the individual as "excessive or unreasonable" (American Psychiatric Association, 1980, p. 228).

As it became more apparent that some persons with social phobia feared many social situations (Liebowitz, Gorman, Fyer, & Klein, 1985), the diagnostic revision of DSM-III (DSM-III-R; American Psychiatric Association, 1987) introduced a generalized subtype of social phobia defined by fear of most social situations. Together with the deletion of the arbitrary DSM-III exclusion of those who met the criteria for avoidant personality disorder, this change broadened the scope of social phobia. In the generalized subtype, persons fear embarrassment or humiliation when engaged in most types of social interaction, including talking to strangers, colleagues, bosses, and even acquaintances. The generalized subtype of social phobia was distinguished from its unnamed complementary subtype, which has since been designated variously as "nongeneralized," "discrete," "specific," or "performance" (Heimberg, Holt, Schneier, Spitzer, & Liebowitz, 1993).

DEVELOPMENT OF DSM-IV CRITERIA FOR SOCIAL PHOBIA

Whereas prior versions of the DSM were based primarily on the judgment of experienced clinicians and researchers, an effort was made by the DSM-IV Task Force to base revisions on empirical data. The greater availability of such data was partly a result of the establishment of operational criteria in prior versions of the DSM. In developing the fourth edition of the DSM (DSM-IV; American Psychiatric Association, 1994), the social phobia subworkgroup identified several ambiguous diagnostic issues for possible revision. Comprehensive and systematic literature reviews were written on these issues, most of which related to defining the relationship of social phobia to several other conditions, including shyness, test anxiety, generalized anxiety disorder (GAD), substance abuse and dependence, avoidant personality disorder, social phobia symptoms secondary to panic disorder, and social phobia symptoms secondary to an embarrassing medical condition. Also considered were alternative subtyping criteria, utility of physiological and biochemical measures, and cross-cultural aspects of diagnosis.

The DSM-IV Task Force's conclusions, summarized below, are discussed in greater detail elsewhere (Schneier, Liebowitz, Beidel, Fyer, et al., in press). Related issues in clinical diagnosis are discussed later in this chapter. For most topics reviewed by the DSM-IV Task Force, empirical data were found to be insufficient to justify changing existing criteria.

Shyness was found to overlap extensively with social phobia, but lack of a broadly accepted definition of shyness prevented delineation of a specific boundary with social phobia. Test anxiety was recognized as a type of performance anxiety (fears that performance on the test would be evaluated negatively by others). Test anxiety was, therefore, included as an example of social phobia in the DSM-IV descriptive text. GAD, which may include social and nonsocial areas of worry, was found to overlap somewhat with social phobia, but there were insufficient data to define a more specific border. Alcohol abuse and dependence were also noted to frequently co-occur with social phobia. Therefore, to assess whether social phobia is an independent diagnosis in comorbid cases, users of the DSM-IV system were encouraged to consider whether social phobic symptoms precede the onset of substance abuse or persist during prolonged periods of abstinence. Avoidant personality disorder was found to overlap extensively with the generalized subtype of social phobia, but there remained insufficient evidence of unity to merge the disorders. In regard to the differential diagnosis of social phobia from panic disorder with agoraphobia, specific criteria were not defined due to the complexity of the issue. Diagnostic guidelines useful in considering this distinction were discussed in the text of DSM-IV.

A review of social anxiety secondary to another embarrassing psychiatric or medical condition (such as stuttering, benign essential tremor, or Parkinson's disease) found evidence for considerable social phobic symptomatology secondary to such conditions. Preliminary evidence for the efficacy of standard social phobia treatments in patients with these conditions exists, but it is limited to case reports (Oberlander, Schneier, & Liebowitz, 1994). In the absence of conclusive empirical validation that secondary social phobia is similar to primary social phobia, it was decided to continue to exclude the diagnosis of social phobia when symptoms are related to another embarrassing condition.

For the issue of subtypes of social phobia, the DSM-III-R distinction of a generalized subtype based on fear of "most social situations" has been partially validated in comparison to nongeneralized social phobia by differences in demographics, social and family background, level of severity and impairment, behavioral and physiological response to behavioral challenge, and possibly by differential response to medications and psychosocial treatments (reviewed in Heimberg et al., 1993). Despite this preliminary support of validity, criticisms of the DSM-III-R subtyping have included the following: (1) unclear definition of the phrase "most social situations"; (2) questionable face validity of basing a categorical distinction on quantity of situations feared rather than on the quality of situations feared, such as a distinction between fear of performance situations versus fear of socially interactive situations; (3) lack of conclusive evidence for a true qualitative distinction between subtypes, as opposed to a continuum of severity; and (4) absence of an intermediate subtype that could be used to describe persons with fear of several, but less than most, interpersonal situations.

The DSM-IV Task Force attempted to address these concerns by examining the reliability and validity of several alternative subtyping systems in a reanalysis of existing data on 229 patients at three research clinics (Schneier, Liebowitz, Beidel, Garfinkel, et al., in press). This study found that performance anxiety without significant fear of any socially interactive situations was present in only 6% of this sample of clinic patients, fear of one or two socially interactive situations was present in 24%, and fear of three or more socially interactive situations was present in 70%. Rates of the generalized subtype alternatively defined by fear of "most situations" and by fear of "3 or more socially interactive situations" did not differ significantly. Reliability and validity of a system based on *qualitative* distinctions was not clearly superior to reliability of the DSM-III-R subtyping system. The DSM-IV Task Force concluded that in the absence of clear superiority for proposed new definitions, the DSM-III-R subtyping system should be retained.

Another consideration in DSM-IV development was a preference for diagnostic continuity from childhood to adulthood. Social phobia has been shown to be a common problem in childhood (Strauss & Last, 1993), and there was concern that use of alternative diagnoses in children, such as avoidant disorder, might obscure the lifetime course of the social phobic syndrome. To address this concern, it was decided to delete the avoidant disorder of childhood diagnosis and to include features specific to children in the DSM-IV social phobia criteria. The DSM-IV criteria specify that, in children, social phobia must be distinguished from social anxiety that is limited to fear of adults. The criteria note that anxiety in children may be expressed differently than in adults (i.e., by children's crying, tantrums, freezing, or withdrawal). Also, children with social phobia, unlike adults with social phobia, may not recognize that their fear is irrational.

Review of the cross-cultural literature showed that cultural differences appear to affect the prevalence and characteristics of social phobia. In Saudi Arabia, social phobia was diagnosed in 13% of 305 patients with "neurotic disorders" seeking treatment at one hospital clinic (Chaleby, 1987). In comparison with other patients in that setting, social phobic patients were more likely to be male (80% vs. 40%), were better educated, and had a higher occupational status. Chaleby attributed what he considers to be a high prevalence of social phobia in Saudi Arabia to the rigidly conformist rules governing social behavior and the tremendous importance of preserving a good reputation in that society.

Social phobia has long been a subject of interest in Japanese psychiatry, where the term *"taijin kyofu-sho"* has been used to describe a spectrum of conditions involving fear of interpersonal relations (Takahashi, 1989). One feature of social phobia in Japan, a feature that received little attention in the West, is the fear that a person's social unease will make *others* uncomfortable. Studies in Japan and Korea have also often grouped social phobic syndromes with referential or delusional social fears, but there was insufficient information on this issue to support the inclusion of delusional social fears in DSM-IV criteria.

The DSM-IV subworkgroup also considered alternative names for social phobia, because of concern that the term "phobia" was inappropriate for the more generalized and pervasive forms of the syndrome. The term "social anxiety disorder" was considered, but there was no clear consensus for its superiority, and changing recently established terminology would be confusing. It was ultimately decided to retain "social phobia" but to also adopt "social anxiety disorder" as an alternative term in DSM-IV (see Table 1.1).

THRESHOLDS FOR THE DIAGNOSIS

The Issue of "Caseness"

Although most studies of social phobia have used clinical samples, recent community studies have found that most persons with social phobia do not seek treatment (Schneier, Johnson, Hornig, Liebowitz, & Weissman, 1992). An even larger pool of persons with extreme fear of embarrassment do not meet criteria for the disorder because their feared situations can be avoided without functional impairment (Pollard & Henderson, 1988). This leads to questions about the appropriate threshold for a definition of caseness within the spectrum of social phobic and social anxiety symptoms. In a recently completed Canadian telephone survey of 526 randomly selected respondents, Stein, Walker, and Forde (1994) examined the effects of different thresholds for determining caseness in persons with social anxiety.

In one condition, caseness was based on extent of impact of social fears. Persons who had reported social anxiety in at least one situation (*n* = 318) were asked if their discomfort or nervousness in their most anxiety-evoking situation had had any negative effect on their life at home, work, or school or had bothered them personally (i.e., caused marked distress, as required in the DSM-III-R social phobia criteria). Of those reporting

TABLE 1.1. DSM-IV Definition of Social Phobia (Social Anxiety Disorder)

A. A marked and persistent fear of one or more social or performance situations in which the person is exposed to unfamiliar people or to possible scrutiny by others. The individual fears that he or she will act in a way (or show anxiety symptoms) that will be humiliating or embarrassing. **Note**: In children, there must be evidence of the capacity for age-appropriate social relationships with familiar people and the anxiety must occur in peer settings, not just in interactions with adults.

B. Exposure to the feared social situation almost invariably provokes anxiety, which may take the form of a situationally bound or situationally predisposed Panic Attack. **Note**: In children, the anxiety may be expressed by crying, tantrums, freezing, or shrinking from social situations with unfamiliar people.

C. The person recognizes that the fear is excessive or unreasonable. **Note**: In children, this feature may be absent.

D. The feared social or performance situations are avoided or else endured with intense anxiety or distress.

E. The avoidance, anxious anticipation, or distress in the feared social or performance situation(s) interferes significantly with the person's normal routine, occupational (academic) functioning, or social activities or relationships, or there is marked distress about having the phobia.

F. In individuals under age 18 years, the duration is at least 6 months.

G. The fear or avoidance is not due to the direct physiological effects of a substance (e.g., a drug of abuse, a medication) or a general medical condition and is not better accounted for by another mental disorder (e.g., Panic Disorder With or Without Agoraphobia, Separation Anxiety Disorder, Body Dysmorphic Disorder, a Pervasive Developmental Disorder, or Schizoid Personality Disorder).

H. If a general medical condition or another mental disorder is present, the fear in Criterion A is unrelated to it, e.g., the fear is not of Stuttering, trembling in Parkinson's disease, or exhibiting abnormal eating behavior in Anorexia Nervosa or Bulimia Nervosa.

Specify if:
  Generalized: if the fears include most social situations (also consider the additional diagnosis of Avoidant Personality Disorder)

Note. From American Psychiatric Association (1994, pp. 416–417). Copyright 1994 by the American Psychiatric Association. Reprinted by permission.

social anxiety 31% (or 19% of the total sample) reported "moderate" or "a great deal" of psychosocial disruption or personal distress. Only 12% of those reporting social anxiety (or 7% of the total sample) met the more stringent threshold criterion of "a great deal" of disruption or distress.

In another approach, caseness was based on the number of situations in which the individual reported experiencing stress: At least one social situation was reported by 69% of the subjects, 40% reported two or more situations, and 18% reported at least three situations. The large proportion of persons fearing only one situation differs from findings in clinical samples, where most patients fear more than one situation (Holt, Heimberg, Hope, & Liebowitz, 1992; Turner, Beidel, Dancu, & Keys, 1986). Fear of multiple situations probably contributes to impairment and to the likelihood of seeking treatment.

The different methods for determining caseness point to the difficulties in setting thresholds for the diagnosis of mental disorders in general and for social phobia in particular. Caseness varies with the cutoff point used to determine significant impairment or distress. In addition, since most social phobic persons in the community fear only one situation, epidemiological screeners must ask about a broad range of situations in order to avoid missing cases. Although social phobic patients seeking treatment are more likely to report multiple feared situations than are nonpatients, it remains important for clinicians to ask about a broad range of situations to define the scope of the problem.

In summary, the distinction between social phobia and subsyndromal social anxiety and distress rests heavily on the assessment of social impairment and distress. This is rarely problematic in clinical settings, where patients have decided to seek relief from impairment and distress. It may be an important source of variability, however, in assessing the prevalence of the diagnosis in community settings and assessing social phobia as a comorbid disorder in clinical studies.

Shyness

Social phobic patients often describe themselves as shy, and it is possible that shyness is a useful descriptor for social phobia. On the other hand, it is unclear where shyness ends and social phobia begins. Since there are no clear clinical criteria for shyness, most studies (recently reviewed by Turner, Beidel & Townsley, 1990) have defined this by subjects' self-attribution as shy or nonshy. The cognitions reported by shy and social phobic groups are very similar; both report a fear of negative evaluation when engaged in social interactions (Ludwig & Lazarus, 1983). Amies, Gelder, and Shaw (1983) and Turner and Beidel (1989) report that somatic arousal symptoms (such as blushing, palpitations, muscle twitching, trembling, and sweating) appear to be similar for shy individuals and social phobics. Both groups also appear to be different from normals on heart rate and blood pressure measures of stress response (Kagan, Reznick, & Snidman, 1988; Turner & Beidel, 1989).

Despite these similarities, self-defined shyness appears to be far more prevalent than social phobia. Prevalence rates for shyness have been reported to be 20–40% among college students (Spielberger, Pollans, &

Wordern, 1984). By contrast, the estimated 12-month population prevalence rate for DSM-III-R social phobia is 7.9%, and the estimated lifetime prevalence for DSM-III-R social phobia is 13.3% (Kessler et al., 1994). Because shyness is also usually self-defined, without specific criteria, it is a more heterogeneous category than social phobia. Shyness may overlap subclinical and mild cases of social phobia, yet it may also extend outside of the social phobia spectrum.

Test Anxiety

Beidel recently reviewed the large literature on test anxiety for the DSM-IV subworkgroup (Schneier, Liebowitz, Beidel, Fyer, et al., in press), selecting a few "classic" papers for more detailed review. Test anxious populations showed elevated levels of social-evaluative anxiety, and a 19% rate of test anxiety was reported in one study of social phobia. Physiological response in test anxious subjects was similar to that reported for social phobics. The social phobia subworkgroup concluded that test anxiety should be considered a form of discrete social phobia if it meets the other required criteria, including the criterion for impairment and distress.

Social Phobia Secondary to Other Psychiatric or Medical Illness

Liebowitz et al. (1985) have described a "secondary social phobia" that can arise when phobic avoidance results from a comorbid psychiatric or medical illness. For example, an individual with benign essential tremor, initially unrelated to social anxiety, may begin to avoid public situations out of fear that it would be embarrassing if others noticed the tremor. For this individual, the social avoidance is secondary to concern about the tremor. Conditions such as stuttering, Parkinson's disease, benign essential tremor, obesity, and severe disfigurement secondary to burns are among those in which related social anxiety has been reported. DSM-IV currently excludes these conditions from the diagnosis of social phobia and places them in the category "anxiety disorder not otherwise specified." Further research in this area is needed to confirm early reports that anxiety in such patients is sometimes responsive to social phobia treatment (Oberlander et al., 1994).

DIFFERENTIAL DIAGNOSIS AND COMORBIDITY

With the development of specific treatments for social phobia, its differential diagnosis from other disorders has taken on greater clinical relevance.

Other mental disorders commonly occur together with social phobia. The Epidemiologic Catchment Area (ECA) study found that 69% of the social phobic persons in the community had comorbid lifetime mental illnesses, and the onset of social phobia occurred first in 77% (Schneier et al., 1992). The relatively early onset of social phobia suggests that it could be an etiological factor, or at least a vulnerability marker of risk, for developing another disorder. The disorders with the highest lifetime prevalence among persons with social phobia in the ECA study were simple phobia (59%), agoraphobia (45%), alcohol abuse (19%), major depression (17%), and drug abuse (13%). All diagnoses examined were significantly more prevalent among persons with social phobia than among persons without social phobia (Schneier et al., 1992).

Panic Disorder with Agoraphobia

This diagnostic distinction is sometimes difficult in a patient with both panic attacks and social anxiety or avoidance. Panic attacks related to fear of social or performance situations may occur as part of the social phobia syndrome. Conversely, fear of social situations may occur in panic disorder, secondary to unexpected panic attacks. Social phobia and panic disorder also co-occur rather frequently. The central issue for this differential diagnosis is to determine the patient's reason for fearing social (or performance) situations. In panic disorder with agoraphobia, social fear occurs secondary to fear of having an unexpected panic attack (or a panic attack cued by a nonsocial stimulus, such as a confined space) in the presence of other people. In social phobia, social situations directly elicit fear of embarrassment. The distinction between these disorders is clinically important because of possible differential efficacy of certain treatments, both pharmacological and psychological.

Mannuzza, Fyer, Liebowitz, and Klein (1990) reviewed group differences between social phobic and agoraphobic patients. First, the mean age of onset for social phobia (midteens) tends to be earlier than the mean age of onset for agoraphobia (early to mid-20s). Second, among patients presenting for treatment, those with agoraphobia are more likely to be female, whereas those with social phobia are more likely to be male or are either equally distributed by gender.

The typical anxiety symptoms reported by the two groups also differ. Studies of symptoms (Amies et al., 1983; Cameron, Thyer, Nesse, & Curtis, 1986; Reich, Noyes, & Yates, 1988) found that blushing and muscle twitching were more common complaints in social phobia, whereas breathing problems, dizziness, palpitations, chest pains, blurry vision, headaches, and ringing in the ears were more common in agoraphobia. In addition,

social phobic patients rarely fear that they will die during an anxiety episode, whereas fears of dying, losing control, or "going crazy" during a
panic attack are classic features of panic disorder with agoraphobia.

The nature of anxiety attacks in the two disorders also differs in that
spontaneous or uncued panic attacks are often observed in patients with
panic disorder but do not occur in social phobia. Similarly, social phobic
patients are not awakened from sleep by nocturnal panic attacks. In persons
with social phobia, a panic attack that is initially reported as unexpected
may, on further probing, be found to relate to thoughts about a social or
performance situation.

While social phobic patients generally report feeling more comfortable
when alone, panic patients feel safer in the company of others. Both groups
may avoid public places, but social phobic patients fear that public scrutiny,
judgment, or humiliation could occur there. Panic disorder patients, by contrast, generally fear being trapped in a closed-in or crowded space from which
they would not be able to escape in the event of a panic attack.

Generalized Anxiety Disorder

The distinction between GAD and social phobia can be unclear when
worries about social situations are present along with other nonsocial fears.
There is a small amount of data suggesting that GAD and social phobia
differ in characteristic symptoms. For example, in one study, insomnia was
found to be more common in GAD than in social phobia (Versiani, Mundim, Nardi, & Liebowitz, 1988). Other studies (Reich et al., 1988; Cameron
et al., 1986) suggest that, compared to patients with GAD, social phobic
patients have fewer headaches, less frequent fear of dying, and more frequent sweating, flushing, and dyspnea. These group differences, however,
are unlikely to be decisive in determining diagnosis. The most important
diagnostic indicator here is whether significant fear of embarrassment or
humiliation is present. If it is present along with other spheres of worry
and the other required criteria, both disorders may be diagnosed.

Depression

Both social phobic and depressed patients exhibit social withdrawal and
avoidance of social situations. The central feature of this diagnostic distinction lies in the assessment of what motivates the withdrawal and avoidance.
Social avoidance, observed in the context of a depressive picture, will
usually be secondary to anhedonia or lack of energy. The same avoidance
in social phobia is associated with a fear of being scrutinized or judged by

others. Unlike depressed patients, social phobic patients believe that if they were able to feel less concerned about the evaluation of others, they would enjoy being in the company of others.

Several research teams have reported evidence for high rates of comorbidity of social phobia and depression. Munjack and Moss (1981), for example, reported that one-third of their social phobic patients had either a past or present history of depression. Another study reported that 5 of 11 unselected social phobic patients met DSM-III-R criteria for major depression past or present (Liebowitz et al., 1985), and depressive symptoms were present in half of the social phobic patients in a third sample (Amies et al., 1983). The "atypical" subtype of depression, which is characterized by hypersensitivity to rejection or criticism, has been noted to bear a similarity to social phobia (Liebowitz et al., 1985), and both conditions may be preferentially responsive to monoamine oxidase inhibitors over tricyclic antidepressant medications (Liebowitz et al., 1992). Other patients with primary depression appear to develop true fear of embarrassment in social situations, but it occurs only during episodes of major depression, and the social fears remit along with the depression (Dilsaver, Qamar, & Del Medico, 1992). Therefore, when social phobia and major depression are comorbid, the diagnosis of social phobia can be made with confidence only if there was a time in the patient's life when social phobic symptoms were present in the absence of major depression. If major depression complicates an already existing social phobic picture, it may be necessary for treatment to address both conditions. Dysthymia may also co-occur with social phobia, but its clinical significance in such cases is unclear, and dysthymia has not been shown to limit the effectiveness of treatment directed at social phobia.

Avoidant Personality Disorder

Several studies have demonstrated high rates of DSM-III-R avoidant personality disorder (50–89%) among patients with the generalized subtype of social phobia but lower rates (21–23%) among patients with the discrete subtype (Herbert, Hope, & Bellack, 1992; Holt, Heimberg, & Hope, 1992; Schneier, Spitzer, Gibbon, Fyer, & Liebowitz, 1991). Additionally, it appears that most patients with avoidant personality disorder also meet criteria for social phobia. This overlap is not surprising, given the similarity of the criteria for the two disorders in DSM-III-R. Compared to persons with generalized social phobia alone, persons with comorbid avoidant personality disorder have been reported to have more severe anxiety, more impairment in functioning, and more comorbidity with other disorders, but no worse social skills or public speaking performance (Herbert et al., 1992;

Holt, Heimberg, & Hope, 1992; Turner, Beidel, & Townsley, 1992). Persons with generalized social phobia with and without avoidant personality disorder appear to differ in the average severity of their social phobia (with the presence of avoidant personality disorder describing more severe psychopathology), but they have not been found to differ *qualitatively* in any substantial way. These findings demonstrate the blurred border between phobic symptomatology and personality traits in the area of social anxiety and avoidance.

The criteria for avoidant personality disorder in DSM-IV are even more similar to those of generalized social phobia than they were in DSM-III-R. These avoidant personality disorder criteria include avoidance of interpersonal activities due to fear of criticism, restraint within intimate relationships due to fear of being ridiculed, preoccupation with rejection in social situations, inhibition in new interpersonal situations, belief that one is socially inept, and reluctance to engage in new activities because they may prove embarrassing.

Rather than attempting differential diagnosis between such similar criteria sets, it seems more useful to consider these patients from the perspectives of both Axis I and Axis II. Generalized social phobia behaves much like a personality disorder. It has a mean age of onset in the preteens or early teens (Holt, Heimberg, & Hope, 1992; Schneier et al., 1991), and its symptoms are chronic and pervasive. Yet while personality disorders have traditionally been considered to be responsive only to intensive psychotherapy, avoidant personality disorder features have been reported to be responsive to treatment with monoamine oxidase inhibitors (Liebowitz et al., 1992) and cognitive-behavioral treatments (see Heimberg & Juster, Chapter 12, this volume). It is important for the clinician planning treatment to consider the co-diagnosis of social phobia in all cases of avoidant personality disorder, as there is now a substantial literature guiding pharmacological and psychosocial treatments for the former.

Schizophrenic Spectrum Disorders

Little research has been done on the relationship of nonpsychotic social fears in social phobia to delusional or paranoid social fears in schizophrenia spectrum disorders. The differential diagnosis of social phobia from schizophrenia, schizotypal personality, and schizoid personality, however, is usually clear. Persons with these disorders usually fear and avoid social situations because of lack of social interest or delusional fears of harm, rather than because of fear of embarrassment. Data from the ECA study suggest that a social phobic syndrome is often present in persons with schizophrenia (Schneier et al., 1992), but the clinical significance of such symptoms is unclear.

Alcoholism

Social phobia is commonly accompanied by alcohol abuse and dependence. Five studies examining alcoholic inpatients found rates of social phobia of 8–56% (Bowen, Cipywnyk, D'Arcy, & Keegan, 1984; Chambless, Cherney, Caputo, & Rheinstein, 1987; Mullaney & Trippett, 1979; Smail, Stockwell, Canter, & Hodgson, 1984; Stravynski, Lamontagne, & Lavallee, 1986), significantly more than the prevalence of DSM-III-R social phobia reported in the general population. Conversely, high rates of alcoholism (16–36%) have been observed among social phobic samples in three reports (Amies et al., 1983; Schneier, Martin, Liebowitz, Gorman, & Fyer, 1989; Thyer, Parrish, Himle, Cameron, Curtis, & Nesse, 1986), although one report found only a 5% rate of alcoholism. The lifetime prevalence of alcoholism in the general population has been reported to be 8–10% in men and 3–5% in women (Schuckit, 1986). The frequent co-occurrence of these disorders highlights the importance of assessment of alcohol use in social phobia and social phobic symptoms in alcoholism.

Order of onset may be helpful in understanding the relationship of the two disorders in an individual. Patients often report that social phobic symptoms preceded the alcohol abuse or dependence (Smail et al., 1984), and alcohol is commonly used to self-medicate social phobia (Turner et al., 1986). Alcohol sometimes provides transient relief of social phobic symptoms, but it can become a costly strategy when it leads to alcohol dependence, which may then become the principal problem. On the other hand, social phobic symptoms often occur as sequelae to alcoholism and may remit completely with the cessation of drinking. Whatever the sequence of onset of these disorders, they frequently become intertwined in the comorbid state. Treatment of just one component of the two may be futile. For example, social phobic symptoms make participation in Alcoholics Anonymous or other group treatments more difficult. Medication or psychotherapeutic interventions focused solely on social phobia are likely to fail and could prove dangerous if problem drinking is not specifically addressed.

SOCIAL PHOBIA SUBTYPES

The generalized subtype of social phobia is currently defined by fear of most social situations, with the remainder of social phobia described by various terms, including "discrete," "circumscribed," "limited," "performance," or "nongeneralized." Persons with discrete social phobia typically fear "performance" situations such as public speaking, eating, or writing in public. Persons with generalized social phobia often complain of similar fears, but they also fear social interactions, such as informal conversation, speaking to authority figures, and attending social gatherings (Mannuzza et al., 1995). To diagnose a social phobia subtype, the clinician must inquire about the patient's feelings and behavior in response to a broad range of social and performance situations. Limiting inquiry to the area of the patient's chief complaint tends to underestimate the breadth of feared situations.

Comparisons of social phobia subtypes have supported their validity. Persons with generalized social phobia have usually been found to have an earlier age of onset, to be less educated, and to be more anxious, depressed, and functionally impaired than persons with discrete social phobia. During social activities in a laboratory behavioral test, they show poorer performance and greater overt anxiety but less heart rate reactivity and no difference in subjective anxiety (Gelernter, Stein, Tancer, & Uhde, 1992; Heimberg, Hope, Dodge, & Becker, 1990.; Holt, Heimberg, & Hope, 1992; Schneier et al., 1991; Turner et al., 1992; also as reviewed by Heimberg et al., 1993).

Mannuzza et al. (1995) reported that the DSM-III-R subtypes could be distinguished reliably in a clinical sample of 129 patients with social phobia, even though the generalized subtype definition (fear of "most social situations") is not fully operationalized. They found that generalized social phobic patients were more often single, had earlier onsets of social phobia, were more often characterized by fear of interpersonal interactions, and had higher rates of major depression and alcoholism and lower rates of panic disorder. Diagnostic interviews of first-degree relatives revealed that over one-third of the families of generalized patients had social phobia, while the prevalence of social phobia in the families of nongeneralized patients did not differ from the rate in the families of controls.

Studies examining subtype differences in response to various treatment modalities are few and, so far, inconclusive (as reviewed by Heimberg et al., 1993). Persons with the generalized subtype have predominated in many treatment studies in social phobia. Further research is needed to clarify the possibility of differential response to specific treatments by subtype.

CONCLUSION

The establishment of operationalized diagnostic criteria for social phobia in 1980 stimulated the growth of research efforts, which have further characterized the disorder and established its validity. DSM-III-R significantly enlarged the scope of the diagnostic category by including the generalized subtype of social phobia, in which most social situations are feared. In the development of DSM-IV, several diagnostic boundary issues for social phobia were assessed systematically, but the empirical data was judged to justify only minor additional revisions. Future research may help clarify a number of diagnostic issues, including the relationship of social phobia to personality factors and to social anxiety caused by another embarrassing condition, such as stuttering, and the validity and clinical utility of social phobia subtypes.

REFERENCES

American Psychiatric Association. (1952). *Diagnostic and statistical manual of mental disorders* (1st ed.). Washington, DC: Author.

American Psychiatric Association. (1968). *Diagnostic and statistical manual of mental disorders* (2nd ed.). Washington, DC: Author.

American Psychiatric Association. (1980). *Diagnostic and statistical manual of mental disorders* (3rd ed.). Washington, DC: Author.

American Psychiatric Association. (1987). *Diagnostic and statistical manual of mental disorders* (3rd ed., rev.). Washington, DC: Author.

American Psychiatric Association. (1994). *Diagnostic and statistical manual of mental disorders* (4th ed.). Washington, DC: Author.

Amies, P. L., Gelder, M. G., & Shaw, P. M. (1983). Social phobia: A comparative clinical study. *British Journal of Psychiatry, 142,* 174–179.

Bowen, R. C., Cipywnyk, D., D'Arcy, C., & Keegan, D. (1984). Alcoholism, anxiety disorders, and agoraphobia. *Alcoholism: Clinical and Experimental Research, 8,* 8–50.

Cameron, O., Thyer, B., Nesse, R., & Curtis, G. (1986). Symptoms profiles of patients with DSM-III anxiety disorders. *American Journal of Psychiatry, 143,* 1132–1137.

Chaleby K. (1987). Social phobia in Saudis. *Social Psychiatry, 22,* 167–170.

Chambless, D. L., Cherney, J., Caputo, G. C., & Rheinstein, B. J. G. (1987). Anxiety disorders and alcoholism: A study with inpatient alcoholics. *Journal of Anxiety Disorders, 1,* 9–40.

Dilsaver, S. C., Qamar, A. B., & Del Medico, V. J.(1992). Secondary social phobia in patients with major depression. *Psychiatry Research, 44,* 33–40.

Freud, S. (1961) Inhibitions, symptoms and anxiety. In J. Strachey (Ed.), *The standard edition of the complete psychological works of Sigmund Freud* (Vol. 20, pp. 87–157). London: Hogarth Press. (Original work published 1926)

Gelernter, C., Stein, M. B., Tancer, M. E., & Uhde, T. W. (1992). An examination of syndromal validity and diagnostic subtypes in social phobia and panic disorder. *Journal of Clinical Psychiatry, 53,* 23–27.

Heimberg, R. G., Holt, C. S., Schneier, F. R., Spitzer, R. L., & Liebowitz, M. R. (1993). The issue of subtypes in the diagnosis of social phobia. *Journal of Anxiety Disorders, 7,* 249–269.

Heimberg, R. G., Hope, D. A., Dodge, C. A., & Becker, R. E. (1990). DSM-III-R subtypes of social phobia: Comparison of generalized social phobics and public speaking phobics. *Journal of Nervous and Mental Disease, 178,* 172–179.

Herbert, J. D., Hope, D. A., & Bellack, A. S. (1992). Validity of the distinction between generalized social phobia and avoidant personality disorders. *Journal of Abnormal Psychology, 101,* 332–339.

Holt, C. S, Heimberg, R. G., & Hope, D. A. (1992). Avoidant personality disorder and the generalized subtype of social phobia. *Journal of Abnormal Psychology, 101*, 318–325.

Holt, C. S., Heimberg, R. G., Hope, D. A., & Liebowitz, M. R. (1992). Situational domains of social phobia. *Journal of Anxiety Disorders, 6*, 63–77.

Janet, P. (1903). *Les obsessions et la psychasthénie*. Paris: F. Alcan.

Kagan, J., Reznick, J. S., & Snidman, N. (1988). Biological bases of childhood shyness. *Science, 240*, 167–171.

Kessler, R. C., McGonagle, K. A., Zhao, S., Nelson, C. B., Hughes, M., Eshelman, S., Wittchen, H., & Kendler, K. S. (1994). Lifetime and 12-month prevalence of DSM-III-R psychiatric disorders in the United States. *Archives of General Psychiatry, 51*, 8–19.

Liebowitz, M. R., Gorman, J. M., Fyer, A. J., & Klein, A. F. (1985). Social phobia: Review of a neglected anxiety disorder. *Archives of General Psychiatry, 42*, 729–736.

Liebowitz, M. R., Schneier, F., Campeas, R., Hollander, E., Hatterer, J., Fyer, A., Gorman, J., Papp, L., Davies, S., Gully, R., & Klein, D. F. (1992). Phenelzine vs. atenolol in social phobia: A placebo-controlled comparison. *Archives of General Psychiatry, 49*, 290–300.

Ludwig, R. P., & Lazarus, P. J. (1983). Relationship between shyness in children and constricted cognitive control as measured by the Stroop color–word test. *Journal of Consulting and Clinical Psychology, 51*, 386–389.

Mannuzza, S., Fyer, A. J., Liebowitz, M. R., & Klein, D. F. (1990). Delineating the boundary of social phobia: Its relationship to panic disorder and agoraphobia. *Journal of Anxiety Disorders, 4*, 41–59.

Mannuzza, S., Schneier, F. R., Chapman, T. F., Liebowitz, M. R., Klein, D. F., & Fyer A. J. (1995). Generalized social phobia: Reliability and validity. *Archives of General Psychiatry, 52*, 230–237.

Marks, I. M. (1969). *Fears and phobias*. New York: Academic Press.

Marks, I. M., & Gelder, M. G. (1966). Different ages of onset in varieties of phobia. *American Journal of Psychiatry, 123*, 218–221.

Mullaney, J. A., & Trippett, C. J. (1979). Alcohol dependence and phobias: Clinical description and relevance. *British Journal of Psychiatry, 135*, 565–573.

Munjack, D. J., & Moss, H. B. (1981). Affective disorder and alcoholism in families of agoraphobics. *Archives of General Psychiatry, 38*, 869–871.

Oberlander, E. L., Schneier, F. R., & Liebowitz, M. R. (1994). Physical disability and social phobia. *Journal of Clinical Psychopharmacology, 14*, 136–143.

Pollard, C. A., & Henderson, J. G. (1988). Four types of social phobia in a community sample. *Journal of Nervous and Mental Disease, 176*, 440–445.

Reich, J., Noyes, R., & Yates, W. (1988). Anxiety symptoms distinguishing social phobia from panic and generalized anxiety disorders. *Journal of Nervous and Mental Disease, 176*, 510–513.

Schneier, F. R., Johnson, J., Hornig, C. D., Liebowitz, M. R., & Weissman, M. M. (1992). Social phobia: Comorbidity and morbidity in an epidemiological sample. *Archives of General Psychiatry, 49*, 282–288.

Schneier, F. R., Liebowitz, M. R., Beidel, D., Fyer, A. J., George, M. S., Heimberg, R. G., Holt, C. S., Klein, A. P., Lydiard, R. B., Mannuzza, S., Martin, L. Y., Nardi, E. G., Roscow, D. B., Spitzer, R. L., Turner, S. M., Uhde, T. W., Vasconcelos, I. L., & Versiani, M. (in press). Social phobia. In T. A. Widiger, A. J. Frances,

H. A. Pincus, M. B. First, R. Ross, & W. Davis (Eds.), *DSM-IV, source book* (Vol. 2). Washington, DC: American Psychiatric Press.

Schneier, F. R., Liebowitz, M. R., Beidel, D., Garfinkel, R., Heimberg, R., Juster, H., Mannuzza, S., Oberlander, E., Turner, S. M., Law, K., Mattia, J., & Orsillo, S. (in press). MacArthur data reanalysis for social phobia. In T. A. Widiger, A. J. Frances, H. A. Pincus, M. B. First, R. Ross, & W. Davis (Eds.), *DSM-IV, source book* (Vol. 2). Washington, DC: American Psychiatric Press.

Schneier, F. R., Martin, L. Y., Liebowitz, M. R., Gorman, J. M., & Fyer, A. J. (1989). Alcohol abuse in social phobia. *Journal of Anxiety Disorders, 3,* 15–23.

Schneier, F. R., Spitzer, R. L., Gibbon, M., Fyer, A. J., & Liebowitz, M. R. (1991). The relationship of social phobia subtypes and avoidant personality disorder. *Comprehensive Psychiatry, 32,* 496–502.

Schuckit, M. A. (1986). Genetic and clinical implications of alcoholism and affective disorder. *American Journal of Psychiatry, 143,* 140–147.

Smail, P., Stockwell, T., Canter, S., & Hodgson, R. (1984). Alcohol dependence and phobic anxiety states. I. A prevalence study. *British Journal of Psychiatry, 144,* 53–57.

Spielberger, C. D., Pollans, C. H., & Wordem, T. J. (1984). Anxiety disorders. In S. M. Turner & M. Hersen (Eds.), *Adult psychopathology and diagnosis* (pp. 263–303). New York: Wiley.

Stein, M., Walker, J., & Ford, D. (1994). Setting diagnostic thresholds for social phobia. *American Journal of Psychiatry, 151,* 408–412.

Strauss, C. C., & Last, C. G. (1993). Social and simple phobias in children. *Journal of Anxiety Disorders, 7,* 141–152.

Stravynski, A., Lamontagne, Y., & Lavallee, Y. J. (1986). Clinical phobias and avoidant personality disorder among alcoholics admitted to an alcoholism rehabilitation setting. *Canadian Journal of Psychiatry, 31,* 714–719.

Takahashi, T. (1989). Social phobia syndrome in Japan. *Comprehensive Psychiatry, 30,* 45–52.

Thyer, B. A., Parrish, R. T., Himle, J., Cameron, O. G., Curtis, G. C., & Nesse, R. M. (1986). Alcohol abuse among clinically anxious patients. *Behaviour Research and Therapy, 24,* 357–359.

Turner, S., & Beidel, D. (1989). Social phobia: Clinical syndrome, diagnosis, and comorbidity. *Clinical Psychology Review, 9,* 3–18.

Turner, S. M., Beidel, D. C., Dancu, C. V., & Keys, D. J.(1986). Psychopathology of social phobia and comparison to avoidant personality disorder. *Journal of Abnormal Psychology, 95,* 389–394.

Turner, S., Beidel, D., & Townsely, R. (1990). Social phobia: Relationship to shyness. *Behaviour Research and Therapy, 28,* 487–505.

Turner, S. M., Beidel, D. C., & Townsley, R. M. (1992). Social phobia: A comparison of specific and generalized subtypes and avoidant personality disorder. *Journal of Abnormal Psychology, 101,* 326–331.

Versiani, M., Mundim, F. D., Nardi, A. E., & Liebowitz, M. R. (1988). Tranylcypromine in social phobia. *Journal of Clinical Psychopharmacology, 8,* 279–283.

CHAPTER TWO

Epidemiology and Family Studies of Social Phobia

TIM F. CHAPMAN
SALVATORE MANNUZZA
ABBY J. FYER

We address two main questions in this chapter: First, *what is the prevalence of social phobia in the general population*? Beginning in the mid-1980s, a number of large-scale surveys from around the world have reported on the prevalence of this disorder, defined according to the criteria of the third edition (DSM-III; American Psychiatric Association, 1980) and the revised third edition (DSM-III-R; American Psychiatric Association, 1987) of the *Diagnostic and Statistical Manual of Mental Disorders*, thus making a comparative inquiry both feasible and informative. Second, *how is social phobia distributed among members of the population*? We examine two sources of evidence: (1) secondary epidemiological data regarding the sociodemographic distribution of the disorder, and (2) family and twin studies, which suggest that social phobia may occur more often among related individuals than chance would predict. As with studies of prevalence, family and twin studies of social phobia have been reported only recently.

EPIDEMIOLOGICAL STUDIES OF PREVALENCE

Table 2.1 summarizes the findings of seven cross-national epidemiological studies from the 1980s, all of which used the Diagnostic Interview Schedule (DIS) in their evaluations (Robins, Helzer, Croughan, & Ratcliff, 1981) and all of which reported on lifetime prevalence of DSM-III social phobia in the general population. Each listed location was the core site for a large-scale psychiatric epidemiology survey. In most studies, stratified probability

TABLE 2.1. Lifetime Prevalence of DIS/DSM-III Social Phobia: Evidence from Cross-National Epidemiological Surveys

| Study/location | Total N | Citation | Lifetime prevalence (%) of DIS/DSM-III social phobia | | |
			All	Males	Females
ECA (four sites)/ United States[a]	13,537	Schneier et al. (1992)	2.4	2.0	3.1
Taipei/Taiwan	5,005	Hwu et al. (1989)	0.6	0.24	0.95
Edmonton/ Canada	3,258	Bland et al. (1988)	1.7	1.4	2.0
Seoul/ South Korea	3,134	Lee et al. (1990)	0.53	0.0	1.03
Puerto Rico/ United States	1,513	Canino et al. (1987)	1.6	1.5	1.6
Christchurch/ New Zealand	1,498	Wells et al. (1989)	3.0	4.3	3.5
Florence/Italy	1,110	Faravelli et al. (1989)	0.99	1.4	0.54

Note. Boxed cells indicate the higher gender-specific rate at each site.

[a] The early version of the DIS used in the New Haven component of the ECA study did not specifically assess social phobia. Hence, the data presented by Schneier et al. (1992) include the data from the remaining four ECA sites only (Baltimore, MD; Los Angeles, CA; St. Louis, MO; and Durham/Piedmont, NC).

sampling methods were employed in identifying target subjects, typically using the methodology of the original Epidemiologic Catchment Area (ECA) study as a model (Eaton et al., 1984; Regier et al., 1984). The aim in each case was to generate a representative sample of the surrounding population, most of which were located in major urban centers.

Each of the studies described in Table 2.1 used approximately equivalent versions of the DIS instrument, translated from the original English-language version where necessary. Their results are, therefore, broadly comparable. The DIS is a detailed, highly structured, interviewer-administered schedule designed for use in psychiatric epidemiology surveys by trained lay persons without extensive clinical expertise. It covers most DSM-III Axis I mental disorder diagnoses and assesses lifetime and current (past 6 months) disorder status.

The initial versions of the DIS used in the New Haven component of the ECA study did not distinguish social phobias from specific (simple) phobias or agoraphobia. Consequently, prevalence data on social phobia are not available from New Haven. Subsequent versions of the DIS used at the other ECA sites (Los Angeles, Baltimore, St. Louis, and Durham/ Piedmont) did ask about a number of social situations in which irrational social fears might be present.

Two observations are noteworthy (Table 2.1): First, in at least some sites, the DIS findings indicate that DIS/DSM-III social phobia is relatively common. The overall ECA lifetime prevalence rate in the United States (2.4%) represents approximately 6 million affected adults. The Christchurch, New Zealand, rate is higher, with almost 1 in 30 individuals in the general population affected. Since significant impairment in occupational and social functioning often accompanies this disorder, and since additional secondary psychiatric comorbidity is frequently present, these prevalence figures suggest at the least that the cumulative effects of social phobia in the population may be considerable (Schneier, Johnson, Hornig, Liebowitz, & Weissman, 1992; see also Davidson, Hughes, George, & Blazer, 1993).

Second, lifetime prevalence rates for the disorder seem to differ across studies. Most obviously, rates in both the East Asian studies (just over 0.5% in each case) are substantially lower than in most other sites. Also of some interest is the fact that, of the seven different locations listed, the three English-speaking sites (Edmonton, ECA, and Christchurch) report the highest lifetime prevalence rates (1.7%, 2.4%, and 3.0% respectively).

The DIS/DSM-III Social Phobia Category

A limitation inherent in these epidemiological studies is that there are various respects in which the DIS social phobia category does not coincide fully with the DSM-III definition. Specifically, the DIS (1) investigates only three types of social situation in which irrational fears might be present, (2) does not require fear of humiliation or embarrassment in the social situation, and (3) does not apply exclusion criteria for secondary social phobia—that is, phobias that may develop after the onset of another embarrassing disorder, such as Parkinson's disease (Schneier et al., 1992).

These discrepancies may affect the accuracy of the DIS estimates of DSM-III social phobia prevalence. But without other evidence, it is not a straightforward task to assess whether DIS social phobia rates are likely to over- or underestimate population rates for the true DSM-III disorder (i.e., the disorder as strictly defined by DSM-III criteria). The restricted number of feared situations asked about in the DIS tends, for example, to decrease the diagnostic sensitivity of the instrument relative to true DSM-III prevalence (i.e., it tends to increase the number of false negatives). By contrast, both the fact that fear of humiliation or embarrassment is not required for the DIS diagnosis to be given and the fact that DSM-III secondary disorder exclusion criteria are not systematically applied by the DIS tend systematically to decrease the diagnostic specificity of the instrument relative to true prevalence (i.e., they tend to increase the number of false positives). All else being equal, the first tendency would result in the DIS estimates being lower than true DSM-III population rates, while the second tendency, by contrast, would result in the DIS estimates being higher than true DSM-III rates. Since the two effects are opposing, their combined effect on the accuracy of DIS estimates of DSM-III social phobia prevalence is hard to predict.

Various other epidemiological studies suggest striking variability in the prevalence of social fears or phobias, and at least some of this variation is clearly due to differences across studies in how the phenomenon of interest is defined. For example, in the pre-DSM-III era, Bryant and Trower (1974) found that 10% of 223 Oxford University undergraduates, particularly those from low socioeconomic backgrounds, manifested strong irrational fears of speaking in public. More recently, Pollard and Henderson (1988) reported an unadjusted lifetime prevalence rate for severe irrational social fears of 22.6% in a random sample of 500 adults in the St. Louis area. As with the ECA studies (and unlike Bryant and Trower), they used a structured interview and applied criteria that were broadly, but not exactly, consistent with DSM-III criteria. They assessed four distinct situations in which social fears may be present (public speaking, eating in public, writing in public, and using public lavatories), only two of which were assessed by the DIS. A high prevalence was reported for situations involving speaking in public (20.6%), suggesting that as many as one in five individuals may have irrational fears in such situations. However, because the DSM-III "marked distress" criterion was not used to define cases, these figures also do not accurately reflect true prevalence for DSM-III social phobia. When this DSM-III criterion *was* applied to Pollard and Henderson's findings, the lifetime disorder rate for social phobia dropped to a much lower 2.0%—that is, a figure more consistent with cross-national DIS estimates (although again, it should be noted that the situations asked about in Pollard and Henderson's study did not coincide entirely with those used in the DIS). Nonetheless, this striking reduction in the overall prevalence reported by Pollard and Henderson (1988) resulted from the strict application of only one criterion inherent in the DSM-III social phobia category.

Stein, Walker, and Forde (1994) provide evidence from a recent Canadian study that even more compellingly demonstrates how much estimates of social phobia prevalence in community samples vary according to different definitions of caseness. Their telephone survey of more than 500 randomly selected inhabitants of Winnipeg indicated that fully 33% of the individuals surveyed reported being "much more nervous than other people" in at least one of the seven social situations they evaluated. In keeping with Pollard and Henderson's (1988) results, by far the most common situation that provoked such anxiety in Stein et al.'s (1994) study was speaking in front of a large audience. When DSM social phobia criteria

(DSM-III-R criteria in this case) were applied, however, specifically including the requirement that "marked interference or distress" accompany the anxiety, the overall prevalence was markedly reduced, to 7.1%.

Differentiation of Social Phobia and Agoraphobia

A second potential problem may affect cross-national DIS-based epidemiological findings of the sort presented in Table 2.1. This concerns the possibility of errors in differential diagnosis resulting from the failure to differentiate social phobia correctly from agoraphobia. This issue has been addressed recently in some detail by Mannuzza, Fyer, Liebowitz, and Klein (1990). Briefly, the problem arises because social phobia may often develop secondary to panic disorder with agoraphobia, particularly if panic attacks occur frequently in social situations and the subject subsequently avoids those situations either because of fear of having another attack or because of the potential for embarrassment that would result from having an attack in that situation. Since the DIS social phobia definition did not apply secondary exclusion criteria in defining social phobia, the possibility exists that some of the social phobia diagnoses enumerated by the DIS should be primary diagnoses of agoraphobia. If so, estimates of prevalence of social phobia may, of course, be too high.

Explaining Cross-National Differences in Social Phobia Prevalence

How can the cross-site differences in overall DIS/DSM-III disorder prevalence shown in Table 2.1 best be explained? Various possible explanations exist, in addition to the possibility of genuine cross-cultural variation in prevalence of social phobia. Among these are (1) random sampling error only, (2) methodological differences across sites in the way the DIS instrument was translated or administered, (3) potential cross-site variation in cultural attitudes about revealing information to interviewers, and (4) cross-site variation in the cultural relevance of the questions asked by the DIS instrument.

The first of these possibilities (random sampling error) seems very unlikely, given the large sample sizes. A direct pairwise comparison of the two largest studies in Table 2.1 (the ECA study [$N = 13,537$] and Taipei [$N = 5,005$]) indicates that the fourfold difference in lifetime rates of social phobia between the two sites is strongly statistically significant (2.4% vs. 0.6%, $\chi^2 = 62.2$, $df = 1$, $p < .001$), and therefore most unlikely to have occurred due to chance factors alone.

Detailed information on the specific questions relating to fears of social situations asked in each study is not included in any of the published reports of the East Asian studies, so assessing the second possibility listed above (that cross-site inconsistencies in translation may account for the variation) is not currently practicable.

Cross-cultural differences in the willingness to reveal information to interviewers may plausibly account for some of this variation, and there seems to be at least some indirect evidence tending to support this conclusion. For example, one of the more conspicuous numbers presented in Table 2.1 is the reported rate for social phobia among males in the Seoul, South Korea, study. This sample included more than 3,000 individuals, of whom approximately half were male, and yet apparently not a single male subject in the entire study reported experiencing social fears of sufficient severity to receive a formal diagnosis.

In a similar vein, the possibility that the differences may derive in part from variation in the cultural relevance of the questions about feared social situations in the DIS is supported by at least some circumstantial evidence. For instance, consider the finding in Table 2.1 that DIS social phobia appears to be significantly more widespread in English-speaking, and more generally, Western cultures than in East Asia and other, non-English-speaking European societies. Since the instrument was originally conceived and developed by researchers in the United States, it is reasonable to argue that this is the pattern one would expect if the cultural relevance argument were true.

The original design and structure of the DIS instrument may have been particularly attuned to those clinical syndromes or patterns of symptomatology that were either of particular interest to American (and more generally, English-speaking) clinicians or were particularly frequently encountered in Western therapeutic settings (e.g., Guarnaccia, Rubio-Stipec, & Canino, 1989). This would be a limitation in cross-cultural studies, if the contexts in which social fears are expressed varies from culture to culture, as seems likely to be the case. In these circumstances, a culturally sensitized instrument is required to test the basic null hypothesis that underlying base prevalence rates of generic social phobia are invariant across all cultures.

Other evidence indirectly supports this idea that generic social phobia prevalence may actually vary less dramatically across cultures than the findings presented in Table 2.1 indicate. For example, although it may not correspond exactly to the typical presentation of social phobia most commonly encountered in Western clinics, a well-documented psychiatric syndrome analogous to this disorder may in fact be quite common in certain East Asian societies (Murphy, 1982, pp. 261–269; Prince, 1993). This syndrome, called in Japanese *"taijin kyofu-sho"* (TKS)—meaning "fear of facing other people"—has long been recognized and extensively described by Japanese psychiatrists and has, moreover, been accorded separate status relative to simple phobias and agoraphobia in Japanese psychiatric nosology since at least the 1920s. Indeed, Prince (1993) argues that the "separation of the social phobias from agoraphobia and the host of simple phobias probably first occurred in the Japanese [psychiatric] literature" (p. 61).

While parallels with the phenomenology of obsessive–compulsive disorder have also been identified, many of the characteristics of TKS seem to parallel those of social phobia as it appears in the West. Seemingly common not just in Japan but also in Korea and possibly other areas of East Asia (Chang, 1984), TKS is characterized by shame about and persistent irrational fears of causing others offense, embarrassment, or even harm, through some perceived personal inadequacy or shortcoming. Feelings of humiliation are apparently integral to the phenomenology of the syndrome (Murphy, 1982). And it is most frequently encountered, at least in treatment settings, among young adult males. Common specific manifestations include fear of blushing (erythrophobia), fear of emitting body odor (dysosmophobia), and fear of displaying unsightly body parts (dysmorphophobia) (Chang, 1984). Other manifestations of TKS are also found, however, including fear of speaking one's thoughts aloud, fear of gaze or facial attitude, and fear of irritating others by "shakiness in the voice or limbs" (Prince, 1993).

While exotic phobias of this sort are not unheard of outside East Asia, they are, nevertheless, only rarely encountered by Western clinicians, and more significantly, they are generally not asked about in the "phobia sections" of Western structured psychiatric assessment instruments. But since a core element of TKS clearly is oriented toward humiliation, shame, and embarrassment engendered by particular *social* interactions, it seems hard to deny its relevance to the DSM social phobia category as encountered in the West.

In summary, therefore, the possibility exists that there may be true cross-national differences in the prevalence of social phobia. However, it is also possible that the differences reported in Table 2.1 are more likely to derive from variation in the cultural contexts in which social fears are most commonly expressed across different societies than from genuine cross-cultural variability. Distinguishing among these possibilities is difficult with current assessment instruments, which generally are not well attuned to the possibility that the cultural relevance of particular questions about symptoms and presentation may vary markedly from one society to another.

Results from the National Comorbidity Survey

The studies reported in Table 2.1 were all undertaken in the mid- to late 1980s, that is, mostly before the publication of DSM-III-R in 1987. Kessler et al.'s recent (1994) preliminary article from the National Comorbidity Survey (NCS) reported on overall lifetime prevalence rates for major DSM-III-R psychiatric disorders (including social phobia), and thus provides a useful supplement to these earlier studies.

Unlike the earlier ECA studies, which used only the urban populations of major metropolitan centers such as Baltimore and Los Angeles, the NCS used a stratified, multistage area probability sample of the entire U.S. population aged 15–54. Over 8,000 subjects were interviewed, using a lay-administered, modified, and updated version of the DIS—the Composite International Diagnostic Interview (CIDI). In this study, the overall lifetime prevalence rate for social phobia in the U.S. population was reported to be 13.3%—one of the highest lifetime rates for any disorder assessed; in fact, only major depressive episodes and alcohol-related diagnoses were more common.

This prevalence rate—13.3%—is clearly so much higher than the DIS/DSM-III rates obtained by the ECA and most other studies conducted in the 1980s that some explanation is called for. One possible reason may be the use of DSM-III-R rather than DSM-III criteria to define morbidity. In particular, the changes from DSM-III to DSM-III-R increased the diagnostic scope of the social phobia category and, therefore, the likely prevalence of social phobia diagnosis. For example, a diagnosis of avoidant personality disorder was considered a primary diagnostic exclusion effectively ruling out a social phobia diagnosis in DSM-III, a convention that was dropped in DSM-III-R. Similarly, DSM-III-R subsumed the generalized social phobia category by explicitly recognizing that people may experience fears in more than a single situation, whereas the DSM-III definition generally focused on "a situation" (Liebowitz, Gorman, Fyer, & Klein, 1985).

Of some interest is the fact that the NCS findings were anticipated in another recent (albeit much smaller-scale) study that used the CIDI in Switzerland. In this study, Wacker, Müllejans, Klein, and Battegay (1992) reported an overall lifetime prevalence rate for DSM-III-R social phobia of 16% in a general population sample of 470 Swiss adults, a rate even higher than that of Kessler et al. (1994). Although somewhat less marked, the findings of Stein et al. (1994), which indicated a 7.1% overall prevalence for DSM-III-R social phobia in a random telephone survey of over 500 residents of Winnipeg, also confirm that DSM-III-R social phobia may be among the most prevalent mental disorders.

DISTRIBUTION OF SOCIAL PHOBIA

We turn now from questions of prevalence to the related topic of how, given its prevalence, social phobia is distributed among members of the general population.

Sociodemographic Findings

In Schneier et al.'s (1992) analysis of the ECA study's aggregated four-site data regarding social phobia, a variety of sociodemographic characteristics were associated with variability in overall social phobia prevalence, including age at interview, gender, socioeconomic status, education, and marital status. Since this study is the largest to have reported on this topic to date, these findings will be considered in some detail below.

In general, Schneier et al. (1992) found that social phobia was more common in individuals who were female, young, poorly educated, of low socioeconomic status, and unmarried (either never married or divorced or separated). These findings are in certain respects consistent with a large body of prior research implicating sociodemographic factors in shaping the population distribution of a number of specific mental disorders. For example, the striking inverse relationship between socioeconomic status and risk for schizophrenia is one of the most robust findings in the social–epidemiological literature (e.g., Faris & Dunham, 1939; Hollingshead & Redlich, 1958; Leaf, Weissman, Myers, Holzer, & Tischler, 1984; Srole, Langner, Michael, Opler, & Rennie, 1962).

Gender Differences in Prevalence

According to the ECA data (Schneier et al., 1992), social phobia is more common in women (3.1% lifetime) than in men (2.0% lifetime) in the general population. This finding does not correspond exactly with studies that suggest a more equal or slightly male-biased gender distribution among subjects in treatment settings (e.g., see Mannuzza et al., 1990, Table 3, for a review of sex-ratio evidence from treatment studies). Nevertheless, it is consistent with prior epidemiologic data regarding other anxiety disorders defined using the DIS (e.g., Robins et al., 1984). Most prevalence studies have indicated that anxiety disorders are relatively less common in males than in females, and that some (e.g., simple phobias and agoraphobia) are very much less so. In both East Asian studies listed in Table 2.1, the female-to-male sex ratio is somewhat more disproportionately skewed than in the ECA study (Hwu, Yeh, & Chang, 1989; Lee et al, 1990). As noted above, in the Seoul, South Korea, study social phobia was completely absent in males. Only the Christchurch, New Zealand, and Florence, Italy, studies reported a sex ratio for social phobia skewed in favor of males.

In the preliminary report on the NCS, a sex ratio for social phobia of approximately 3:2 female-to-male was also reported by Kessler et al. (1994). Females reported a 15.5% lifetime prevalence and males an 11.1%

prevalence. Despite the dramatic differences in the absolute magnitude of these rates, this 3:2 ratio is consistent with previous ECA findings.

The study by Pollard and Henderson (1988) indicated a similar 3:2 female-to-male sex ratio among subjects with broadly defined social anxiety (i.e., defined ignoring the DSM-III "significant distress" criterion). However, an almost exactly *reversed* sex ratio (2:3) was found when the distress criterion was strictly applied. This finding is of some interest. It is consistent with various reports of a predominance of males in treatment settings (Mannuzza et al., 1990). But it also raises the possibility that certain *types* of social phobia may be characterized by particular sex ratios in the general population. For example, if phobias of asking directions were disproportionately prevalent in males, then variation across studies in reported sex ratios for overall social phobia would obviously not be unexpected if fears relating to this sort situation were not evaluated consistently. Pollard and Henderson did assess a somewhat different range of phobic situations from those assessed by the ECA, and hence the discrepancy in their sex ratio findings may result at least in part from characteristic population-level sex ratios for particular types of social anxiety.

Marital Status

In keeping with data from clinical settings, the ECA data also indicate that individuals who receive a social phobia diagnosis are more likely to be unmarried than are individuals who do not receive such a diagnosis. This finding remained strongly significant in the ECA sample even after controlling statistically for study site, subject age, gender, socioeconomic status, and race (Schneier et al., 1992).

Given the characteristic phenomenology of the disorder, the association seems reasonable. For example, fears of attending social gatherings or parties, talking to strangers, and especially, dating are all common manifestations of social anxiety in individuals with generalized DSM-III-R social phobia. And such fears may obviously have markedly detrimental effects on a young, unmarried individual's ability to participate successfully in marriage markets. First, it may be the case that, specifically because of their social anxiety, individuals systematically avoid attending the sorts of social gatherings at which potential marriage partners are likely to be encountered. Alternatively, even if such avoidance is not systematic, pervasive social anxiety may appear to be a somewhat undesirable trait in a potential partner. Either of these two effects may reduce the likelihood of marriage for individuals suffering from severe social anxiety in marriage market contexts.

There is also some preliminary evidence that when individuals with histories of DSM-III-R social phobia do marry, they may tend to mate assortatively, tending to marry others with similar histories (Chapman, 1993). This phenomenon may also result from the effects of severe social anxiety on overall patterns of marriage market participation in unmarried individuals. Socially anxious individuals may systematically avoid informal unstructured events at which face-to-face social interaction is expected, such as parties or social gatherings, but nevertheless participate actively in less anxiety-provoking social contexts, such as church groups. All else being equal, potential spouses encountered in such settings may themselves be disproportionately likely to suffer from similar types of social anxiety.

Age-at-Interview Differences

The ECA data indicate a strong and approximately inverse linear relationship between social phobia prevalence and the age of the interviewee, with the highest lifetime rate of disorder (3.6%) found in the youngest individuals (those aged 18–29 at the time of the interview) and the lowest rate (1.8%) found in the oldest individuals (those aged 65 or older). Schneier et al. (1992) note that this finding is unexpected and somewhat difficult to interpret. At least two plausible interpretations are possible. The first is that the result reflects birth cohort-level fluctuations in social phobia prevalence, with individuals in more recent birth cohorts disproportionately likely to develop the disorder, relative to those born in earlier cohorts. This possibility is supported by ECA data on post-World War II birth cohort variation in major depression prevalence (Weissman, 1987; Wickramaratne, Weissman, Leaf, & Holford, 1989), which suggest that age-specific rates of depressive illness have increased over the last 60 years. Similar cohort effects for social phobia may account for the findings reported by Schneier et al. (1992).

The second potential interpretation of this finding, however, is that there is either poor recall or reduced reporting accuracy on the part of older subjects (Ruben, 1986). Since social phobia is frequently characterized by early first onsets (e.g., Schneier et al., 1992 indicate that the modal category of age at onset for social phobia in the ECA data was 11–15 years), it may simply be more difficult for older subjects to accurately recall specific constellations of childhood or teenage phobic symptomatology than it is for younger individuals. Hence, the rates of lifetime diagnosis in these older individuals may be disproportionately reduced (see also Cohen, 1988). This explanation may, of course, be less apt in the case of chronic social phobias, which affect individuals for their entire lives.

Education and Socioeconomic Status

As noted above, epidemiological studies have frequently found inverse associations between socioeconomic status and mental disorder prevalence (see Dohrenwend, 1990, for a summary review). This negative relationship has been most apparent for certain severe and impairing forms of mental illness, such as schizophrenia, and for alcohol and substance abuse. The ECA social phobia prevalence findings reported by Schneier et al. (1992) are clearly analogous, since they indicate that the highest rates of social phobia are found among the lowest socioeconomic groups and among the most poorly educated.

As with other mental disorders for which associations of this sort have been reported in the past, explaining this association is not straightforward. Both selection and causation arguments are plausible explanations (Dohrenwend et al., 1992; Schwartz & Link, 1991). In the first case (selection), impairment in occupational and educational functioning resulting directly from the disorder itself (e.g., an inability to complete a college degree because of a pervasive phobia of speaking in classroom settings or of dealing with authority figures such as teachers or professors) may tend to lower the ultimate achieved socioeconomic status of individuals with this disorder relative to otherwise similar individuals who do not suffer from the disorder (i.e., social phobia directly results in selection into low-status jobs, etc.). In the second case (causation), low socioeconomic status may itself be etiologically implicated for some reason in the development of the disorder.

THE FAMILIAL NATURE OF SOCIAL PHOBIA

We turn now to evidence from family and twin studies, which investigate the question of whether genetic factors play a role in the etiology of social phobia. Twin studies compare monozygotic and dizygotic twin pairs for the presence of the trait or illness in question (Faraone & Santangelo, 1992). Monozygotic (i.e., identical) twin pairs share 100% of their genetic information, whereas dizygotic (i.e., nonidentical) twins are no more closely related to each other than ordinary first-degree siblings (i.e., 50% of their genetic information is shared); differences between the two types of twin pairs in particular traits can thus provide clues about the relative contributions of genetic versus environmental influences on the expression of those traits.

In family studies, the analogous question addressed is whether illness tends to aggregate within family units (cf. different types of twin pairs) more systematically than would be expected were chance factors alone to determine illness status among members of all families in the population. And as with twin studies, biological/genetic, environmental, and gene–

environment interaction models can be invoked as potential explanations if familial aggregation is observed (Faraone & Santangelo, 1992; King, Rotter, & Motulsky, 1992).

Family Studies

Information on the organization of and typical methodology used in psychiatric family studies can be found in the review by Weissman et al. (1986). Family studies can be thought of as complementing the twin study approach to illness etiology. Within specific family units, particular focal individuals, that is, "probands," are of crucial methodological significance in family studies. A case–control design variant is adopted at the level of probands (Weissman et al., 1986). Case probands are by definition ill—meaning that the disorder of interest is currently (or was at some point in the past) present in the individual concerned. Control probands, by contrast, are always by definition not-ill with respect to the disorder of interest, although whether the cases and controls share the same status with respect to illnesses *other than* the one of interest varies from study to study (Tsuang, Fleming, Kendler, & Gruenberg, 1988). Typically, family studies attempt to assess the first-degree biological relatives (i.e., the biological parents, full siblings, and children) of the proband. Proband spouses (if any) are also frequently assessed even though they are (usually) not directly related other than by marriage to the proband.

Weissman (1985) observed that "the familial nature of anxiety disorders was noted over a century ago . . . and subsequent writers have frequently cited the occurrence of additional cases within a patient's family. . . . Hence, the notion that anxiety disorders are familial is not new" (p. 285). (For summary reviews of this literature, see Carey & Gottesman, 1981, and Weissman et al., 1986.)

Recent family and twin studies of specific anxiety disorders—for example, panic disorder (Noyes et al., 1986), obsessive–compulsive disorder (Lenane et al., 1990), and simple phobias (Fyer et al, 1990) (see also Torgerson, 1983)—have, moreover, consistently tended to confirm these findings of familial aggregation. For the most part, these results have been interpreted as indicating the likely existence of heritable contributions to the etiology of these disorders.

Family study evidence of this sort pertaining to social phobia has, however, become available only recently (Reich & Yates, 1988; Fyer, Mannuzza, Chapman, Liebowitz, & Klein, 1993; Mannuzza et al., 1995). The relevant studies are described below.

Reich and Yates (1988) studied 17 probands with a diagnosis of DSM-III social phobia recruited from an anxiety treatment clinic. Also studied were 88 probands with panic disorder and 10 not-ill control subjects. Family history information on first-degree relatives was provided by each of these probands (i.e., relatives were not interviewed directly). According to these family history assessments, the rates of social phobia were higher in the 76 relatives of the social phobia probands (rate = 6.6%) than in either the 46 relatives of control subjects (2.2%) or the 471 relatives of the panic disorder probands (0.4%).

Rates of major depression were also higher in the relatives of the social phobia probands than in the control relatives. Conversely, panic disorder, generalized anxiety disorder, and alcohol abuse were all more common in the panic disorder relatives than in the social phobia relatives.

In the only other study focusing specifically on the familial transmission of social phobia, Fyer et al. (1993) studied 30 probands with social phobia and 77 never mentally ill controls and their respective first-degree family members. As with the study of Reich and Yates (1988), social phobia probands were recruited from an anxiety treatment clinic; none had any form of additional lifetime anxiety disorder comorbidity (i.e., they had no anxiety diagnoses other than social phobia). Control probands were recruited using a modification of the "acquaintanceship" procedure (Mannuzza et al., 1992). In this study, both probands and relatives were directly interviewed using the same semistructured assessment instrument, applying DSM-III-R social phobia criteria. In the case of relative interviews, interviewers were also blind to proband diagnostic status.

While absolute rates of illness among relatives were higher than in Reich and Yates's (1988) study—probably due either to the low sensitivity of informant-only data (Andreasen, Rice, Endicott, Reich, & Coryell, 1986), or to the fact that DSM-III-R rather than DSM-III diagnostic criteria were applied (see above)—the overall pattern of results obtained by Fyer et al. (1993) was relatively similar to those of Reich and Yates. Social phobia was present in 13 of 83 relatives of social phobia probands (16%), compared to 12 of 231 of relatives of control subjects (5%). Rates of social phobia were similar for male and female relatives, but the disorder was more common among siblings of social phobia probands than among parents. No elevation in rates of other (i.e., non-social phobia) DSM-III-R diagnoses were apparent in the social phobia relatives compared to relatives of not-ill controls.

Taken together, these two studies both indicate a significant, approximately threefold elevation in rates of social phobia among relatives of probands with social phobia compared to the relatives of not-ill control subjects. They suggest that social phobia may indeed be a familial disorder, and also that it may breed true (i.e., that it is not associated with increased liability for *other* anxiety disorders in addition to social phobia in relatives).

In a recent extension of Fyer et al.'s (1993) study, which used an overlapping sample but did not control for non-social phobia anxiety disorder comorbidity in probands, Mannuzza et al. (1995) investigated familial transmission of the generalized versus nongeneralized forms of DSM-III-R social phobia. Results indicated that social phobia was significantly more common in relatives of 33 outpatient probands with generalized social phobia (15 out of 96 relatives, or 16%) than in the relatives of 30 probands with the nongeneralized form of the disorder (5 out of 88 relatives, or 6%). Since the rate of illness in the relatives of probands with nongeneralized social phobia was similar to the rate in the control sample in this study, the finding tends both (1) to confirm the validity of the generalized versus nongeneralized distinction in social phobia, and (2) to raise the possibility that familial transmission may be more likely in the generalized form of the disorder.

Twin Studies

Family studies alone cannot adequately assess the possible respective contributions of environmental and genetic influences in explaining results such as these. To address this issue more fully, twin and adoption studies are necessary. To date, no adoption studies of DSM-III or DSM-III-R social phobia are available. In the only available twin study of DSM-III social phobia, Kendler, Neale, Kessler, Heath, and Eaves (1992) examined 2,163 female twin pairs identified from the Virginia twin registry. Their results indicated a 24.4% concordance rate on DSM-III social phobia for monozygotic twins, versus a 15.3% concordance rate for dizygotic twins. Overall, the heritability index for social phobia in this study was estimated to be moderate, at approximately 30%; the best-fitting univariate and multivariate genetic models indicated that environmental influences were also likely to be influential in determining liability to the disorder.

Analogue twin studies examining social *fears* (variously defined; cf. true DSM-III social phobia) produced estimates of heritability of similar or somewhat higher magnitude, ranging from a high of 50% (Torgersen, 1983) to a low of 22% (Phillips, Fulker, & Rose, 1987). Overall, this series of results supports the hypothesis that a genetic component accounts at least in part for the tendency for social phobia to aggregate within family units (see also Horn, Plomin, & Rosenman, 1976; Rose & Ditto, 1983).

SUMMARY

The purpose of this chapter has been to provide a summary overview of recent epidemiological and family study evidence regarding the DSM-III and DSM-III-R social phobia categories. The discussion suggests the following conclusions:

1. Early epidemiological studies of prevalence of DSM-III social phobia conducted in the 1980s indicated that social phobia was not uncommon. Exact estimates of prevalence, however, varied markedly depending on how the disorder was defined. More recent findings, in particular those from the NCS, which assessed the disorder according to DSM-III-R criteria, indicate that social phobia may affect upward of 10% of the population and may thus be among the most prevalent of all psychiatric disorders in the general population. More than 20% of the population may experience significant irrational fears of social situations that do not meet full DSM-III-R criteria, particularly fears of public speaking.

2. Cross-cultural differences in overall social phobia prevalence may exist. This appears particularly likely when comparing East Asian and English-speaking cultures; the highest prevalence rates have typically been reported in studies undertaken in English-speaking countries (e.g., the United States, Canada, and New Zealand). One possible explanation is that social phobia as currently identified in the West may be an instance of a culture-bound syndrome. It is likely, however, that a more culturally inclusive definition of the disorder may reduce apparent discrepancies in prevalence rates. Comparative evidence does indicate that social phobia-like syndromes occur in Asian cultures at greater frequency than is typically reported by studies that use standardized psychiatric assessment instruments, most of which were developed in the West. Further epidemiological research using culturally sensitized instruments is needed to clarify this issue.

3. Consistent with prior sociological and epidemiological evidence regarding other mental disorders, current evidence suggests that sociodemographic factors are associated in various ways with the overall distribution of social phobia in the general population. Specifically, the disorder appears to be disproportionately common in females, in young people, in unmarried individuals, and in individuals from poorly educated, low-status socioeconomic groups.

4. Recent family study evidence also suggests that the disorder aggregates within families more often than chance would predict, and that social phobia may breed true. Consistent with the social epidemiological evidence, however, twin studies of DSM-III social phobia and analogue studies of social fears suggest that shared environmental as well as genetic factors contribute at least in part to this familial tendency.

REFERENCES

American Psychiatric Association. (1980). *Diagnostic and statistical manual of mental disorders* (3rd ed.). Washington, DC: Author.

American Psychiatric Association. (1987). *Diagnostic and statistical manual of mental disorders* (3rd ed., rev.). Washington, DC: Author.

Andreasen, N. C., Rice, T., Endicott, J., Reich, T., & Coryell, W. (1986). The family history approach to diagnosis: How useful is it? *Archives of General Psychiatry, 43,* 421−429.

Bland, R. C., Orn, H., & Newman, S. C. (1988). Lifetime prevalence of psychiatric disorders in Edmonton. *Acta Psychiatrica Scandinavica, 77,* 24−32.

Bryant, B., & Trower, P. E. (1974). Social difficulty in a student sample. *British Journal of Educational Psychology, 44,* 13−21.

Canino, G. J., Bird, H. R., Shrout, P. E., Rubio-Stipec, M., Bravo, M., Martinez, R., Sesman, M., & Guevara, L. M. (1987). The prevalence of specific psychiatric disorders in Puerto Rico. *Archives of General Psychiatry, 44,* 727−735.

Carey, G., & Gottesman, I. (1981). Twin and family studies of anxiety, phobic, and obsessive disorders. In D. F. Klein & J. G. Rabkin (Eds.), *Anxiety: New research and changing concepts* (pp. 117−136). New York: Raven Press.

Chang, S. C. (1984). [English-language review of Yamashita, I, *Taijin-Kyofu.* Tokyo: Kenehara (in Japanese)]. *Transcultural Psychiatry Review, 21,* 283−288.

Chapman, T. F. (1993). *Assortative mating and mental illness.* Unpublished doctoral dissertation, Yale University, New Haven, CT.

Cohen, P. (1988). The effects of instruments and informants on ascertainment. In D. L. Dunner, E. S. Gershon, & J. E. Barrett (Eds.), *Relatives at risk for mental disorder* (pp. 31−52). New York: Raven Press.

Davidson, J. R. T., Hughes, D. L., George, L. K., & Blazer D. G. (1993). The epidemiology of social phobia: Findings from the Duke Epidemiologic Catchment Area study. *Psychological Medicine, 23,* 709−718.

Dohrenwend, B. P. (1990). Socioeconomic status (SES) and psychiatric disorders: Are the issues still compelling? *Social Psychiatry and Psychiatric Epidemiology, 25,* 41−47.

Dohrenwend, B. P., Levav, I., Shrout, P. E., Schwartz, S., Naveh, G., Link, B. G., Skodol, A. E., & Stueve, A. (1992). Socioeconomic status and psychiatric disorders: The causation-selection issue. *Science, 255,* 946−951.

Eaton, W. W., Holzer III, C. E., von Korff, M., Anthony, J. C., Helzer, J. E., George, L., Burman, M. A., Boyd, J. H., Kessler, L. G., & Locke, B. Z. (1984). The design of the Epidemiologic Catchment Area surveys: The control and measurement of error. *Archives of General Psychiatry, 41,* 942−948.

Faraone, S. V., & Santangelo, S. L. (1992). Methods in genetic epidemiology. In M. Fava & J. F. Rosenbaum (Eds.), *Research designs and methods in psychiatry* (pp. 93−118). New York: Elsevier.

Faravelli, C. B., Innocenti, G. D., & Giardinelli L. (1989). Epidemiology of anxiety disorders in Florence. *Acta Psychiatrica Scandinavica, 79,* 308−312.

Faris, R. E. L., & Dunham, H. W. (1939). *Mental disorders in urban areas: An ecological study of schizophrenia and other psychoses.* Chicago: University of Chicago Press.

Fyer, A. J., Mannuzza, S., Chapman, T. F., Liebowitz, M. R., & Klein, D. F. (1993). A direct interview family study of social phobia. *Archives of General Psychiatry, 50,* 286−293.

Fyer, A. J., Mannuzza, S., Gallops, M. S., Martin, L. Y., Aaronson, C., Gorman, J. M., Liebowitz, M. R., & Klein, D. F. (1990). Familial transmission of simple phobias and fears: A preliminary report. *Archives of General Psychiatry, 47,* 252−256.

Guarnaccia, P. J., Rubio-Stipec, M., & Canino, G. (1989). *Ataques de nervios* in the Puerto Rican Diagnostic Interview Schedule: The impact of cultural categories on psychiatric epidemiology. *Culture, Medicine, and Psychiatry, 13*, 275–295.

Hollingshead, A. B., & Redlich, F. C. (1958). *Social class and mental illness.* New York: Wiley.

Horn, J. M., Plomin, R., & Rosenman, R. (1976). Heritability of personality traits in adult male twins. *Behavior Genetics, 6*, 17–30.

Hwu, H., Yeh, E. K., & Chang, L. Y. (1989). Prevalence of psychiatric disorders in Taiwan defined by the Chinese Diagnostic Interview Schedule. *Acta Psychiatrica Scandinavica, 79*, 136–147.

Kendler, K. S., Neale, M. C., Kessler, R. C., Heath, A. C., & Eaves, L. J. (1992). The genetic epidemiology of phobias in women: The interrelations of agoraphobia, social phobia, situational phobia, and simple phobia. *Archives of General Psychiatry, 49*, 273–281.

Kessler, R. C., McGonagle, K., Zhao, S., Nelson, C., Hughes, M., Eschlemann, S., Wittchen, H.-U., & Kendler, K. S. (1994). Lifetime and 12-month prevalence of DSM-III-R psychiatric disorders in the United States: Results from the National Comorbidity Survey. *Archives of General Psychiatry, 51* 8–19.

King, R. A., Rotter, J. I., & Motulsky, A. G. (1992). The approach to genetic bases of common diseases. In R. G. King, J. I. Rotter, & A. G. Motulsky (Eds.) *The genetic basis of common diseases* (pp. 3–70). New York: Oxford University Press.

Leaf, P. J., Weissman, M. M., Myers, J. K., Holzer, C. E., & Tischler, G. L. (1984). Social factors related to psychiatric disorder: The Yale Epidemiologic Catchment Area study. *Social Psychiatry, 19*, 53–61.

Lee, C.-K., Kwak, Y.-S., Yamamoto, J., Rhee, H., Kim, Y. S., Han, J. H., Choi, J. O., & Lee, Y. H. (1990). Psychiatric epidemiology in Korea: I. Gender and age differences in Seoul. *Journal of Nervous and Mental Disease, 178*, 242–246.

Lenane, M. C., Swedo, S. E., Leonard, H., Pauls, D. L., Sceery, W., & Rapoport, J. (1990). Psychiatric disorders in first degree relatives of children and adolescents with obsessive compulsive disorder. *Journal of the American Academy of Child and Adolescent Psychiatry, 29*, 407–412.

Liebowitz, M. R., Gorman, J. M., Fyer, A. J., & Klein, D. F. (1985). Social phobia: Review of a neglected anxiety disorder. *Archives of General Psychiatry, 42*, 729–735.

Mannuzza, S., Fyer, A. J., Endicott, J., Gallops, M. S., Martin, L. Y., Reich, T., & Klein, D. F. (1992). An extension of the acquaintanceship procedure in family studies of mental disorder. *Journal of Psychiatric Research, 26*, 45–57.

Mannuzza, S., Fyer, A. J., Liebowitz, M. R., & Klein, D. F. (1990). Delineating the boundaries of social phobia: Its relationship to panic disorder and agoraphobia. *Journal of Anxiety Disorders, 4*, 41–59.

Mannuzza, S., Schneier, F. R., Chapman, T. F., Liebowitz, M. R., Klein, D. F., & Fyer, A. J. (1995). Generalized social phobia: Reliability and validity. *Archives of General Psychiatry, 52*, 230–237.

Murphy, H. B. M. (1982). *Comparative psychiatry.* Berlin: Springer Verlag.

Noyes, R., Crowe, R. R., Harris, E. L., Hamra, B. J., McChesney, C. M., & Chaudry, D. R. (1986). The relationship between panic disorder and agoraphobia: A family study. *Archives of General Psychiatry, 43*, 227–232.

Phillips, K., Fulker, D. W., & Rose, R. J. (1987). Path analysis of seven fear factors in adult and sibling pairs and their children. *Genetic Epidemiology, 4,* 343–355.

Pollard, C. A., & Henderson, J. G. (1988). Four types of social phobia in a community sample. *Journal of Nervous and Mental Disease, 176,* 440–445.

Prince, R. H. (1993). Culture bound syndromes: The example of social phobias. In A. Ghadirian & H. E. Lehman (Eds.), *Environment and psychopathology* (pp. 55–72). New York: Springer.

Regier, D. A., Myers, J. K., Kramer, M., Robins, L. N., Blazer, D. G., Hough, R. L., Eaton, W. W., & Locke, B. Z. (1984). The NIMH Epidemiologic Catchment Area program: Historical context, major objectives and study population characteristics. *Archives of General Psychiatry, 41,* 934–941.

Reich, J. H., & Yates, W. (1988). Family history of psychiatric disorders in social phobia. *Comprehensive Psychiatry, 29,* 72–75.

Robins, L. N., Helzer, J. E., Croughan, J., & Ratcliff, K. S. (1981). National Institute of Mental Health Diagnostic Interview Schedule: Its history, characteristics and validity. *Archives of General Psychiatry, 38,* 381–389.

Robins, L. N., Helzer, J. E., Weissman, M. M., Orvaschel, H., Gruenberg, E., Burke, J. D., & Regier, D. A. (1984). Lifetime prevalence of specific psychiatric disorders in three sites. *Archives of General Psychiatry, 41,* 949–958.

Rose, R. J., & Ditto, W. B. (1983). A developmental–genetic analysis of common fears from early adolescence to early adulthood. *Child Development, 54,* 361–368.

Ruben, D. C. (Ed.). (1986). *Autobiographical memory.* New York: Cambridge University Press.

Schneier, F. R., Johnson, J., Hornig, C. D., Liebowitz, M. R., & Weissman, M. M. (1992). Social phobia: Comorbidity and morbidity in an epidemiologic sample. *Archives of General Psychiatry, 49,* 282–288.

Schwartz, S., & Link, B. G. (1991). Sociological perspectives on mental health: An integrative approach. In D. Offer & M. Sabshin (Eds.), *The diversity of normal behavior* (pp. 239–274). New York: Basic Books.

Srole, L., Langner, T. S., Michael, S. T., Opler, M. K., & Rennie, T. A. C. (1962). *Mental health in the metropolis: The midtown study* (Vol. 1). New York: McGraw-Hill.

Stein, M. B., Walker, J. R., & Forde, D. R. (1994). Setting diagnostic thresholds for social phobia: Considerations from a community survey of social anxiety. *American Journal of Psychiatry, 151,* 408–412.

Torgersen, S. (1983). Genetic factors in anxiety disorders. *Archives of General Psychiatry, 40,* 1085–1089.

Tsuang, M. T., Fleming, J. A., Kendler, K. S., & Gruenberg, A. S. (1988). Selection of controls for family studies: Biases and implications. *Archives of General Psychiatry, 45,* 1006–1008.

Wacker, H. R., Müllejans, R., Klein, K. H., & Battegay, R. (1992). Identification of cases of anxiety disorders and affective disorders in the community according to ICD 10 and DSM-III-R by using the Composite International Diagnostic Interview (CIDI). *International Journal of Methods in Psychiatric Research, 2,* 91–100.

Weissman, M. M. (1985). The epidemiology of anxiety disorders: Rates, risks and familial patterns. In A. H. Tuma & J. D. Maser (Eds.), *Anxiety and the anxiety disorders* (pp. 275–296). Hillsdale, NJ: Erlbaum.

Weissman, M. M. (1987). Advances in psychiatric epidemiology: Rates and risks for major depression. *American Journal of Public Health, 4,* 445–451.

Weissman, M. M., Merikangas, K. R., John, K., Wickramaratne, P., Prusoff, B. A., & Kidd, K. K. (1986). Family genetic studies of psychiatric disorders: Developing technologies. *Archives of General Psychiatry, 43,* 1104–1116.

Wells, J. E., Bushnell, J. A., Hornblow, A. R., Joyce, P. R., & Oakley-Browne, M. A. (1989). Christchurch Psychiatric Epidemiology Study: Methodology and lifetime prevalence for specific psychiatric disorders. *Australian and New Zealand Journal of Psychiatry, 23,* 315–326.

Wickramaratne, P .J., Weissman, M. M., Leaf, P. J., & Holford, T. R. (1989). Age, period and cohort effects on the risk of major depression: Results from five United States communities. *Journal of Clinical Epidemiology, 42,* 333–343.

CHAPTER THREE

Descriptive Psychopathology of Social Phobia

RONALD M. RAPEE

Many of the descriptive aspects of social phobia are very similar to those of the other anxiety disorders, thus clearly supporting the inclusion of social phobia in the anxiety cluster. However, the validity of considering social phobia as a unique diagnostic entity is supported by a number of descriptive features that are relatively specific to this disorder. This chapter will provide an overview of the descriptive psychopathology of social phobia. While specific theories of social phobia will not be discussed, it should be recognized that any theoretical model of a disorder must be consistent with its descriptive features. It is impossible to avoid some overlap with issues of diagnosis and theory. However, as much as possible, this chapter will adhere to a simple description of the key features of social phobia.

SHYNESS AND SOCIAL PHOBIA

The term "social phobia" was first used consistently by British researchers in the 1960s (e.g., Marks, 1969). However, it was not until 1980 that the term received "official" status in the third edition of the *Diagnostic and Statistical Manual of Mental Disorders* (DSM-III; American Psychiatric Association, 1980). Thus, research relating to the specific disorder social phobia has been conducted primarily since the mid-1980s, leading one group to describe it as recently as 1985 as a "neglected anxiety disorder" (Liebowitz, Gorman, Fyer, & Klein, 1985, p. 729).

In contrast to the neglected status of social phobia, there has been a vast literature, conducted mainly among social and counseling psychologists, investigating specific personality features described variously as "social anxiety," "heterosocial anxiety," "embarrassability," "dating anxiety," "love shyness," and "shyness." In most ways, the individuals identified in these studies are very similar to individuals technically diagnosed with social phobia. It is not the purpose of this chapter to provide a comprehensive discussion of this issue. However, it is important to note that studies that have directly compared "shy" college students with clinical social phobics have failed to find major differences between these groups on behavioral, cognitive, or physiological parameters (Turner, Beidel, & Larkin, 1986; Turner, Beidel, & Townsley, 1990). Thus, the difference between the concepts of shyness and social phobia may be more quantitative than qualitative, centering on such issues as degree of functional impairment and extent of avoidance (see Bruch & Cheek, Chapter 8, this volume).

For the purposes of this chapter, it will be assumed that shyness and social phobia are two largely overlapping phenomena. In this way, studies conducted on subjects described as "shy," "socially anxious," and so on, can be used to provide additional information on the descriptive psychopathology of social phobia. However, wherever possible, individuals will still be referred to in the terms used in the original studies.

FEARED EVENTS

Types of Fears

By definition, social phobics fear and avoid situations in which they are "exposed to unfamiliar people or to possible scrutiny by others" (American Psychiatric Association, 1994, p. 416; see also Table 1.1), in other words, situations that involve other people. Some of the most commonly feared situations include attending social gatherings, meeting new people, formal performance situations, and assertiveness situations. Studies that have compared the potential of various situations to elicit fear have found public speaking to be the most commonly feared situation (Holt, Heimberg, Hope, & Liebowitz, 1992; Rapee, Sanderson, & Barlow, 1988; Schneier, Johnson, Hornig, Liebowitz, & Weissman, 1992; Turner, Beidel, Dancu, & Keys, 1986; Turner, Beidel, & Townsley, 1992), closely followed by situations such as parties, meetings, and speaking to authority figures (Rapee et al., 1988). Most social phobics report fear of a number of social situations, and it is the exception for fear to be specific to one (Holt, Heimberg, Hope, & Liebowitz, 1992; Rapee et al., 1988; Turner, Beidel, Dancu, & Keys, 1986).

One question that has interested researchers in the field is whether the types of feared situations reported by social phobics can be formed into meaningful clusters. One potential distinction has been suggested between concerns related to performance (e.g., eating or working in front of others) and concerns related to social interaction (e.g., meeting new people, talking on the telephone) (Liebowitz, 1987; Mattick & Clarke, 1989; Turner et al., 1992). This distinction has been reflected in some questionnaire and clinician measures of social phobia that have been developed to assess fears of each type of situation (Liebowitz, 1987; Mattick & Clarke, 1989). Unfortunately, the distinction between situation types reflected in these measures has not been based on empirical discrimination. In fact, one study that subjected the Liebowitz Social Anxiety Scale to factor analysis failed to find support for the suggested two-factor structure (Slavkin, Holt, Heimberg, Jaccard, & Liebowitz, 1990), although other work has provided some support for the construct validity of the two separate Mattick and Clarke scales (Heimberg, Mueller, Holt, Hope, & Liebowitz, 1992). Thus, empirical support for the performance−interaction distinction is unclear at present and considerably more work needs to be conducted before conclusions can be drawn.

Subtypes of Social Phobia

Some authors have suggested that the different types of situations feared by people with social phobia (performance concerns vs. social interaction concerns) may characterize independent subgroups of social phobia (e.g., Turner et al., 1992). In other words, it may be that certain individuals are primarily concerned about performance situations and are hardly bothered by social interaction situations, while other individuals have the opposite characteristic.

Along similar lines, in the shyness literature, there has been an attempt to specify two subgroups of shy persons: "fearful" and "self-conscious" (Buss, 1980). Fearful shys respond primarily to novel social situations and the intrusiveness of other people, while self-conscious shys respond to situations in which they are the focus of scrutiny. Thus, there is a marked similarity between the distinction evidenced by these subgroups and the performance−interaction distinction in social phobia. To date, at least one study has provided evidence consistent with Buss's predictions (e.g., an earlier age of onset for fearful shys)(Bruch, Giordano, & Pearl, 1986), but the data can also be interpreted to suggest that the two groups differ in degree rather than quality. Given that there is currently little empirical evidence for the performance−interaction distinction based purely on feared situations (see above), it is difficult to argue convincingly for such a distinction between individuals.

A related, but not identical, issue refers to the number of situations feared by individuals with social phobia. This issue is reflected in the specification in the revised third (DSM-III-R) and fourth (DSM-IV) editions of the *Diagnostic and Statistical Manual of Mental Disorders* (American Psychiatric Association, 1987, 1994) of a generalized subtype of social phobia that is presumably distinct from other types of social phobia (often referred to as "nongeneralized" in the literature). The issue is somewhat related to the previous one because it is often believed that individuals who are more concerned about performance situations are likely to have a narrower range of fears (i.e., nongeneralized) (Heimberg, Hope, Dodge, & Becker, 1990; Turner et al., 1992).

In recent years, a number of studies have attempted to identify differences between these two subtypes of social phobia. The results have been largely consistent in indicating that generalized social phobics score higher on a broad range of social anxiety and other self-report measures than do nongeneralized social phobics (Heimberg, Hope, et al., 1990; Holt, Heimberg, & Hope, 1992; Turner et al., 1992). Generalized social phobics have also been shown to display greater life interference and general clinical severity than do nongeneralized social phobics (Heimberg, Hope, et al., 1990; Holt, Heimberg, & Hope, 1992; Turner et al., 1992). These findings suggest that the generalized subtype of social phobia specified in DSM-III-R and DSM-IV may differ from other types of social phobia primarily in degree. Only one set of findings has indicated a possible qualitative difference between these groups. In one study, public speaking phobics (nongeneralized) were found to have a significantly lower heart rate reactivity to an individualized behavioral challenge than did generalized social phobics (Heimberg, Hope, et al., 1990). This finding was substantially replicated by Levin et al. (1993), who reported that public speaking phobics had significantly higher heart rates than did generalized social phobics or normal controls in response to a speech task, but this finding may be accounted for by higher baseline (prespeech) heart rates among the public speaking phobics and also by the fact that the task (speech) was, by definition, the most feared situation for the public speaking phobics but may not have been so for the generalized social phobics. Notably, generalized social phobics and normal controls did not differ from each other in heart rate. However, a study by Turner et al. (1992) found that heart rate in response to a standardized behavioral test did not differ between generalized and nongeneralized social phobic subjects and that, in fact, there was a slight tendency for generalized social phobics to have a higher heart rate in response to the challenge. Thus, while the data on heart rate reactivity in response to behavioral challenge provide the only potential evidence for a qualitative difference between subtypes at present, the evidence is mixed and the results are far from conclusive. Further, even if a difference in heart rate reactivity is found, it remains to be demonstrated whether this has any implications for classification. Presumably, classification is based on assumed differences in etiology, nature, and treatment. A difference on a single physiological subsystem is hardly grounds for making such a distinction.

A final issue that has been discussed fervently in the social phobia literature is the question of the relationship between social phobia and the Axis II diagnosis of avoidant personality disorder. Avoidant personality disorder has been found to be the most common Axis II correlate of social phobia (Turner, Beidel, Borden, Stanley, & Jacob, 1991) and has been found to be more frequently associated with generalized social phobia than with nongeneralized social phobia (Schneier, Spitzer, Gibbon, Fyer, & Liebowitz, 1991). However, studies have failed to find qualitative differences between social phobics with and without avoidant personality disorder. Rather, individuals with social phobia and avoidant personality disorder have been found to score higher on most measures of social anxiety, general psychopathology, and overall severity than do individuals with social phobia but without avoidant personality disorder (Herbert, Hope, & Bellack, 1992; Holt, Heimberg, & Hope, 1992; Turner et al., 1992: see also Heimberg, Holt, Schneier, Spitzer, & Liebowitz, 1993).

Thus, there is currently little conclusive empirical support for a qualitative distinction between subtypes of social phobia or between social phobia and avoidant personality disorder. While it is possible that qualitative differences will be demonstrated in the future, the evidence to date may be interpreted most parsimoniously in terms of a quantitative rather than a qualitative difference between these groups (Heimberg, Hope, et al., 1990; Holt, Heimberg, & Hope, 1992; Turner et al., 1992). For example, one study that looked at the number of situations feared by social phobic individuals failed to find evidence for a bimodal distribution of number of feared situations; rather, it found a relatively linear decrease in numbers as the number of feared situations increased (Holt, Heimberg, Hope, & Liebowitz, 1992). As noted by Turner et al. (1992), the core feature of social phobia is a fear of negative evaluation, and this feature appears to be the essential issue in all types of social phobia and in avoidant personality disorder. Presumably, individuals differ in the degree of their fear of negative evaluation and in the degree of general neuroticism (or negative affectivity), suggesting that trying to distinguish subtypes may simply reflect arbitrary cutoffs along a continuum.

Moderating Variables

A final issue related to situational fear in social phobia concerns the moderating influences on the degree of fear experienced. It is generally believed that the degree of fear experienced in social situations can be influenced by a number of parameters. These parameters include the size, gender, and social status of the audience and the implicit rules (formality) of the situation. To date, there have been few empirical tests of these effects, but a number of hints can be drawn from related research. In one study, social phobic subjects were more likely to report distress and avoidance related to formal rather than to informal speaking situations (Turner, Beidel, Dancu, & Keyes, 1986). In a study using self-report diaries of daily interactions, socially anxious subjects were found to engage in fewer interactions with the opposite sex than were low anxious subjects (Dodge, Heimberg, Nyman, & O'Brien, 1987). Similarly, in studies using standardized behavioral tasks, greater responsivity was demonstrated to opposite-sex interactions than to same-sex interactions on cognitive, physiological, and social skills measures (Beidel, Turner, & Dancu, 1985; Turner, Beidel, & Larkin, 1986). (Unfortunately, sexual orientation of the subjects was not assessed.) It would be of value to the future understanding of social phobia to more clearly identify the general environmental variables which influence levels of social fear.

Summary

In summary, people with social phobia are characterized by a tendency to fear and avoid a variety of situations having in common a potential for scrutiny or evaluation by others. The degree of fear experienced in these situations can be influenced by a number of general parameters, such as the formality of the situations or the gender of the observer. There is also some possibility that the feared situations may cluster into two broad types: those characterized by performance in front of others and those characterized by verbal interaction. In turn, there is considerable speculation that social phobia can be better conceptualized as consisting of a number of subtypes, most widely accepted being a generalized subtype (the person with this subtype of social phobia fears most social situations, both performance and social interaction) versus a nongeneralized subtype (the person with this type of social phobia fears more specific situations, generally performance related). To date, however, there is little evidence for a qualitative difference between these subtypes, and most findings of differences can be easily explained by positing an arbitrary distinction between individuals differing in the degree of their social phobia.

SOMATIC FEATURES

The physiological symptoms reported by social phobics are essentially those reported by most anxious groups. They include sweating, shaking, hot flushes, palpitations, and nausea. Few studies have directly compared the physical symptoms reported by social phobics with those reported by individuals with other disorders. Two studies, however, have indicated that social phobics are more likely than are panic disorder subjects to report blushing, twitching, and stammering (Amies, Gelder, & Shaw, 1983; Solyom, Ledwidge, & Solyom, 1986), and another has indicated that social phobics are more likely to report a dry mouth (Reich, Noyes, & Yates, 1988).

In studies using physiological measures, social phobics show the increased arousal typical of most anxious subjects on exposure to their feared stimuli (Beidel et al., 1985; Turner, Beidel, & Larkin, 1986). Similarly, habituation to auditory stimuli has been found to be slower in social phobics than in normal controls or specific phobics but faster than in persons with "anxiety states" and mixed anxiety/depression (Lader, 1980). This finding fits with self-report studies showing social phobics to have lower trait anxiety scores than do subjects with panic disorder, obsessive–compulsive disorder, or generalized anxiety disorder but to have higher scores than do simple phobics (Rapee, Brown, Antony, & Barlow, 1992; Turner, McCann, Beidel, & Mezzich, 1986).

PERFORMANCE AND SOCIAL SKILLS

Test Anxiety

One of the most formal and threatening evaluation situations is the academic test. Not surprisingly then, many social phobics report being anxious in test situations. Empirically, fears of tests, failure, and lack of success tend to load with social fears in factor analytic studies (Bernstein & Allen, 1969; Lovibond & Rapee, 1993; B. M. Rubin, Katkin, Weiss, & Efran, 1968). Given these findings, it would be expected that subjects who seek treatment for test anxiety and tend to do poorly on tests would often meet criteria for a diagnosis of social phobia. Indeed, this appears to be the case. In one study of 8- to 12-year-old children who scored high on a measure of test anxiety, social phobia was the most frequently assigned DSM-III-R diagnosis (Beidel & Turner, 1988). In terms of performance, there is a considerable body of evidence to suggest that test anxiety is negatively related to academic performance (Seipp, 1991). Of course the direction of this relationship is not clear, but it is certainly possible that the greater anxiety experienced by test anxious individuals may in turn cause decrements in test performance (see below).

Cognitive Task Performance

The link between high levels of anxiety and poor task performance has long been recognized. A vast literature attests to the fact that excessive levels of anxiety can interfere with the adequate performance of complex tasks (Eysenck, 1979; Seipp, 1991). The evidence appears to be especially strong for cognitive tasks, with anxiety seeming to have less detrimental effect on motor tasks (Eysenck, 1979).

Significantly, there is considerable evidence to suggest that interference with task performance is not an effect of the entire phenomenon of anxiety but, rather, is a specific effect of the mental component (worry) (Morris, Davis, & Hutchings, 1981). Theories of the mechanism by which anxiety produces a decrease in performance tend to center on the role of self-focused attention and self-evaluative concerns (Eysenck, 1979; Wine, 1971), which, in turn, utilize space in working memory (Eysenck, 1985; Rapee, 1993). Given the prominence of both of these features in social phobia (see the next section), it may be expected that social phobics could be especially prone to interference with performance on cognitive tasks. On the other hand, it has been suggested that subjects whose performance is adversely affected by anxiety may compensate for this interference through increased motivation (Eysenck, 1979). Thus, it is also possible that social phobics may be characterized by increased effort on cognitive tasks. Certainly with respect to academic performance, social phobics do not appear to be different from nonanxious individuals in overall educational attainment or school grades (Ludwig & Lazarus, 1983), and they may attain a higher level of education than do agoraphobics (Solyom et al., 1986). However, on at least one specific task, performance on Stroop color-naming, levels of shyness have been found to be inversely related to task performance in both children and college students (Arnold & Cheek, 1986; Ludwig & Lazarus, 1983). Similarly, social phobics have been found to generally perform more poorly on Stroop tasks than do nonanxious subjects (Mattia, Heimberg, & Hope, 1993).

Social Skills

Whereas the performance of social phobics in academic situations has not been the focus of much research, their performance in social situations has. A number of studies have examined the question of whether socially anxious subjects perform more poorly in social-evaluative situations than do nonanxious subjects. The results have been far from consistent. Some studies have found socially anxious subjects to be significantly worse on a number of social performance indicators than are nonanxious subjects, as measured by independent raters (Pilkonis, 1977b; Twentyman & McFall, 1975). (It should be noted that in the study by Pilkonis, significant differences were only found on a few measures and for only one task.) In contrast, a number of studies have found no difference between the performance of nonanxious subjects and subjects with social anxiety or DSM-III-R diagnosed social phobia on public speaking (Pilkonis, 1977b; Rapee & Lim, 1992) or interaction with an opposite-sex confederate (Clark & Arkowitz, 1975; Glasgow & Arkowitz, 1975). Finally, an intermediate position has been demonstrated in some studies that failed to find many differences between socially anxious and nonanxious subjects on specific skills measures (e.g., eye contact), but that found worse performance in socially anxious subjects on broader, more global measures of performance (Arkowitz, Lichtenstein, McGovern, & Hines, 1975; Beidel et al., 1985; Borkovec, Stone, O'Brien, & Kaloupek, 1974).

The issue of social performance in social phobics is complex. Even in studies that have found a difference between anxious and nonanxious subjects, it is not clear whether this reflects a lack of skills or a skills inhibition. Certainly, most data do not seem to be consistent with a lack of specific, basic skills. However, whether more global measures of social skills are reduced in socially anxious subjects seems to vary between studies, perhaps reflecting the influence of as yet unidentified parameters. If so, this would suggest that social skills, when reduced, are inhibited rather than deficient in social phobia, a suggestion that is consistent with the anxiety and performance literature. In support of this conclusion, it has been found that shy and nonshy subjects appear to be relatively similar in their knowledge of appropriate social behaviors, but shy subjects are less willing to use these behaviors and do not believe that they have the ability to do so (Hill, 1989). Similarly, one study has provided some empirical evidence for the importance of anxiety levels in inhibiting performance in a public speaking situation (Rapee & Hilton, 1993). In this study, groups of subjects who differed in levels of state anxiety were also found to differ in their public speaking performance in an "inverted-U" fashion. The worst performance (as measured by independent raters) was provided by both high socially anxious subjects who were made to feel extra anxious (and thus had very high levels of state anxiety) and low socially anxious subjects who were made to feel extra relaxed (and thus had very low levels of state anxiety). Better performance was demonstrated by both high socially anxious subjects who were made to feel relaxed and low socially anxious subjects who were made to feel anxious (both groups had similar, intermediate levels of state anxiety). Thus, high socially anxious subjects appear to have adequate abilities but their abilities may be inhibited by increased state anxiety in threatening situations. A similar finding was reported in another study that found that recall of social information was disrupted by a low anxiety condition for low socially anxious subjects but by a high anxiety condition for high socially anxious subjects (Hope, Heimberg, & Klein, 1990). This study also indicated that self-focused attention (see below) was positively correlated with omission of information in a recall task in socially anxious subjects.

Summary

While some theories of social phobia assume a lower level of abilities in these individuals, the evidence to date is mixed. It is very likely that socially anxious individuals will perform worse on certain (usually complex, cognitive) tasks than do nonanxious individuals, probably because of the effects of anxiety on working memory capacity. Thus, increasing state social anxiety in a given situation will probably initially enhance and eventually disrupt performance in an inverted-U relationship. Whether social phobic individuals actually lack social abilities is less clear. However, the evidence to date does not require an explanation in terms of lesser social abilities among social phobics. Rather, an inhibition of social skills because of excessive state anxiety can adequately explain the data.

COGNITIVE FEATURES

The cognitive features of social phobics have been examined in terms of both content and process. Content has been assessed using self-report instruments, self-monitoring diaries, and continuous recording. Process has been assessed using self-report measures of perceived attentional focus as well as more experimental information-processing tasks. (The reader is referred to Elting & Hope, Chapter 11, this volume, for a more detailed review of these issues.)

Cognitive Content

On broad, self-report measures of cognitive content, social phobics and high socially anxious subjects have been found to report more negative and fewer positive thoughts than non-clinical or low anxious subjects during social interactions (Beidel et al., 1985; Cacioppo, Glass, & Merluzzi, 1979; Halford & Foddy, 1982; Turner, Beidel, & Larkin, 1986). There is some indication, however, that it is negative thoughts that are more closely related to levels of anxiety and phobic severity (Dodge, Hope, Heimberg, & Becker, 1988).

More specifically, social phobics have been found to engage in a number of thoughts related to negative evaluation, lack of ability, and concerns about appearance. One of the most widely used assessment instruments with social phobics is the Fear of Negative Evaluation Scale (Watson & Friend, 1969), which is characterized by items relating to concerns over looking foolish, making a bad impression on others, and being thought of badly. Social phobics have consistently been found to score higher on this instrument than do subjects with other psychopathology, other anxiety disorders, or no mental disorder (Heimberg, Hope, Rapee, & Bruch, 1988). Thus, some authors have suggested that fear of negative evaluation is the central concern in social phobia (Butler, 1985; Turner et al., 1992). On the other hand, there appear to be other types of concerns that also characterize social phobics. Hartman (1984) conducted a factor analysis of 21 items assessing social-evaluative concerns. Four factors were generated relating to concerns about social inadequacy, others' awareness of distress, fear of negative evaluation, and autonomic arousal. In addition, shy subjects have been found to perceive themselves as less physically attractive than nonshy subjects perceive themselves (Bruch et al., 1986), although there is some evidence that this may be a somewhat realistic appraisal (Pilkonis, 1977b).

Cognitive Process

The process of social phobics' cognition has been primarily characterized by an increase in self-focused attention (Hope, Heimberg, & Klein, 1990; Ingram, 1990). One particular construct, public self-consciousness, has been defined as a tendency to view the self as a social object (Fenigstein, Scheier, & Buss, 1975), implying an excessive degree of attention devoted to external aspects of the self. This construct has been empirically distinguished from private self-consciousness (Fenigstein et al., 1975), which is more related to the degree of attention devoted to internal physiological changes and feeling states. Social anxiety has been found to correlate positively with public self-consciousness (Bruch, Gorsky, Collins, & Berger, 1989; Fenigstein et al., 1975; Pilkonis, 1977a) and has been found to be more strongly correlated with this construct than with private self-consciousness (Hope & Heimberg, 1988). In addition, shy subjects and social phobics have been found to score higher than nonshy or agoraphobic subjects on measures of public self-consciousness (Bruch, Heimberg, Berger, & Collins, 1989; Pilkonis, 1977a). Bruch and Heimberg (1994) have shown a similar difference between social phobic and nonclinical subjects. In one experimental test of attentional focus, the percentage of time spent focusing on the self during a social interaction (measured by self-report) was found to be positively correlated with degree of shyness (Melchior & Cheek, 1990).

In addition to self-focused attention, social phobics presumably also display the excessive attentional allocation to environmental threat displayed by most anxious subjects (Dalgleish & Watts, 1990). For example, it has been demonstrated that anxious subjects with primarily social concerns tend to allocate extra attentional resources to the specific detection of social threat (Mathews & MacLeod, 1985). Similarly, a number of studies have demonstrated that social phobics show a greater interference in cognitive tasks such as modified Stroop color-naming or lexical decisions when words are related to social threat (typically negative evaluation) than when words are related to physical threat or are neutral (Cloitre, Heimberg, Holt, & Liebowitz, 1992; Hope, Rapee, Heimberg, & Dombeck, 1990; Mattia et al., 1993).

In contrast to findings on attentional allocation, there have been mixed results with respect to encoding and retrieval biases in social phobics. In an early study, it was demonstrated that socially anxious subjects tend to interpret ambiguous feedback more negatively than do low anxious subjects (Smith & Sarason, 1975). However, there have been few attempts to replicate this finding, and at least one study with clinical social phobics has not supported this result (Rapee, McCallum, Melville, Ravenscroft, & Rodney, 1994). On the other hand, an investigation of the interpretation of ambiguous sentences by anxious subjects indicated that they were more likely than nonanxious subjects to interpret ambiguous sentences in a threatening fashion, and that this was equally the case for both subjects suffering from physical and social concerns (Eysenck, Mogg, May, Richards, & Mathews, 1991).

With respect to memory, at least one study has provided data to suggest that socially anxious subjects are more likely to recall social threat information than are low anxiety subjects (O'Banion & Arkowitz, 1977). However, it has been pointed out that the results of this study are far from clearly interpreted (Rapee et al., 1994), and a series of studies with clinical social phobics has failed to find any support for biased retrieval using explicit, implicit, or autobiographical tasks (Rapee et al., 1994).

In contrast to the results with encoding and retrieval, a particularly robust finding in social phobics has been their tendency to inaccurately perceive their own performance. The typical paradigm involves having subjects perform a particular task (e.g., public speaking, heterosocial interaction) and then asking the subjects themselves, as well as independent judges, to rate the quality of the performance on a number of parameters. It has been consistently found that social phobics rate their own performance considerably worse than judges rate their performance, and that this discrepancy is significantly larger than for nonclincal subjects (Clark & Arkowitz, 1975; Glasgow & Arkowitz, 1975; Rapee & Hilton, 1993; Rapee & Lim, 1992). Interestingly, this distortion only seems to occur for ratings of subjects' own performance, since social phobics and nonphobics are equally accurate in rating other people's performance (Curran, Wallander, & Fischetti, 1980; Rapee & Lim, 1992).

Summary

Cognitively, social phobics appear to be characterized by an excess of negative thoughts, particularly related to their own perceived inadequacy and others' evaluations. In social performance situations, they demonstrate biases in perception of their own (but not of others') performance and underestimate their own abilities. Finally, there is some evidence that social phobic individuals allocate considerable attentional resources to external threat and to monitoring their own appearance. However, current data are mixed as to the existence of other information-processing biases.

DEMOGRAPHIC FEATURES

Age at Onset

It has been consistently reported that the onset of social phobia occurs later than is found for many specific phobias (e.g., small animal phobias) but considerably earlier than is found for panic disorder (Marks & Gelder, 1966; Öst, 1987; Thyer, Parrish, Curtis, Nesse, & Cameron, 1985). The mean age of onset has generally been placed around the mid to late teens (Mannuzza, Fyer, Liebowitz, & Klein, 1990). However, the pattern of onset appears to be considerably skewed (Amies et al., 1983; Schneier et al., 1992), suggesting that a median age of onset (in the early teens) may be a better estimate. However, even a median age of onset may not adequately reflect the data, since a number of social phobics report experiencing the disorder all their life (Schneier et al., 1992). As many as 47% have been found to report a lifelong disorder or, at least, onset prior to age 10 (Schneier et al., 1992). In addition, age of onset is typically measured by retrospective self-report and thus depends on recall of specific instances of the disorder. Naturally, this may be highly inaccurate.

An alternative way to estimate age of onset is from a developmental perspective. It could be argued that social phobia cannot begin until children have an awareness of others and of themselves as objects of evaluation. Along these lines, it has been found that self-consciousness and concerns about negative evaluation from others develops in children at around

8 years of age (Bennett & Gillingham, 1991; Crozier & Burnham, 1990). In contrast, some research has demonstrated that the majority of children are quite capable of showing embarrassment (reflected in certain behaviors) by 3 years of age (Lewis, Stanger, Sullivan, & Barone, 1991). From a more theoretical stance, Buss (1980) has suggested that self-conscious shyness cannot begin until children develop a sense of themselves as social objects, but that fearful shyness can develop before this stage primarily because of greater emotional reactivity. Indeed, there is some evidence that so-called fearful shys are more likely to report being shy "all their lives," while self-conscious shys more commonly report an age of onset after the beginning of school (Bruch et al., 1986).

Social phobia is also commonly diagnosed in children and can often be diagnosed below the age of 10 (Beidel, 1991). Consistent with these clinical data, questionnaire assessment of nonclinical children indicates that concern over social-evaluative negative outcomes (such as being laughed at) can be found in children as young as 6 years and does not significantly increase with age (La Greca, Kraslow Dandes, Wick, Shaw, & Stone, 1988; Campbell & Rapee, 1994). This is in contrast to some data examining fears of social stimuli (such as giving a talk) that do seem to increase with age (King et al., 1989). Finally, behaviors have been identified in children as young as 21 months that are indicative of strong social fears, and that predict an increased incidence of social phobia in later years (Rosenbaum, Biederman, Hirshfeld, Bolduc, & Chaloff, 1991).

Based on these developmental data, it appears that the precise age of onset of social phobia will depend integrally on the definition used. It is likely that fears of social situations can occur from early infancy (Bennett & Gillingham, 1991; Crozier & Burnham, 1990; Garcia-Coll, Kagan, & Reznick, 1984). However, the often cited central feature of adult social phobia, fear of negative evaluation by others, may not develop until somewhat later in life (Bennett & Gillingham, 1991; Crozier & Burnham, 1990). Given the above confusion, the age of onset in social phobia can at best be said to be unclear. However, it seems that it may well be earlier than the average determined by retrospective studies. Further, it is likely that at least a tendency toward social reticence may be evident from infancy (K. H. Rubin & Asendorpf, 1993).

Age at Presentation

Social phobics present for treatment at a typically earlier age than do individuals with other anxiety disorders (Amies et al., 1983; Rapee et al., 1988; Solyom et al., 1986). The mean age of presentation appears to be around 30 years (Butler, Cullington, Munby, Amies, & Gelder, 1984;

Heimberg, Dodge, et al., 1990; Rapee et al., 1988). Given the early age of onset, this suggests that social phobics present for treatment, on average, between 15 to 25 years after the onset of their disorder. This is considerably slower than is found in subjects with panic disorder (Solyom et al., 1986), which may be explained by the relative distress caused by these disorders, by lesser public awareness of social phobia as a treatable disorder, or by the fact that social phobics are more likely to view their disorder as an intractable component of their personality.

Course of the Disorder

Compared with concerns about physical threat, concern over social threat appears to be relatively stable across the lifespan (Campbell & Rapee, 1994; Lovibond & Rapee, 1993). This suggests that untreated social fears should have a fairly chronic course. Indeed, this has been reported by several studies. From a retrospective perspective, Solyom et al. (1986) have found that social phobics most commonly report a constant static course to their disorder. Similar results are indicated by prospective data. In a study of shy individuals covering approximately 30 years, shyness in childhood appeared to persist fairly consistently into adulthood (Caspi, Elder, & Bem, 1988). Extreme social reticence in early childhood has been also reported to be relatively stable up to at least 7.5 years of age (Rosenbaum et al., 1991).

Gender Distribution

One of the most obvious differences between social phobia and the other anxiety disorders lies in the gender ratio of presenting patients. In contrast to the marked female predominance in most of the anxiety disorders, social phobics presenting to clinics show an equal distribution across sex or even a slight preponderance of males (Rapee et al., 1988; Solyom et al., 1986). However, it may be that this greater proportion of males reflects presentation differences rather than actual diagnostic differences. Epidemiological data from the National Institute of Mental Health study indicate a greater number of females meeting criteria for social phobia than males, in the ratio of around 2:1 (Schneier et al., 1992). Similar results are indicated in questionnaire studies, in which females report greater social fears and shyness than males (La Greca et al., 1988; Lovibond & Rapee, 1993).

Thus, it seems that, consistent with other anxiety disorders, females report more social anxiety than males, but that males are more likely to seek treatment. The reasons for this discrepancy are not clear, but they may reflect societal influences. For example, in traditional Western society, where the man is generally expected to initiate romantic contact, have higher career aspirations, and be more assertive than the woman, social concerns are likely to produce greater life interference for males than for females. In line with this suggestion, one study found twice as many females than males meeting DSM-III criteria for social phobia without the criterion of "significant distress" (Pollard & Henderson, 1988). When significant distress was included as a criterion, the proportion of each gender became more similar.

Family Factors

There is very little direct evidence relating to the family backgrounds of social phobics. Anxious subjects are generally characterized by having anxious families, and this appears to be the case for social phobics (Amies et al., 1983). Compared to other disorders, the first-degree relatives of social phobics have been found to have a higher degree of social phobia (Fyer, Mannuzza, Chapman, Liebowitz, & Klein, 1993; Reich & Yates, 1988). In one of the few adoption studies to date, shy children were found to have both biological and adoptive mothers who were more socially anxious and less sociable than those of nonshy children (Plomin & Daniels, 1986). Similarly, social phobics retrospectively rate their parents as being more socially anxious and less sociable and as stressing the opinions of others to a greater extent than do agoraphobics or nonclinical subjects (Bruch, 1989; Bruch & Heimberg, 1994; Bruch, Heimberg, et al., 1989). Interestingly, on a variety of retrospectively rated parental variables, nongeneralized social phobics score midway between generalized social phobics and nonclinical subjects (Bruch & Heimberg, 1994), supporting the suggestion made earlier in this chapter that these subtypes of social phobia may differ more quantitatively than qualitatively.

In terms of mediating constructs, social phobic subjects retrospectively rate their parents as more rejecting and overprotective and less emotionally warm than do nonclinical subjects, although differences with other anxiety disorders are inconclusive (Arrindell, Emmelkamp, Monsma, & Brilman, 1983; Parker, 1979). Similarly, it has been found that levels of shyness are related to decreased maternal acceptance and increased maternal control (Eastburg & Johnson, 1990). It is unfortunate that prospective studies have not been conducted to confirm these retrospective reports. One study of children who were high in fear of failure found that the parents of these children were less likely to provide reinforcement for appropriate behaviors, less likely to respond to expressions of insecurity in the child, and more likely to express tension and irritation than parents of low anxious children (Hermans, ter Laak, & Maes, 1972).

ASSOCIATED FEATURES

Comorbidity

It is the exception for subjects with anxiety disorders to meet the criteria for only a single disorder (Sanderson, Di Nardo, Rapee, & Barlow, 1990), and social phobia is no different. Additional disorders have been found in around 50% of individuals with social phobia (de Ruiter, Rijken, Garssen, van Schaik, & Kraaimaat, 1989; Sanderson et al., 1990; Turner et al., 1991). Most common among these additional disorders have been other anxiety disorders (especially panic disorder and simple phobia), mood disorders, and substance abuse (de Ruiter et al., 1989; Sanderson et al., 1990; Schneier et al., 1992; Turner et al., 1991). Two of these disorders, substance abuse and depression, will be discussed in more detail below.

Substance Abuse

According to the tension reduction theory of alcohol abuse, alcohol consumption is reinforcing because of its ability to reduce tension and anxiety (Kingham, 1958). Further, it has been demonstrated that consumption of alcohol is particularly effective in reducing the response to social threat (Higgins & Marlatt, 1975). Thus, it would be expected that social phobics would be especially at risk for alcohol abuse.

Indeed, it has been found that rates of excessive alcohol consumption are higher in social phobics than in subjects with most other anxiety disorders (Amies et al., 1983; Kushner, Sher, & Beitman, 1990; Turner, Beidel, Dancu, & Keyes, 1986) and that the presence of social phobia increases the risk for alcohol abuse in panic disorder patients (Otto, Pollack, Sachs, O'Neill, & Rosenbaum, 1992). However, data on formal diagnoses of alcohol abuse have been mixed. Approximately 19% of a community sample of social phobics have been found to meet criteria for an additional diagnosis of alcohol abuse (Schneier et al., 1992). In contrast, in clinical settings this figure has varied from around 2% (Herbert et al., 1992; Turner et al., 1991, 1992) to 16% (Schneier, Martin, Liebowitz, Gorman, & Fyer, 1989). This discrepancy may be partly a result of the exclusion of individuals with severe alcohol problems from many anxiety units. From the opposite perspective, it has been found that a considerable proportion of individuals in alcohol detoxification units meet the criteria for social phobia (Kushner et al., 1990). In the majority of cases, alcohol abuse appears to begin after onset of the social phobia, and alcohol is reported to be used as a form of self-medication (Kushner et al., 1990).

Abuse of other substances has not been widely studied among social phobics. In one study using college students, shy students were more likely than nonshy students to use cocaine, marijuana, and hallucinogens (Page, 1990). A formal diagnosis of substance (drug) abuse has also been found in 13% of community social phobics (Schneier et al., 1992) but has not been found to be especially common among clinical social phobics (Amies et al., 1983; Herbert et al., 1992). However, a sizable proportion of clinical social phobics report using daily anxiolytic medication (Sanderson et al., 1990).

Depression

Depression and anxiety are highly related, and overlapped constructs and depressive disorders are a common concomitant of anxiety disorders (Brady & Kendall, 1992; Barlow, Di Nardo, Vermilyea, Vermilyea, & Blanchard, 1986). In addition, social phobia has a high degree of associated life interference, especially interference with interpersonal relationships (see below). Thus, it is not surprising that a large proportion of social phobics meet the criteria for major depression or dysthymic disorder (Sanderson et al., 1990; Schneier et al., 1992; Stein, Tancer, Gelernter, Vittone, & Uhde, 1990). In addition, when present, the mood disorder has been found to begin after the onset of the social phobia in the majority of cases (Schneier et al., 1992; Stein et al., 1990). Further, suicidal ideation has been found to occur frequently among social phobics (Schneier et al., 1992), while there is some, weaker, evidence that the frequency of suicidal attempts is also higher than normal (Amies et al., 1983; Schneier et al., 1992).

Interpersonal Relationships

Social phobia, by its very nature, interferes with both romantic and nonromantic relationships. In a longitudinal study over 30 years, shy males were found to get married and have a first child around three years later than did nonshy males (Caspi et al., 1988). This was not the case for females, which may relate to the different social roles for the two genders. In studies of clinical populations, social phobics are consistently found to be less likely to be married than are persons with other anxiety disorders (Amies et al., 1983; Sanderson et al., 1990; Solyom et al., 1986), and this is also the case in community samples (Schneier et al., 1992).

Studies of nonromantic relationships are less common than are studies of romantic relationships, but one study found that 69% of a group of social phobics believed that their anxiety interfered with social relationships (Turner, Beidel, Dancu, & Keyes, 1986). An inverse relationship has also been reported between shyness and sociability (Bruch, Gorsky, et al., 1989; Pilkonis, 1977a), and shy children are rated by their teachers as less friendly and sociable (Caspi et al., 1988). Shyness has also been found to correlate positively with loneliness (Anderson & Harvey, 1988; Lamm & Stephan, 1987), and, according to daily diary ratings, shy students engage in significantly fewer social interactions than do nonshy students (Dodge et al., 1987).

Career Functioning

Over 90% of a group of social phobics reported that their anxiety interfered significantly with occupational functioning, and 85% reported interference with academic functioning (Turner, Beidel, Dancu, & Keyes, 1986). In the longitudinal study described earlier, shy males were found to enter a steady career around three years later than do nonshy males, which, in turn, increased the chance that shy males would change careers and achieve less in their career (Caspi et al., 1988). Similarly, shy females were less likely to have either entered the workforce or to have reentered it after childbirth than were nonshy females. In addition, among college students, shyness has been found to be negatively related to a number of behaviors that are predicted to be important in establishing a career, such as information seeking and career decidedness (Phillips & Bruch, 1988). Socially anxious students were also apparently more restricted in their career choice, being less likely to choose careers with an interpersonal orientation (Phillips & Bruch, 1988; Bruch et al., 1986). Overall, despite the apparent subtle interferences in career functioning noted above, social phobic individuals in general have not been found to be more financially dependent than individuals without social phobia, although there is some evidence that individuals with uncomplicated social phobia (i.e., without other comorbid diagnoses) may be more financially dependent than others (Schneier et al., 1992).

CONCLUSION

There is a common perception among clinicians that social phobia is a minimal and relatively unimportant problem in sufferers' lives. In turn, this perception may explain the relative lack of research into the clinical form of this disorder. On the contrary, the present review of the descriptive features of social anxiety and social phobia points to the tremendous influence that social concerns can have on an individual's life. Social fears are characterized by restricted behavioral functioning, increased somatic symptomatology, and negative and interfering cognitive style. Social phobic individuals are at a disadvantage with respect to task performance, their career, and interpersonal and romantic relationships. They are also at increased risk for substance abuse, depression, and suicidal ideation. Furthermore, social fears appear to be extremely chronic and may be present throughout most of an individual's life. There is no better argument for urging increased research into and understanding of this debilitating disorder.

ACKNOWLEDGMENTS

Preparation of this chapter was supported by Australian Research Council Grant No. A79231562 to Ronald M. Rapee.

REFERENCES

American Psychiatric Association. (1980). *Diagnostic and statistical manual of mental disorders* (3rd ed.). Washington, DC: Author.

American Psychiatric Association. (1987). *Diagnostic and statistical manual of mental disorders* (3rd ed., rev.). Washington, DC: Author.

American Psychiatric Association. (1994). *Diagnostic and statistical manual of mental disorders* (4th ed.). Washington, DC: Author.

Amies, P. L., Gelder, M. G., & Shaw, P. M. (1983). Social phobia: A comparative clinical study. *British Journal of Psychiatry, 142,* 174–179.

Anderson, C. A., & Harvey, R. J. (1988). Discriminating between problems in living: An examination of measures of depression, loneliness, shyness, and social anxiety. *Journal of Social and Clinical Psychology, 6,* 482–491.

Arkowitz, H., Lichtenstein, E., McGovern, K., & Hines, P. (1975). The behavioral assessment of social competence in males. *Behavior Therapy, 6,* 3–13.

Arnold, A. P., & Cheek, J. M. (1986). Shyness, self-preoccupation and the Stroop Color and Word Test. *Personality and Individual Differences, 7,* 571–573.

Arrindell, W. A., Emmelkamp, P. M. G., Monsma, A., & Brilman, E. (1983). The role of perceived parental rearing practices in the aetiology of phobic disorders: A controlled study. *British Journal of Psychiatry, 143,* 183–187.

Barlow, D. H., Di Nardo, P. A., Vermilyea, B. B., Vermilyea, J., & Blanchard, E. B. (1986). Comorbidity and depression among the anxiety disorders: Issues in diagnosis and classification. *Journal of Nervous and Mental Disease, 174,* 63–72.

Beidel, D. C. (1991). Social phobia and overanxious disorder in school-age children. *Journal of the American Academy of Child and Adolescent Psychiatry, 30,* 545–552.

Beidel, D. C., & Turner, S. M. (1988). Comorbidity of test anxiety and other anxiety disorders in children. *Journal of Abnormal Child Psychology, 16,* 275–287.

Beidel, D. C., Turner, S. M., & Dancu, C. V. (1985). Physiological, cognitive and behavioral aspects of social anxiety. *Behaviour Research and Therapy, 23,* 109–117.

Bennett, M., & Gillingham, K. (1991). The role of self-focused attention in children's attributions of social emotions to the self. *Journal of Genetic Psychology, 152,* 303–309.

Bernstein, D. A., & Allen, G. J. (1969). Fear survey schedule (II): Normative data and factor analyses based upon a large college sample. *Behaviour Research and Therapy, 7,* 403–407.

Borkovec, T. D., Stone, N. M., O'Brien, G. T., & Kaloupek, D. G. (1974). Evaluation of a clinically relevant target behavior for analog outcome research. *Behavior Therapy, 5,* 503–513.

Brady, E. U., & Kendall, P. C. (1992). Comorbidity of anxiety and depression in children and adolescents. *Psychological Bulletin, 111,* 244–255.

Bruch, M. A. (1989). Assessing familial and developmental antecedents of social phobia: Issues and findings. *Clinical Psychology Review, 9,* 37–47.

Bruch, M. A., Giordano, S., & Pearl, L. (1986). Differences between fearful and self-conscious shy subtypes in background and current adjustment. *Journal of Research in Personality, 20,* 172–186.

Bruch, M. A., Gorsky, J. M., Collins, T. M., & Berger, P. A. (1989). Shyness and sociability reexamined: A multicomponent analysis. *Journal of Personality and Social Psychology, 57,* 904–915.

Bruch, M. A., & Heimberg, R. G. (1994). Differences in perceptions of parental and personal characteristics between generalized and nongeneralized social phobics. *Journal of Anxiety Disorders, 8,* 155–168.

Bruch, M. A., Heimberg, R. G., Berger, P., & Collins, T. M. (1989). Social phobia and perceptions of early parental and personal characteristics. *Anxiety Research, 2,* 57–65.

Buss, A. H. (1980). *Self-consciousness and social anxiety.* San Francisco: Freeman.

Butler, G. (1985). Exposure as a treatment for social phobia: Some instructive difficulties. *Behaviour Research and Therapy, 23,* 651–657.

Butler, G., Cullington, A., Munby, M., Amies, P., & Gelder, M. (1984). Exposure and anxiety management in the treatment of social phobia. *Journal of Consulting and Clinical Psychology, 52,* 642–650.

Cacioppo, J. T., Glass, C. R., & Merluzzi, T. V. (1979). Self-statements and self-evaluations: A cognitive-response analysis of heterosocial anxiety. *Cognitive Therapy and Research, 3,* 249–262.

Campbell, M. A., & Rapee, R. M. (1994). The nature of feared outcome representations in children. *Journal of Abnormal Child Psychology, 22,* 99–111.

Caspi, A., Elder, G. H., Jr., & Bem, D. J. (1988). Moving away from the world: Life-course patterns of shy children. *Developmental Psychology, 24,* 824–831.

Clark, J. V., & Arkowitz, H. (1975). Social anxiety and self-evaluation of interpersonal performance. *Psychological Reports, 36,* 211–221.

Cloitre, M., Heimberg, R. G., Holt, C. S., & Liebowitz, M. R. (1992). Reaction time to threat stimuli in panic disorder and social phobia. *Behaviour Research and Therapy, 30,* 609–618.

Crozier, W. R., & Burnham, M. (1990). Age-related differences in children's understanding of shyness. *British Journal of Developmental Psychology, 8,* 179–185.

Curran, J. P., Wallander, J. L., & Fischetti, M. (1980). The importance of behavioral and cognitive factors in hetero-social anxiety. *Journal of Personality, 48,* 285–292.

Dalgleish, T., & Watts, F. N. (1990). Biases of attention and memory in disorders of anxiety and depression. *Clinical Psychology Review, 10,* 589–604.

de Ruiter, C., Rijken, H., Garssen, B., van Schaik, A., & Kraaimaat, F. (1989). Comorbidity among the anxiety disorders. *Journal of Anxiety Disorders, 3,* 57–68.

Dodge, C. S., Heimberg, R. G., Nyman, D., & O'Brien, G. T. (1987). Daily heterosocial interactions of high and low socially anxious college students: A diary study. *Behavior Therapy, 18,* 90–96.

Dodge, C. S., Hope, D. A., Heimberg, R. G., & Becker, R. E. (1988). Evaluation of the Social Interaction Self-Statement Test with a social phobic population. *Cognitive Therapy and Research, 12,* 211–222.

Eastburg, M., & Johnson, W. B. (1990). Shyness and perceptions of parental behavior. *Psychological Reports, 66,* 915–921.

Eysenck, M. W. (1979). Anxiety, learning, and memory: A reconceptualization. *Journal of Research in Personality, 13,* 363–385.

Eysenck, M. W. (1985). Anxiety and cognitive task performance. *Personality and Individual Differences, 6,* 579–586.

Eysenck, M. W., Mogg, K., May, J., Richards, A., & Mathews, A. (1991). Bias in interpretation of ambiguous sentences related to threat in anxiety. *Journal of Abnormal Psychology, 100,* 144–150.

Fenigstein, A., Scheier, M. F., & Buss, A. H. (1975). Public and private self-consciousness: Assessment and theory. *Journal of Consulting and Clinical Psychology, 43,* 522–527.

Fyer, A. J., Mannuzza, S., Chapman, T. F., Liebowitz, M. R., & Klein, D. F. (1993). A direct interview family study of social phobia. *Archives of General Psychiatry, 50,* 286–293.

Garcia-Coll, C., Kagan, J., & Reznick, J. S. (1984). Behavioral inhibition in young children. *Child Development, 55,* 1005–1019.

Glasgow, R. E., & Arkowitz, H. (1975). The behavioral assessment of male and female social competence in dyadic heterosexual interactions. *Behavior Therapy, 6,* 488–498.

Halford, K., & Foddy, M. (1982). Cognitive and social skills correlates of social anxiety. *British Journal of Clinical Psychology, 21,* 17–28.

Hartman, L. M. (1984). Cognitive components of social anxiety. *Journal of Clinical Psychology, 40,* 137–139.

Heimberg, R. G., Dodge, C. S., Hope, D. A., Kennedy, C. R., Zollo, L. J., & Becker, R. E. (1990). Cognitive behavioral group treatment for social phobia: Comparison with a credible placebo control. *Cognitive Therapy and Research, 14,* 1–23.

Heimberg, R. G., Holt, C. S., Schneier, F. R., Spitzer, R. L., & Liebowitz, M. R. (1993). The issue of subtypes in the diagnosis of social phobia. *Journal of Anxiety Disorders, 7,* 249–269.

Heimberg, R. G., Hope, D. A., Dodge, C. S., & Becker, R. E. (1990). DSM-III-R subtypes of social phobia: Comparison of generalized social phobics and public speaking phobics. *Journal of Nervous and Mental Disease, 178,* 172–179.

Heimberg, R. G., Hope, D. A., Rapee, R. M., & Bruch, M. A. (1988). The validity of the Social Avoidance and Distress Scale and the Fear of Negative Evaluation Scale with social phobic patients. *Behaviour Research and Therapy, 26,* 407–410.

Heimberg, R. G., Mueller, G. P., Holt, C. S., Hope, D. A., & Liebowitz, M. R. (1992). Assessment of anxiety in social interaction and being observed by others: The Social Interaction Anxiety Scale and the Social Phobia Scale. *Behavior Therapy, 23,* 53–73.

Herbert, J. D., Hope, D. A., & Bellack, A. S. (1992). Validity of the distinction between generalized social phobia and avoidant personality disorder. *Journal of Abnormal Psychology, 101,* 332–339.

Hermans, H. J. M., ter Laak, J. J. F., & Maes, P. C. J. M. (1972). Achievement motivation and fear of failure in family and school. *Developmental Psychology, 6,* 520–528.

Higgins, R. L., & Marlatt, G. A. (1975). Fear of interpersonal evaluation as a determinant of alcohol consumption in male social drinkers. *Journal of Abnormal Psychology, 84,* 644–651.

Hill, G. J. (1989). An unwillingness to act: Behavioral appropriateness, situational constraint, and self-efficacy in shyness. *Journal of Personality, 57,* 871–890.

Holt, C. S., Heimberg, R. G., & Hope, D. A. (1992). Avoidant personality disorder and the generalized subtype of social phobia. *Journal of Abnormal Psychology, 101,* 318–325.

Holt, C. S., Heimberg, R. G., Hope, D. A., & Liebowitz, M. R. (1992). Situational domains of social phobia. *Journal of Anxiety Disorders, 6,* 63–77.

Hope, D. A., & Heimberg, R. G. (1988). Public and private self-consciousness and social phobia. *Journal of Personality Assessment, 52,* 626–639.

Hope, D. A., Heimberg, R. G., & Klein, J. F. (1990). Social anxiety and the recall of interpersonal information. *Journal of Cognitive Psychotherapy: An International Quaterly, 4,* 185–195.

Hope, D. A., Rapee, R. M., Heimberg, R. G., & Dombeck, M. J. (1990). Representations of the self in social phobia: Vulnerability to social threat. *Cognitive Therapy and Research, 14,* 177–189.

Ingram, R. E. (1990). Self-focused attention in clinical disorders: Review and a conceptual model. *Psychological Bulletin, 107,* 156–176.

King, N. J., Ollier, K., Iacuone, R., Schuster, S., Bays, K., Gullone, E., & Ollendick, T. H. (1989). Fears of children and adolescents: A cross-sectional Australian study using the Revised-Fear Survey Schedule for Children. *Journal of Child Psychology and Psychiatry, 30,* 775–784.

Kingham, R. J. (1958). Alcoholism and the reinforcement theory of learning. *Quarterly Journal of Studies on Alcohol, 19,* 320–330.

Kushner, M. G., Sher, K. J., & Beitman, B. D. (1990). The relation between alcohol problems and the anxiety disorders. *American Journal of Psychiatry, 147,* 685–695.

La Greca, A. M., Kraslow Dandes, S., Wick, P., Shaw, K., & Stone, W. L. (1988). Development of the Social Anxiety Scale for Children: Reliability and concurrent validity. *Journal of Clinical Child Psychology, 17,* 84–91.

Lader, M. H. (1980). The psychophysiology of anxiety. In H. M. van Pragg, M. H. Lader, O. J. Rafaelson, & E. J. Sachar (Eds.), *Handbook of biological psychiatry:*

Part II. Brain mechanisms and abnormal behavior—psychophysiology (pp. 225–247). New York: Dekker.

Lamm, H., & Stephan, E. (1987). Loneliness among German university students: Some correlates. *Social Behavior and Personality, 15,* 161–164.

Levin, A. P., Saoud, J. B., Strauman, T., Gorman, J. M., Fyer, A. J., Crawford, R., & Liebowitz, M. R. (1993). Responses of "generalized" and "discrete" social phobics during public speaking. *Journal of Anxiety Disorders, 7,* 207–222.

Lewis, M., Stanger, C., Sullivan, M. W., & Barone, P. (1991). Changes in embarrassment as a function of age, sex and situation. *British Journal of Developmental Psychology, 9,* 485–492.

Liebowitz, M. R. (1987). Social phobia. *Modern Problems in Pharmacopsychiatry, 22,* 141–173.

Liebowitz, M. R., Gorman, J. M., Fyer, A. J., & Klein, D. F. (1985). Social phobia: Review of a neglected anxiety disorder. *Archives of General Psychiatry, 42,* 729–736.

Lovibond, P. F., & Rapee, R. M. (1993). The representation of feared outcomes. *Behaviour Research and Therapy, 31,* 595–608.

Ludwig, R. P., & Lazarus, P. J. (1983). Relationship between shyness in children and constricted cognitive control as measured by the Stroop color–word test. *Journal of Consulting and Clinical Psychology, 51,* 386–389.

Mannuzza, S., Fyer, A. J., Liebowitz, M. R., & Klein, D. F. (1990). Delineating the boundaries of social phobia: Its relationship to panic disorder and agoraphobia. *Journal of Anxiety Disorders, 4,* 41–59.

Marks, I. M. (1969). *Fears and phobias.* London: Heinemann.

Marks, I. M., & Gelder, M. G. (1966). Different ages of onset in varieties of phobias. *American Journal of Psychiatry, 123,* 218–221.

Mathews, A., & MacLeod, C. (1985). Selective processing of threat cues in anxiety states. *Behaviour Research and Therapy, 23,* 563–569.

Mattia, J. I., Heimberg, R. G., & Hope, D. A. (1993). The revised Stroop color–naming task in social phobics. *Behaviour Research and Therapy, 31,* 305–313.

Mattick, R. P., & Clarke, J. C. (1989). *Development and validation of measures of social phobia scrutiny fear and social interaction anxiety.* Unpublished manuscript.

Melchior, L. A., & Cheek, J. M. (1990). Shyness and anxious self-preoccupation during a social interaction. *Journal of Social Behavior and Personality, 5,* 117–130.

Morris, L. W., Davis, M. A., & Hutchings, C. H. (1981). Cognitive and emotional components of anxiety: Literature review and a revised worry–emotionality scale. *Journal of Educational Psychology, 73,* 541–555.

O'Banion, K., & Arkowitz, H. (1977). Social anxiety and selective memory for affective information about the self. *Social Behavior and Personality, 5,* 321–328.

Öst, L. G. (1987). Age of onset in different phobias. *Journal of Abnormal Psychology, 96,* 223–229.

Otto, M. W., Pollack, M. H., Sachs, G. S., O'Neill, C. A., & Rosenbaum, J. F. (1992). Alcohol dependence in panic disorder patients. *Journal of Psychiatric Research, 26,* 29–38.

Page, R. M. (1990). Shyness and sociability: A dangerous combination for illicit substance use in adolescent males? *Adolescence, 25,* 803–806.

Parker, G. (1979). Reported parental characteristics of agoraphobics and social phobics. *British Journal of Psychiatry, 135*, 555–560.

Phillips, S. D., & Bruch, M. A. (1988). Shyness and dysfunction in career development. *Journal of Counseling Psychology, 35*, 159–165.

Pilkonis, P. A. (1977a). Shyness, public and private, and its relationship to other measures of social behavior. *Journal of Personality, 45*, 585–595.

Pilkonis, P. A. (1977b). The behavioral consequences of shyness. *Journal of Personality, 45*, 596–611.

Plomin, R., & Daniels, D. (1986). Genetics and shyness. In W. H. Jones, J. M. Cheek, & S. R. Briggs (Eds.), *Shyness: Perspectives on research and treatment* (pp. 63–80). New York: Plenum Press.

Pollard, C. A., & Henderson, J. G. (1988). Four types of social phobia in a community sample. *Journal of Nervous and Mental Disease, 176*, 440–445.

Rapee, R. M. (1993). The utilisation of working memory by worry. *Behaviour Research and Therapy, 31*, 617–620.

Rapee, R. M., Brown, T. A., Antony, M. M., & Barlow, D. H. (1992). Response to hyperventilation and inhalation of 5.5% carbon dioxide-enriched air across the DSM-III-R anxiety disorders. *Journal of Abnormal Psychology, 101*, 538–552.

Rapee, R.M., & Hilton, D. E. (1993). *Self evaluation of performance in social anxiety: The influence of state anxiety.* Unpublished manuscript.

Rapee, R. M., & Lim, L. (1992). Discrepancy between self and observer ratings of performance in social phobics. *Journal of Abnormal Psychology, 101*, 727–731.

Rapee, R. M., McCallum, S. L., Melville, L. F., Ravenscroft, H., & Rodney, J. M. (1994). Memory bias in social phobia. *Behaviour Research and Therapy, 32*, 89–99.

Rapee, R. M., Sanderson, W. C., & Barlow, D. H. (1988). Social phobia features across the DSM-III-R anxiety disorders. *Journal of Psychopathology and Behavioral Assessment, 10*, 287–299.

Reich, J., Noyes, R., & Yates, W. (1988). Anxiety symptoms distinguishing social phobia from panic and generalized anxiety disorders. *Journal of Nervous and Mental Disease, 176*, 510–513.

Reich, J., & Yates, W. (1988). Family history of psychiatric disorders in social phobia. *Comprehensive Psychiatry, 29*, 72–75.

Rosenbaum, J. F., Biederman, J., Hirshfeld, D. R., Bolduc, E. A., & Chaloff, J. (1991). Behavioral inhibition in childhood: A possible precursor to panic disorder or social phobia. *Journal of Clinical Psychiatry, 52*(Suppl.), 5–9.

Rubin, B. M., Katkin, E. S., Weiss, B. W., & Efran, J. S. (1968). Factor analysis of a fear survey schedule. *Behaviour Research and Therapy, 6*, 65–75.

Rubin, K. H., & Asendorpf, J. B. (Eds.). (1993). *Social withdrawal, inhibition, and shyness, in childhood.* Hillsdale, NJ: Erlbaum.

Sanderson, W. C., Di Nardo, P. A., Rapee, R. M., & Barlow, D. H. (1990). Syndrome co-morbidity in patients diagnosed with a DSM-III-Revised anxiety disorder. *Journal of Abnormal Psychology, 99*, 308–312.

Schneier, F. R., Johnson, J., Hornig, C. D., Liebowitz, M. R., & Weissman, M. M. (1992). Social phobia: Comorbidity and morbidity in an epidemiologic sample. *Archives of General Psychiatry, 49*, 282–288.

Schneier, F. L., Martin, L. Y., Liebowitz, M. R., Gorman, J. M., & Fyer, A. J. (1989). Alcohol abuse in social phobia. *Journal of Anxiety Disorders, 3,* 15–23.

Schneier, F. L., Spitzer, R. L., Gibbon, M., Fyer, A. J., & Liebowitz, M. R. (1991). The relationship of social phobia subtypes and avoidant personality disorder. *Comprehensive Psychiatry, 32,* 496–502.

Seipp, B. (1991). Anxiety and academic performance: A meta-analysis of findings. *Anxiety Research, 4,* 27–41.

Slavkin, S. L., Holt, C. S., Heimberg, R. G., Jaccard, J. J., & Liebowitz, M. R. (1990, November). *The Liebowitz Social Phobia Scale: An exploratory analysis of construct validity.* Paper presented at the 24th annual meeting of the Association for Advancement of Behavior Therapy, San Francisco, CA.

Smith, R. E., & Sarason, I. G. (1975). Social anxiety and the evaluation of negative interpersonal feedback. *Journal of Consulting and Clinical Psychology, 43,* 429.

Solyom, L., Ledwidge, B., & Solyom, C. (1986). Delineating social phobia. *British Journal of Psychiatry, 149,* 464–470.

Stein, M. B., Tancer, M. E., Gelernter, C. S., Vittone, B. J., & Uhde, T. W. (1990). Major depression in patients with social phobia. *American Journal of Psychiatry, 147,* 637–639.

Thyer, B. A., Parrish, R. T., Curtis, G. C., Nesse, R. M., & Cameron, O. G. (1985). Ages of onset of DSM-III anxiety disorders. *Comprehensive Psychiatry, 26,* 113–122.

Turner, S. M., Beidel, D. C., Borden, J. W., Stanley, M. A., & Jacob, R. G. (1991). Social phobia: Axis I and II corelates. *Journal of Abnormal Psychology, 100,* 102–106.

Turner, S. M., Beidel, D. C., Dancu, C. V., & Keys, D. J. (1986). Psychopathology of social phobia and comparison to avoidant personality disorder. *Journal of Abnormal Psychology, 95,* 389–394.

Turner, S. M., Beidel, D. C., & Larkin, K. T. (1986). Situational determinants of social anxiety in clinic and nonclinic samples: Physiological and cognitive correlates. *Journal of Consulting and Clinical Psychology, 54,* 523–527.

Turner, S. M., Beidel, D. C., & Townsley, R. M. (1990). Social phobia: Relationship to shyness. *Behaviour Research and Therapy, 28,* 497–505.

Turner, S. M., Beidel, D. C., & Townsley, R. M. (1992). Social phobia: A comparison of specific and generalized subtypes and avoidant personality disorder. *Journal of Abnormal Psychology, 101,* 326–331.

Turner, S. M., McCann, B. S., Beidel, D. C., & Mezzich, J. E. (1986). DSM-III classification of the anxiety disorders: A psychometric study. *Journal of Abnormal Psychology, 95,* 168–172.

Twentyman, C. T., & McFall, R. M. (1975). Behavioral training of social skills in shy males. *Journal of Consulting and Clinical Psychology, 43,* 384–395.

Watson, D., & Friend, R. (1969). Measurement of social-evaluative anxiety. *Journal of Consulting and Clinical Psychology, 33,* 448–457.

Wine, J. (1971). Test anxiety and the direction of attention. *Psychological Bulletin, 76,* 92–104.

PART II

Theoretical and Empirical Approaches

CHAPTER FOUR

A Cognitive Model
of Social Phobia

DAVID M. CLARK
ADRIAN WELLS

In the absence of treatment, social phobia can persist for years or even decades. Why? What is it that keeps social phobia going? In this chapter we attempt to answer this question by outlining a cognitive model of social phobia that pays particular attention to the factors that prevent social phobics from changing their negative beliefs about the danger inherent in certain social situations. The model draws heavily on the writings of earlier theorists, especially those of Beck, Emery, and Greenberg (1985), Butler (1985), Hartman (1983), Heimberg and Barlow (1988), Leary (1983), Salkovskis (1991), Teasdale and Barnard (1993), and Trower and Gilbert (1989). However, the model is distinct in the particular synthesis it provides.

AN OUTLINE OF THE COGNITIVE MODEL

The core of social phobia appears to be a strong desire to convey a particular favorable impression of oneself to others and marked insecurity about one's ability to do so. Figure 4.1 (below) illustrates the processes that we suggest occur when a social phobic enters a feared social situation. As a consequence of previous experience interacting with innate behavioral predispositions, social phobics develop a series of assumptions about themselves and their social world that make them prone to believe that they are in danger in one or more social situations. In particular, they believe that when they enter such situations, (1) they are in danger of behaving in an inept and unacceptable fashion, *and* (2) that such behavior will have disastrous consequences in terms of loss of status, loss of worth, and rejection. Once the social phobic perceives a social situation in this way, an "anxiety program" is automatically and reflexively activated. The anxiety program is a complex constellation of cognitive, somatic, affective, and behavioral changes that are probably inherited from our evolutionary past and were originally designed to protect us from harm in objectively dangerous primitive environments (see Trower & Gilbert, 1989). However, when the danger is more imagined than real, these anxiety responses are largely inappropriate. Instead of serving a useful function, they often become further sources of perceived danger and in this way contribute to a series of vicious circles that tend to maintain or exacerbate social anxiety. First, the somatic and behavioral symptoms of anxiety become further sources of perceived danger and anxiety (e.g., blushing is interpreted as evidence that one is making a fool of oneself; a racing heart is interpreted as evidence of impending loss of control). Second, social phobics become preoccupied with their somatic responses and negative social-evaluative thoughts, and this preoccupation interferes with their ability to process social cues, an effect that they notice and take as further evidence of social threat and failure. Third, some of the ways in which social phobics behave when anxious (e.g., appearing less warm and outgoing) may then elicit less friendly behavior from others and partly confirm the phobics' fears. Finally, some of the behavioral symptoms directly produce further feared sensations (e.g., talking quickly is accompanied by hyperventilation and results in further increased heart rate, dizziness, and blurred vision; cf. Salkovskis, Clark, & Jones, 1986).

Having given a general outline of the cognitive model, we will now discuss in more detail four processes that prevent social phobics from disconfirming their negative beliefs about the danger inherent in social situations and that hence maintain their social anxiety. Three of the processes are things social phobics do when in a feared situation, while the fourth is concerned with what they do before entering and after leaving the situation.

Self-Focused Attention and the Construction of an Impression of Oneself as a Social Object

One of the most significant changes that occurs when a social phobic enters a feared situation is a shift in attentional focus. When social phobics think they are in danger of negative evaluation by others, they shift their attention to detailed monitoring and observation of themselves. As pointed out above, this attentional shift is problematic because it produces an enhanced awareness of feared anxiety responses and interferes with processing the situation and other people's behavior. In addition, and perhaps more important for understanding maintenance, social phobics appear to use the interoceptive information produced by self-focus to construct an impression of themselves that they then assume reflects what other people actually notice and think about them. This concept is perhaps best introduced by example. Many social phobics complain that in a social situation, they often feel they are the center of attention and that they find this highly aversive. When asked what makes them think that they are the center of attention, they rarely answer, "I could see that everyone was looking at me." Instead, they are more likely to say, "I don't know, I just *felt* I was the center of attention." Instead of observing other people more closely in order to gain clues about what they think about him or her, the social phobic appears to turn attention inwards, notice how he or she feels, and then automatically assume that this information is relevant to others' evaluation. In a process that has variously been called "emotional reasoning" (Burns, 1980), "ex-consequentia reasoning" (Arntz, Rauner, & van den Hout, 1994), and "processing of felt sense" (Teasdale & Barnard, 1993), the social phobic equates feeling humiliated with being humiliated, feeling out of control with being (observably) out of control, and feeling anxious with being noticeably anxious. This equation can lead to quite marked distortions. For example, a patient may have a strong shaky feeling and assume that others must be able to see his or her hand shaking violently, when all that can be observed by others is a mild tremor or nothing at all. Often the negative impression that social phobics construct of their observable self is best described as a "compelling feeling," but sometimes it is also accompanied by images in which the phobics are able to see themselves as though from other people's point of view. Such images contain visible exaggerations (such as hands shaking or humiliated posture). In some cases, the exact content of the image varies from situation to situation, whereas in other cases, a more general image is triggered whenever a particular feeling is experienced. For example, a salesman who was worried that he would visibly sweat when talking to clients reported that a warm feeling on his forehead would trigger a vivid image of how his face looked in the mirror after a strenuous aerobics workout. In the image, his face was running with sweat. Irrespective of whether the impression is accompanied by an image or is simply a feeling, it seems self-evidently true. In the case of images, this is easy to understand. The image is from an observer's perspective, so it is not surprising that it can be mistaken for what the observer sees and thinks. In the case of impressions without images, the impression probably seems true because it fits with a preexisting belief.

Figure 4.1 graphically represents (by lines of varying thickness) the idea that much of social phobics' evidence for their negative beliefs comes from their own impression of how they appear to others, rather than from

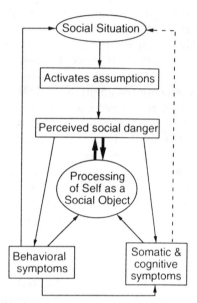

FIGURE 4.1. A model of the processes that are hypothesized to occur when a social phobic enters a feared social situation.

observation of others' responses. The greater importance of the former process is signified by broad lines between *Perceived social danger* and *Processing of self as a social object* and by thin lines, between *Perceived social danger* and the *Social situation*. Clinically, the importance of this processing bias is that it prevents social phobics from getting maximum benefit from their everyday experience with social situations or from the exposure exercises used in behavior therapy treatment programs. When in feared social situations, social phobics process the negative feelings generated by their fear of the situation, but they do not check out what is really happening. Stopa and Clark (1993) have hypothesized that this is a fundamental difference between shyness and social phobia. People who are shy may enter social situations with many of the same anticipatory concerns as social phobics have, but they notice that other people are responding in an interested way and decide that in this situation, at least, they are not being boring, thus terminating the sequence of negative thoughts and anxiety. Social phobics, on the other hand, may fail to do this checking and thus keep the sequence of negative thoughts and anxiety going.

If the processing style outlined above is maladaptive, why do social phobics use it? There are two possible explanations. First, in normal social interactions there are very few cues that provide unambiguous information about how other people view us. For the non-socially anxious person, this is not a great problem. Such individuals presumably either feel fairly confident that other people will accept them as they are or that, if they do not, it doesn't matter. In contrast, social phobics are greatly threatened by the possibility that other people will evaluate them negatively and as a consequence are strongly motivated to search for information that gives them clues about how others view them. Research in social psychology (Kenny & DePaulo, 1993) indicates that everyone's impression of how others view them is partly based on self-perceptions, and social phobics' greater need to know what others think will enhance this type of processing. Second, many of the things that individuals can do in order to gain more information about how others view them (increasing eye contact, asking for reactions to what one has said, disclosing more personal information) are too threatening for social phobics because they are perceived as further increasing the risk of negative evaluation. For example, increased eye contact while speaking to another person would help social phobics decide whether the other person is interested in what they are saying, but avoidance of eye contact is often a strategy that social phobics use to feel less vulnerable and more in control of the interaction.

The Role of In-Situation Safety Behaviors in Maintaining Negative Beliefs and Anxiety

While in social situations, social phobics engage in a wide range of behaviors that are intended to reduce the risk of negative evaluation. Often there are quite precise links between specific safety behaviors and feared outcomes. For example, one patient, who was concerned about the possibility that her hand might shake while drinking, would half fill her wine glass and then grip the glass very tightly while drinking. Another patient, who was concerned about the possibility of fainting in public, tensed his leg muscles and leaned against the nearest solid object when he felt dizzy. A patient who was concerned that people would think he was anxious and evaluate him negatively if he paused during a speech rehearsed the speech in great detail and spoke quickly. As Salkovskis (1991) and Wells et al. (1995) have pointed out, such safety behaviors are problematic for two reasons. First, they prevent social phobics from experiencing an unambiguous disconfirmation of their unrealistic beliefs about feared behaviors (e.g., shaking) or the consequences of these behaviors (e.g., being humiliated and rejected). Second, in some instances, they can make feared behaviors more likely. For example, the woman who grasped her wine glass very tightly discovered during therapy that this made her hand more likely to shake.

Anxiety-Induced Performance Deficits and Their Effects on Other People's Thinking and Behavior

In most anxiety disorders, the things that patients fear rarely occur. For example, despite panic disorder patients' conviction to the contrary, the breathlessness and palpitations experienced in a panic attack do not lead to a heart attack and sudden death. Similarly, social phobics overestimate how negatively other people evaluate their performance (Rapee & Lim, 1992; Stopa & Clark, 1993) and the consequences of such evaluation. However, some of social phobics' fears about the way anxiety will affect their behavior are partly justified. Anxiety can produce blushing, an unsteady voice, sweating, or shaky hands. In addition, preoccupation with monitoring one's performance and safety behaviors such as gaze avoidance and avoidance of self-disclosure are likely to mean that social phobics behave in a less friendly, warm, and outgoing fashion when anxious. Such behavioral deficits are likely to make other people somewhat less friendly and hence produce a negative interaction pattern that further contributes to the maintenance of social phobia.

Anticipatory and Postevent Processing

Social phobics often report considerable anticipatory anxiety. Prior to a social event, they review in detail what they think might happen. As they start to think about the situation, they become anxious and their thoughts tend to be dominated by recollections of past failures, by negative images of themselves in the situation, and by other predictions of poor performance and rejection. Sometimes these ruminations lead the phobic to completely avoid the situation. If this does not happen and the phobic enters the situation, he or she is likely to already be in a self-focused processing mode, to expect failure, and to be less likely to notice any signs of being accepted by other people.

Leaving or escaping from a social situation does not necessarily bring to an immediate end the social phobic's negative thoughts and distress. There is no longer an immediate social danger, and so anxiety rapidly declines. However, as we have mentioned above, the nature of social interactions is such that the social phobic is unlikely to have received from others unambiguous signs of social approval, and for this reason it is not uncommon for him or her to conduct a "postmortem" of the event. The interaction is reviewed in detail. During this review, the patient's anxious feelings and negative self-perception are likely to figure particularly prominently because they were processed in detail while the patient was in the situation and hence were strongly encoded in memory. The unfortunate consequence of this is that the patient's review is likely to be dominated by his or her negative self-perception, and the interaction is likely to be seen as much more negative than it really was. This may explain why some social phobics report a sense of shame that persists for a while after the anxiety has subsided. A further aspect of the postmortem is the retrieval of other instances of perceived social failure. The recent interaction is then added to the list of past failures, with the consequence that an interaction that may have looked entirely neutral from an outside observer's perspective will have strengthened the patient's belief in his or her social inadequacy. Heimberg (1991) gives a graphic and tragic example of postevent processing. During a therapy session a woman role-played being a cocktail party hostess. Everything went very well except that she spilled one drop of someone's drink. When discussing the role-play immediately afterward she was pleased with her performance, but after thinking about it more on her own that evening she attempted suicide.

Assumptions and Self-Schemata in Social Phobia

The cognitive model assumes that social phobics' tendency to interpret social situations in a threatening fashion is the consequence of a series of dysfunctional beliefs (assumptions) that they hold about themselves and the way they should behave in social situations. Three categories of dysfunctional beliefs can be distinguished: excessively high standards for social performance, conditional beliefs concerning social evaluation, and unconditional beliefs about the self.

Excessively High Standards for Social Performance

Examples of these are "I must get everyone's approval"; "I must not show any signs of weakness"; "I must not let anyone see I am anxious"; and "I must appear intelligent and witty." High standards generate anxiety because they are difficult, if not impossible, to achieve, and as a consequence social phobics are constantly concerned that they may fail to convey their desired, favorable impression.

Conditional Beliefs Concerning Social Evaluation

Examples of these are "If I show feelings (or make mistakes) others will reject me"; "If others really get to know me, they won't like me"; "If I disagree with someone, they will think I'm stupid/will reject me"; and "If someone doesn't like/approve of me, it must be my fault (e.g., it's because I am worthless, stupid, unattractive, or uninteresting)." The last conditional belief is often itself a consequence of the assumption that "What people think about me (or more accurately, what I think they think about me) must be the truth about me."

Unconditional Beliefs about the Self

Like depressed patients, many social phobics have negative beliefs about their worth and value. Examples are "I'm odd/peculiar"; "I'm different"; "I'm a nerd"; "I'm unacceptable"; "I'm stupid"; "I'm unattractive"; "I'm vulnerable"; or "I'm inadequate." However, there is an important difference between the self-schemata of depressed patients and those of (nondepressed) social phobics. The self-schemata in depressives are relatively stable and persist throughout depressive episodes. In contrast (nondepressed) social phobics are characterized by unstable self-schemata. When in social situations, they have an uncertain, negative view of themselves, but they often have a more positive view of themselves when alone or in situations that they do not find threatening. This point can be readily illustrated by asking social phobics whether they would still think that they were worthless, stupid, inadequate, peculiar, and so on if they were alone on a desert island. Usually they either say no or that their negative view of themselves would be much less marked. Often social phobics also report that they have a positive view of themselves when they are with their families and with other people with whom they feel comfortable. The feeling that they are different, odd, and inadequate is mainly triggered, and seems compelling, when they are with people who they think may be evaluating them.

Although all three sets of beliefs are usually present in social phobics seeking treatment, the way in which the beliefs develop and interact in the early stages of the disorder is quite varied. Some individuals report feeling comfortable in social situations during adolescence, though they tended to be a little introverted. Social phobia developed later and quickly after a social interaction that they thought went wrong or almost went wrong. For these individuals, only the excessively high standards and conditional beliefs outlined above antedate the onset of the social phobia. That is to say they initially believed that one must always appear poised and perform well in key social interactions but were confident about their ability to do so. An event that undermined this confidence then triggered the social phobia and doubts about their public self (unconditional assumptions). For example, a young newspaper editor had an exceptional early career and was awarded a prize as the nation's most promising newcomer. He greatly enjoyed the gala dinner at which the prize was awarded but drank too much before being asked to give his acceptance speech. As he started speaking, he noticed he had difficulty finding some words and was sweating. He became convinced that other people noticed these "failings" and rapidly developed a public speaking phobia. He then feared that he would be in danger of sweating profusely and forgetting his words whenever he spoke in public. When describing his problem to his therapist, he emphasized the ego-dystonic nature of his new situational and negative self-image. In contrast to these late and fairly rapid onset cases, many other social phobics report always being unconfident about their public self-image and having been shy from childhood. These individuals tend to find it difficult to date the onset of their social phobia and present for treatment when the problem starts to severely interfere with the attainment of personally important goals. In such cases, unconditional beliefs about the self develop early and are less likely to seem ego-dystonic. Excessively high standards and conditional beliefs often develop later as a part of a compensatory or protective strategy. For example, someone might believe that they are boring (unconditional belief) and develop this protective (conditional) assumption: "If (and only if) I can *appear* witty and intelligent will people accept me." In general, it appears that social phobics who fall into the generalized subtype are more likely to show the pattern in which unconditional beliefs and social anxiety develop early, whereas those who fall into the specific/nongeneralized subtype are more likely to have a later onset following a social event in which they failed to meet, or thought they were in danger of failing to meet, their high standards for acceptable social behavior.

A Clinical Case Series

The cognitive model presented here was based in part on a series of interviews with 12 patients who met the criteria for social phobia of the revised third edition of the *Diagnostic and Statistical Manual of Mental Disorders* (DSM-III-R; American Psychiatric Association, 1987). In order to give the reader more examples of the processes involved in the model, Table 4.1 summarizes for each patient the main negative thoughts, about self and about others, that occurred in feared situations, the information the patient used to construct an impression of him- or herself as a social object, the safety behaviors used in feared situations, and the patient's main assumptions about self and about others.

A BRIEF REVIEW OF RESEARCH

Having outlined a cognitive model of social phobia, we will now briefly review the literature on social phobia to determine whether existing research is broadly consistent with the model.

TABLE 4.1. Cognitive and Behavioral Characteristics of 12 Consecutive Cases of Social Phobia

Patient number and sex	Feared situation(s)	Negative self-evaluation (in situation)	Negative thoughts about others	Information used to infer others' reaction	Safety behaviors	Assumptions and self-schemata[a]
1M	Speaking to a group. Serving drinks.	I'm making a fool of myself. I'm losing control. I can't get the words out.	They'll think I'm stupid. People will stare. They'll think I'm not confident.	Shaking. Subjective difficulty talking. Image of self losing control.	Distraction. Use mugs. Avoid situation. Say less. Mentally rehearse sentences. Avoid eye contact. Don't talk about self.	I'm vulnerable (u).
2F	Administering chalice in church.	I'll lose control and shake. My hands are paralyzed. I'll spill the wine. I always get things wrong. Idiot-woman, why do I always mess up?	They'll see me shake. They'll criticize me. They'll think I can't do it.	Shaking. Image of self losing control. Negative feeling of some parishioners about women priests.	Take beta blockers. Control breathing. Grip chalice tightly. Move hands slowly. Focus on hands. Don't overfill chalice.	I have to get everything right or I'll be rejected (s). If someone dislikes me, I'm a failure (c). If people don't accept me, I'm worthless (c). I'm worthless (u). I'm powerless (u). I'm a failure (u).
3F	Being in formal meetings.	I'll lose control. I'll break down and cry. Panic will take over.	They won't respect me. They won't like me. They'll pity me.	Feeling of wanting to cry. Blushing. Someone joked about blushing. Image of self in anxious situation.	Avoid situation. Say less. Avoid eye contact.	If people think badly of me, then I am bad (c). I'm weak (u).
4F	Drinking in front of others.	I'm going to pieces. I'll shake and lose control.	People will stare. They'll think I'm stupid.	Focus on shaking (observing self).	Distraction. Hold cup with both hands. Leave saucer on table. Sit down to drink. Try to relax. Positive self-talk?	?
5F	Attracting attention.	I'll knock things over. I'll make a noise. I'll get things wrong. They're better than me.	They think I'm a fool. They'll look at me. They don't like the way I look.	Monitor own behavior. Blushing sensations. Work colleagues try to embarrass her.	Deep breathing. Keep still. Distraction. Avoid eye contact.	I must not show any signs of weakness (s). If people see me blush, they'll put me down (c). If they see me blush, they'll know I'm not as tough as they are (c). If they see I'm anxious, they'll be better than me (c). I'm different (u). I'm the odd one out (u). I'm inferior (u).

6F	Eating in public. Talking in groups.	I'll vomit. I'll get my words wrong.	People will notice. They'll think badly of me. I'll be the center of attention.	Stomach churning. Own embarrassment at vomiting in a pub. Negative self-evaluation projected onto others.	Avoid eating. Break food up. Nibble food. Drink a lot. Cough. Smoke cigarette. Rehearse sentences in mind. Talk quickly. Distraction. Change the subject.	?
7F	Reading in group. New social situations.	I'll go red. I'm unable to talk. I'll lose bladder control. I'll look stupid. I'll totally clam up. I'll shake.	They'll reject me. People don't like me.	Imagines how people will react in advance of situation. Focuses on sensations.	Slow breathing. Distraction. Talk/read slowly. Stand still. Try to look confident. Positive self-talk.	I must get everyone's approval (s). If people see me shake, it means I'm inferior to them (c). If people see how I feel, it means I'm different (c). Being different means I'll end up alone, rejected, isolated (c). I'm odd/peculiar (u). I'm different (u).
8M	Making and serving drinks at work.	I'll shake uncontrollably. I'll get tongue-tied. It's going to escalate.	They'll think I'm inadequate. They'll know I'm anxious. They'll think I'm mentally ill.	"In my mind it looks really bad." Images in situation and before-hand. Projected negative self-evaluation.	Avoid situation. Use two hands. Try to control self. Do not pick up cup and saucer together.	My personal adequacy depends on not showing any signs of weakness or flawed performance (s). I need to be liked by everyone (s). If people don't like me it must be my fault, i.e., I'm boring, not talkative (c). If I shake I'm inadequate (c). I'm incapable (u).
9M	Walking in crowded shops/places.	My legs are giving way. I'll collapse. I can't walk straight. I'll shake.	People will stare.	?	Avoid crowds. Hold onto things. Deep breathing. Sing to self. Look for exit. Sit down. Crouch down. Stiffen legs. Avoid eye contact. Leave situation.	?

(Table continues on next page.)

TABLE 4.1. (Continued)

Patient number and sex	Feared situation(s)	Negative self-evaluation (in situation)	Negative thoughts about others	Information used to infer others' reaction	Safety behaviors	Assumptions and self-schemata[a]
10M	One-to-one social encounters.	I'll say the wrong thing. I won't be able to talk. I'm paralyzed. I'll freeze. I'll choke. I haven't got anything worthwhile to say.	They'll criticize me. They think I'm boring. They don't want to know me.	Visualizes things going wrong. Postmortem.	Do not think about self. Self-monitor thoughts. Talk less.	I have to say something witty, intelligent, and interesting or people won't like me (s). If I'm quiet, people will think I'm boring (c). I'm inadequate (u).
11F	Drinking in public. Making group conversation.	I'll lose control and rush out. I'll shake uncontrollably. I'll say or do the wrong thing.	They'll think I'm inferior. They'll think I'm less than whole. They'll think I'm odd. They won't think I'm credible. They'll see I'm weak. People will stare.	Projected negative self-evaluation.	Pick up drink quickly. Avoid cups and saucers. Relax and stiffen arms. Drink quickly.	Everyone has to think good of me (s). I'm a strong, dependable, in-control person and this problem will spoil that (c). If I shake, I'll lose my own and others' belief in myself as a worthy, acceptable person (c). If people think I'm worthless, that means I am worthless (c). I'm a failure (u). My potential is wasted (u).
12F	Making conversation with strangers. Being in crowds. Pervasive social anxiety.	I'll talk funny. I'll do something silly. I'll say the wrong thing. I'm being boring. I'll get muddled. I'll make a mess of talking.	They think I'm stupid. They think I'm different. They don't like me. They think I'm silly. They're staring at me. They think I'm boring.	If I *feel* stupid, then I'll act stupid.	Talk less. Deep breaths. Tense muscles. Ignore others. Avoid eye contact. Do not talk about self. Let mind wander. "Blank out mind."	I must not make mistakes (s). If I act foolishly, no one will want to talk to me, people won't like me and I'll end up alone (c). If I feel stupid, then I'll act stupid (c). I'm foolish (u). I'm stupid (u). I'm inadequate (u). I'm ugly (u).

[a] s, excessively high standards; c, conditional beliefs; u, unconditional beliefs.

Interpretation of Social Situations

Cognitive models assume that social phobics interpret social situations in a more threatening fashion than do non-social phobics. Clark and Stopa (1994) used modified versions of the Ambiguous Events Questionnaire developed by Butler and Mathews (1993) to investigate this assertion. Social phobics, other anxiety disorder patients, and nonpatient controls completed two questionnaires. One questionnaire contained ambiguous social situations (e.g., "You have visitors round for a meal and they leave sooner than expected") and ambiguous nonsocial situations (e.g., "A letter marked urgent arrives at your home"). Social phobics were significantly more likely to choose negative interpretations of the ambiguous social situations than were either other anxious patients or nonpatient controls, but they did not differ from these two groups in their interpretation of nonsocial ambiguous situations. The second questionnaire contained mildly negative social events (e.g., "You have been talking to someone for a while and it becomes clear that they're not really interested in what you're saying") and was used to assess catastrophic interpretations. Consistent with the cognitive model, social phobics were more likely to choose catastrophic interpretations of mildly negative social events (e.g., "It means I am a boring person") than were other anxious patients or nonpatient controls.

Investigations of thoughts in actual social situations using various thought-listing procedures have produced results consistent with the questionnaire data on hypothetical social situations. Stopa and Clark (1993) reported an experiment in which social phobics, other anxious patients, and nonpatient controls were asked to have a brief conversation with an attractive, female stooge. The stooge was instructed to behave in a reserved but not unfriendly manner. After the conversation, subjects listed their thoughts and rated the extent to which they had shown a variety of positive and negative behaviors. Independent assessors rated the same behaviors. Analysis of the thoughts data revealed that social phobics reported more negative self-evaluative thoughts than did either the other anxious patients or the nonpatient controls. Similarly, Dodge, Hope, Heimberg, and Becker (1988) found that, among a group of patients seeking treatment for fear and avoidance of social interactions, negative thoughts were significantly correlated with degree of anxiety in a social situation.

The cognitive model assumes that social phobics' negative evaluations of their performance are at least partly distorted. To investigate this, Rapee and Lim (1992) compared self-ratings and observer ratings of public speaking performance. When compared to the observers' ratings, social phobics underestimated their performance, while nonpatients were relatively accurate. Stopa and Clark (1993) reported a similar finding. Social phobics gave their behavior significantly higher negative ratings and significantly lower positive ratings than did the observer. In contrast, other anxious patients did not differ from the observer in ratings of their positive behaviors but gave themselves significantly lower negative behavior ratings than did the observer.

Self-Focused Attention and the Construction of an Impression of Oneself as a Social Object

A key component of our model is the idea that social phobics use interoceptive information to construct an impression of themselves, which they assume reflects what other people observe, and that this information is relatively more important than observation of others' actual behavior. No studies have directly investigated this hypothesis. However, a number of studies have reported findings that are consistent with various aspects of the hypothesis.

First, several studies have suggested that social phobics' belief that others are evaluating them negatively is not based on detailed information about others' responses to them. Stopa and Clark (1993) found that social phobics reported more negative self-evaluative thoughts (e.g., "I'm boring") than did controls during a conversation with a stooge but did not report more negative thoughts that explicitly mentioned evaluation by the stooge (e.g., "She thinks I'm boring"). Winton, Clark, and Edelmann (1995) investigated accuracy in detecting negative emotion in briefly presented slides of different emotional expressions. Slides of negative and neutral facial expressions were presented for 60 milliseconds, followed by a pattern mask. Students scoring high on the Fear of Negative Evaluation Scale (FNE; Watson & Friend, 1969) correctly identified more negative facial expressions than did low FNE students, but a signal detection analysis revealed that this was due to a negative response bias. That is to say, high FNE students were more likely to rate a briefly presented face as negative in the absence of having abstracted more affective information from the face.

Second, Kimble and Zehr (1982), Daly, Vangelisti, and Lawrence (1989) and Hope, Heimberg, and Klein (1990) found that, compared to low socially anxious subjects, high socially anxious subjects had poorer memory for the details of a recent social interaction. However, Stopa and Clark (1993), using a slightly different methodology, failed to replicate this effect.

Third, Johansson and Öst (1982) investigated awareness of heart rate changes in social phobics and controls. Social phobics were particularly accurate in estimating their heart rate changes in social situations, suggesting enhanced awareness of interoceptive information in such situations.

Fourth, McEwan and Devins (1983), Bruch, Gorsky, Collins, and Berger (1989), and Arntz et al. (1994) have all reported results that suggest social phobics' estimates of the dangerousness of social situations are partly based on the perception of their own emotional response. McEwan and Devins (1983) asked high and low socially anxious individuals to rate themselves on a checklist of behavioral signs of anxiety and asked a peer who knew the subject well to rate the subject on the same checklist. High socially anxious individuals overestimated the extent to which their anxiety was observable, whereas low socially anxious individuals' ratings of the observability of their anxiety agreed with ratings made by a peer. Bruch et al. (1989) also compared self-ratings and observer ratings of anxiety visibility. Compared to individuals low in shyness, those with high shyness scores overestimated the visibility of their anxiety. Arntz et al. (1994) presented subjects with scripts describing hypothetical social situations in which they were participants. The scripts varied along two dimensions: the presence of objective danger or safety information and whether the subject felt anxious or nonanxious. After imagining being in the scripted situation, subjects were asked to rate how dangerous they thought the situation was. Controls' estimates of danger were only influenced by the presence of objective danger information, but social phobics' estimates were also influenced by anxiety response information.

Fifth, in a preliminary study, Yuen (1994) recently obtained results that suggest that high social anxiety may be associated with an attentional bias *away* from negative social cues. In a modified version of MacLeod, Mathews, and Tata's (1986) dot-probe task, high and low FNE subjects were presented with two faces, one above the other. The faces were presented for one second and then followed by a dot that appeared in the spatial location of either the top or bottom face. On crucial trials, one facial expression was negative and the other was neutral. High FNE subjects were slower at locating the dot if it appeared in the location where the negative face had been than if it appeared in the location where the neutral face had been. Low FNE subjects showed no difference in reaction times for the two locations. Interestingly, this pattern of results is the exact opposite of that shown by social phobics in another recent dot-probe experiment that used words rather than faces as stimuli. Asmundson and Stein (1994) found that, compared to nonpatient controls, social phobics were quicker at locating dots that followed social threat words (e.g., "foolish") than dots following either neutral words or physical threat words. Hope, Rapee, Heimberg, and Dombeck (1990) and Mattia, Heimberg, and Hope (1993) obtained essentially similar results in earlier word-processing studies that used the modified Stroop paradigm to assess attentional bias. Compared to controls, social phobics showed increased color-naming times for social threat words but not for physical threat words.

One way in which the apparent discrepancy in results between attentional bias studies using faces and words could be explained would be to suppose that the face-processing studies are modeling attention to actual social cues, while the word-processing studies are more closely related to mental preoccupation (see Wells & Matthews, 1994). That is to say, social phobics show an attentional bias to social threat words not because they are hypervigilant for negative cues in a social interaction but because they are preoccupied with thoughts concerning negative self-evaluation. An alternative explanation would be that anxious individuals show an initial attentional bias toward negative real-life social threat cues followed by avoidance (Williams, Watts, MacLeod, & Mathews, 1988) and that the longer presentation time used in the face dot-probe experiment (1 second vs. 500 milliseconds in the word dot-probe experiments) is responsible for the differences in results. Further research is required to resolve this issue. The current ambiguity about whether social phobics show an initial attentional bias toward real-life social cues is reflected by the use of a dotted line to represent this process in Figure 4.1.

In-Situation Safety Behaviors

Wells et al. (1995) tested the hypothesis that in-situation safety behaviors play a role in maintaining social phobia by comparing one session of exposure to a feared social situation with one session of similar exposure accompanied by the intentional dropping of safety behaviors. Although the two procedures did not differ in patients' credibility ratings, exposure plus dropping of safety behaviors produced significantly greater reductions in anxiety and belief ratings for feared outcomes in a behavior test administered before and after the intervention.

How Believing Another Dislikes You Affects the Way That Person Thinks about You

We hypothesized that social phobics' fears that others will evaluate them negatively may be partially self-fulfilling because the safety behaviors and self-focused attention generated by the fears are likely to have a negative effect on the way social phobics appear to others. An ingenious experiment by Curtis and Miller (1986) provides an elegant demonstration that this can happen. Students had a brief conversation with another person. After the conversation, they were given false feedback indicating that the other person either liked or disliked them. They then had a second conversation with the same person. At the end of this conversation, that person was asked to rate the student. Students who were led to believe that the other person disliked them after the first conversation were rated as less warm, self-disclosing, and friendly after the second conversation and were less well liked.

Several other studies have documented negative effects of social anxiety on social behavior and the way it is perceived by others. Bond and Omar (1990) found that high, but not low, socially anxious subjects showed impaired recall of neutral words presented immediately before they were due to speak to an audience. Stopa and Clark (1993) found that independent observers judged social phobics' performance in a conversation more negatively than that of other anxiety disorder patients or nonpatient controls. However, as mentioned above, social phobics' ratings of their own behavior were significantly more negative than were the independent observers' ratings of their behavior.

Postevent Processing

We have hypothesized that social phobics conduct a postmortem on their social encounters and that this tends to reinforce their negative beliefs about their own performance and other peoples' evaluation of them. To date, few studies have investigated postevent processing. Two studies have looked at whether high anxious subjects selectively recall negative information about a social interaction after it has happened. O'Banion and Arkowitz (1977) asked women to have a brief conversation with a male confederate. After the conversation, high and low socially anxious women were given identical feedback about their personality characteristics, as rated by the confederate. A subsequent recognition test indicated that the high socially anxious subjects had better memory for negative information about themselves than did low socially anxious subjects and that the two groups did not differ in memory for positive information about themselves. However, the crucial group by type of feedback interaction failed to reach significance. Rapee, McCallum, Melville, Ravenscroft, and Rodney (1994, Study 3) reported a study that was similar except that the social interaction was imagined, rather than real. Social phobics did not show enhanced recall of hypothetical negative feedback. This finding is difficult to interpret because additional analyses suggested that the social phobics did not find the imaginal task particularly threatening. Clearly, further investigation of postevent processing is required. Future studies should bear in mind (1) the importance of encoding material in a public self-referent fashion when testing for memory biases (see Smith, Ingram, & Brehm, 1983), (2) the importance of creating an affective state similar to that involved in naturally occurring anticipatory and postevent rumination, and (3) the likelihood that most of the more destructive postevent processing involves reviewing and drawing negative conclusions from remembered interoceptive information and from ambiguous aspects of the social interaction.

IMPLICATIONS FOR TREATMENT

The model outlined above has several implications for treatment. First, it helps explain the relative ineffectiveness of exposure alone as a treatment for social phobia (Butler, Cullington, Munby, Amies, & Gelder, 1984). In particular, it suggests that exposure often fails to lead to substantial cognitive change because patients are not really processing what is happening in the social situation, are engaging in safety behaviors that prevent disconfirmation, and are using their own impression of themselves as the main evidence for the idea that other people are negatively evaluating them. Second, it suggests that the effectiveness of cognitive-behavioral treatment could be improved by formulating cases in terms of the maintenance processes outlined in the model, helping patients to become aware of these processes and the way in which they maintain the problem, and teaching them how to overcome them. Below we outline some of the interventions that we have found helpful in achieving these goals.

Selling the Model

At the start of treatment, the therapist reviews with the patient a series of recent episodes of social anxiety with the aim of eliciting examples of each of the elements in the model and drawing out an idiosyncratic version of Figure 4.1. In the process, a considerable part of the discussion is devoted to helping the patient to see how these processes maintain the problem. For example, patients who fear that they will be unable to think of something interesting to say in a social situation are likely to report that while listening to what other people say they are also mentally rehearsing and censoring the things that they might say. The therapist enquires whether this helps the patient to follow the conversation and generate appropriate responses to it. This line of questioning helps patients see that their safety behaviors are counterproductive and that they are focusing internally, generating criticisms of themselves, rather than focusing on the interaction itself. In this way it is possible to illustrate the key idea that they are operating within a closed system in which their belief in the danger of negative evaluation is strengthened by internally generated information and opportunities for disconfirmation are neglected or avoided. This point can be confirmed by a behavioral experiment, such as role playing a conversation with the therapist under two conditions. In the first condition, the patient is instructed to mentally rehearse what he or she is about to say and to evaluate the possibilities that come to mind while simultaneously engaging in the conversation. In the second condition, the patient is instructed to focus on what the therapist says, not rehearse sentences and not censor them.

Manipulating Safety Behaviors

Safety behaviors are problematic because they can cause or exaggerate some of the symptoms that social phobics fear (e.g., holding a cup tightly to prevent spillage can increase unsteadiness and tremor) and because they prevent social phobics from disconfirming their belief that certain symptoms and behaviors will be negatively evaluated by other people. Systematic manipulation of safety behaviors is, therefore, an important component of therapy (Wells et al., 1995). First, the therapist identifies the patient's key safety behaviors and the way in which they are linked to specific beliefs. The feared catastrophe is identified by asking, "When you are in the situation and you feel particularly anxious, what is the worst that you think could happen?" Once a catastrophe has been identified, safety behaviors are elicited by asking, "Is there anything you do in that situation to try and prevent it from happening?" When asking the latter question, it is important to focus on mental strategies (e.g., dissociating) as well as behavioral strategies. Next, the therapist helps the patient to see how each safety behavior may be exacerbating symptoms and/or preventing disconfirmation of beliefs. Finally, this suggestion is tested by intentionally manipulating the safety behaviors. A patient who grips a cup too tightly will be asked to grip loosely and will then find that this produces a steadier feeling. A patient who speaks quickly and avoids pauses because he thinks others will notice any hesitancy and think badly of him will be asked to intentionally add a pause in his speech and to carefully observe others' responses (by observing their facial expressions at the time and asking them afterward). Invariably what happens is that a pause that is viewed as agonizingly long by the patient either is not noticed by others or, if it is, is viewed as a sign of thoughtfulness.

Shifting to Externally Focused Processing

As social phobics habitually focus internally, a large number of strategies have been developed to help them shift to an external focus and detailed processing of the situation itself. For example, it is common for social phobics to have the feeling that they are the center of attention. This is often an exaggerated perception that increases self-consciousness. It can be dealt with by a behavioral experiment in which patients are asked to estimate, on the basis of their felt sense, how many people are systematically observing them and then to scan the situation to check out the extent to which their estimates are correct. Invariably they find that fewer people are observing them than they think and that those who are looking at them often do so fleetingly with little interest. This exercise can be followed up by a second experiment in which the patient challenges the felt sense of being the center of attention by intentionally trying to increase this feeling and then observing whether this maneuver causes people to look at them more. Despite a marked increase in the subjective sense of being the center of attention, they discover that there has been no change in the extent to which other people are observing them. This nicely illustrates the misleading nature of their appraisals of themselves. In appropriate cases, Socratic questioning can further establish this point by helping them to consider the paradox that they often think others are not interested in them and simultaneously believe that everyone chooses to focus on them rather than on others.

A shift away from internal focus can be greatly facilitated by encouraging patients to engage in visual-interrogation tasks such as detecting the color of other people's eyes, deciding whether they have a good fashion sense, and deciding what mood they are in.

Video feedback is a useful technique for correcting distorted beliefs about how visible anxiety symptoms are to other people. This is illustrated by the case of a businessman with public speaking anxiety who feared that his colleagues would see that he was anxious while giving a presentation and would cease to respect him as a consequence. His belief that because he *felt* anxious others must be able to see that he was anxious was tested by asking him to give a short speech while being videotaped. Immediately after the speech, he was asked to image how he believed he appeared to other people. This constructed image was then compared with the videotape. In his image, his anxiety was highly visible, but to his amazement, he was unable to detect any visible signs of anxiety when viewing the videotape. The intermediate step of constructing an image of how the patient thought he appeared before viewing the videotape helped solve a problem we encountered in our early attempts with this procedure. The problem was that for some patients the videotape triggered images of how they thought they appeared and these became confused with what was being seen on the videotape. Of course, some patients do show visible signs of anxiety, but video feedback is often still helpful because it demonstrates that these signs are overestimated.

Manipulating Self-Image

Various exercises involving the manipulation of self-image in feared social situations can be used to help patients challenge their erroneous belief that the negative image that they have constructed based on interoceptive information represents what others see and think. For example, the businessman described above recalled the more positive and realistic image of himself that he had observed on the videotape and used this when constructing his public self-image in subsequent feared situations. Other patients have found it useful to remind themselves of positive social accomplishments and their positive personal qualities (by the use of self-statements) both before and during exposure to social situations. A further useful strategy is to encourage patients to try out different scripts or personae as though they were actors in a play. Obviously, care must be taken to ensure that these strategies do not themselves become safety behaviors. Some patients who successfully manipulate scripts argue that the new scripts do not represent how they really are. The therapist can counter this by using questioning to establish the unrealistic nature of their existing public self-image.

Testing Predictions about Negative Evaluation by Others

Normal social interactions provide only limited opportunities to test patients' distorted beliefs about the consequences of behaving in ways that they perceive as inept. This problem can be partly overcome by asking patients to intentionally perform behaviors that they falsely believe will lead to negative evaluation. For example, a secretary feared that if she spilled her drink in a local bar, people that she knew would think that she was an alcoholic and would reject her. The first step in challenging this belief was to ask her how she thought the other people would react if they thought spilling her drink meant she was an alcoholic. She said that they would stare at her and start whispering. This was then tested by intentionally spilling a drink in a conspicuous fashion. To her amazement, no one showed any interest apart from the barman, who briefly glanced in her direction but hardly paused in his conversation. Similarly, patients can be asked to experiment with introducing boring topics into conversations, stammering, and expressing opinions that they know others will disagree with.

Dealing with the Postmortem

Because normal social interactions rarely provide patients with unambiguous feedback on how well they have performed and on how others perceive them, social phobics often conduct postmortems of their social interactions. In these postmortems, the patients' anxious feelings and negative self-perceptions figure particularly prominently, and so the postmortems provide further, incorrect, evidence of social failure. This point needs to be established with the patient, and then the postmortem is banned.

Modifying Assumptions

The assumptions that lead social phobics to interpret social situations in a threatening fashion can be modified by the use of Socratic questioning. For example, the assumption "If someone doesn't like me, it means I am inadequate" can be modified by questions such as these: "How do you know that someone doesn't like you?"; "Are there any reasons why someone might not respond well to you other than your adequacy, such as their mood, you reminding them of someone else, their mind being elsewhere, etc.?"; "Can you think of any examples in which someone wasn't liked yet they were not inadequate, for example, Jesus and the Pharisees?"; "If one person doesn't like you and another does, who is right?"; "If one person doesn't like you, does that write you off as a person?"

SUMMARY AND CONCLUSIONS

We have proposed a cognitive model of social phobia that suggests that the problem persists because patients are not really processing what is happening in the social situation, are engaging in safety behaviors that prevent disconfirmation, are negatively influencing other people's behavior, and are using their own impression of themselves as the main evidence for the idea that other people are negatively evaluating them. Existing research is consistent with the model, but further investigation is required. In the meantime, the model suggests several ways in which existing cognitive-behavioral treatments could be made more effective.

ACKNOWLEDGMENTS

Preparation of this chapter and our experimental work was supported by the Wellcome Trust. We would like to thank Richard Heimberg for helpful comments on an earlier version.

REFERENCES

American Psychiatric Association. (1987). *Diagnostic and statistical manual of mental disorders* (3rd ed., rev.). Washington, DC: Author.

Arntz, A., Rauner, M., & van den Hout, M. A. (1994). "If I feel anxious, there must be danger": The fallacy of ex-consequentia reasoning in inferring danger in anxiety disorders. Manuscript submitted for publication.

Asmundson, G. J. G., & Stein, M. B. (1994). Selective attention for social threat in patients with generalized social phobia: Evaluation using a dot-probe paradigm. *Journal of Anxiety Disorders, 8*, 107–117.

Beck, A. T., Emery, G., & Greenberg, R. L. (1985). *Anxiety disorders and phobias: A cognitive perspective.* New York: Basic Books.

Bond, C. F., & Omar, A. S. (1990). Social anxiety, state dependence and the next-in-line effect. *Journal of Experimental Social Psychology, 26*, 185–198.

Bruch, B. A., Gorsky, J. M., Collins, T. M., & Berger, P. A. (1989). Shyness and sociability reexamined: A multicomponent analysis. *Journal of Personality and Social Psychology, 57*, 904–915.

Burns, D. D. (1980). *Feeling good: The new mood therapy.* New York: William Morrow.

Butler, G. (1985). Exposure as a treatment for social phobia: Some instructive difficulties. *Behaviour Research and Therapy, 23*, 651–657.

Butler, G., Cullington, A., Munby, M., Amies, P., & Gelder, M. (1984). Exposure and anxiety management in the treatment of social phobia. *Journal of Consulting and Clinical Psychology, 59*, 167–175.

Butler, G., & Mathews, A. M. (1993). Cognitive processes in anxiety. *Advances in Behaviour Research and Therapy, 5*, 51–63.

Clark, D. M., & Stopa, L. (1994). *Social phobia and the interpretation of ambiguous and mildly negative social events.* Manuscript in preparation.

Curtis, R. C., & Miller, K. (1986). Believing another likes or dislikes you: Behaviors making the beliefs come true. *Journal of Personality and Social Psychology, 51*, 284–290.

Daly, J. A., Vangelisti, A. L., & Lawrence, S. G. (1989). Self-focused attention and public speaking anxiety. *Personality and Individual Differences, 10*, 903–913.

Dodge, C. S., Hope, D. A., Heimberg, R. G., & Becker, R. E. (1988). Evaluation of the Social Interaction Self-Statement Test with a social phobic population. *Cognitive Therapy and Research, 12*, 211–222.

Hartman, L. M. (1983). A metacognitive model of social anxiety: Implications for treatment. *Clinical Psychology Review, 3*, 435–456.

Heimberg, R. G. (1991). *Cognitive behavioral treatment of social phobia in a group setting: A treatment manual.* Unpublished manuscript, State University of New York at Albany.

Heimberg, R. G., & Barlow, D. H. (1988). Psychosocial treatments for social phobia. *Psychosomatics, 29*, 27–37.

Hope D. A., Heimberg, R. G., & Klein, J. F. (1990). Social anxiety and the recall of interpersonal information. *Journal of Cognitive Psychotherapy, 4*, 185–195.

Hope, D. A., Rapee, R. M., Heimberg, R. G., & Dombeck, M. J. (1990). Representations of the self in social phobia: Vulnerability to social threat. *Cognitive Therapy and Research, 14*, 177–189.

Johansson, J., & Öst, L. G. (1982). Perception of autonomic reactions and actual heart rate in phobic patients. *Journal of Behavioral Assessment, 4,* 133–143.

Kenny, D. A., & DePaulo, B. M. (1993). Do people know how others view them? An empirical and theoretical account. *Psychological Bulletin, 114,* 145–161.

Kimble, C. E., & Zehr, H. D. (1982). Self-consciousness, information load, self-presentation, and memory in a social situation. *Journal of Social Psychology, 118,* 39–46.

Leary, M. R. (1983). *Understanding social anxiety.* Beverly Hills, CA: Sage.

MacLeod, C., Mathews, A., & Tata, P. (1986). Attentional bias in emotional disorders. *Journal of Abnormal Psychology, 95,* 15–20.

Mattia, J. I., Heimberg, R. G., & Hope. D. A. (1993). The revised Stroop color-naming task in social phobics. *Behaviour Research and Therapy, 31,* 305–313.

McEwan, K. L., & Devins, G. M. (1983). Is increased arousal in social anxiety noticed by others? *Journal of Abnormal Psychology, 92,* 417–421.

O'Banion, K., & Arkowitz, H. (1977). Social anxiety and selective memory for affective information about the self. *Social Behavior and Personality, 5,* 321–328.

Rapee, R. M., & Lim, L. (1992). Discrepancy between self- and observer ratings of performance in social phobics. *Journal of Abnormal Psychology, 101,* 728–731.

Rapee, R. M., McCallum, S. L., Melville, L. F., Ravenscroft, H., & Rodney, J. M. (1994). Memory bias in social phobia. *Behaviour Research and Therapy, 32,* 89–99.

Salkovskis, P. (1991). The importance of behaviour in the maintenance of anxiety and panic: A cognitive account. *Behavioural Psychotherapy, 19,* 6–19.

Salkovskis, P. M., Clark, D. M., & Jones, D. R. O. (1986). A psychosomatic mechanism in anxiety attacks: The role of hyperventilation in social anxiety and cardiac neurosis. In H. Lacey & J. Sturgeon (Eds.), *Proceedings of the 15th European Conference in Psychosomatic Medicine* (pp. 239–245). London: John Libbey.

Smith, T. W., Ingram, R. E., & Brehm, S. S. (1983). Social anxiety, anxious preoccupation, and recall of self-relevant information. *Journal of Personality and Social Psychology, 44,* 1276–1283.

Stopa, L., & Clark, D. M. (1993). Cognitive processes in social phobia. *Behaviour Research and Therapy, 31,* 255–267.

Teasdale, J. D., & Barnard, P. J. (1993). *Affect, cognition and change.* Hove, UK: Erlbaum.

Trower, P., & Gilbert, P. (1989). New theoretical conceptions of social anxiety and social phobia. *Clinical Psychology Review, 9,* 19–35.

Watson, D., & Friend, R. (1969). Measurement of social-evaluative anxiety. *Journal of Consulting and Clinical Psychology, 33,* 448–457.

Wells, A., Clark, D. M., Salkovskis, P., Ludgate, J., Hackmann, A., & Gelder, M. G. (1995). Social phobia: The role of in-situation safety behaviors in maintaining anxiety and negative beliefs. *Behavior Therapy, 26,* 153–161.

Wells, A., & Matthews, G. (1994). *Attention and emotion: A clinical perspective.* Hove: Lawrence Erlbaum.

Williams, J. M. G., Watts, F. N., MacLeod, C., & Mathews, A. (1988). *Cognitive psychology and emotional disorders.* Chichester, UK: Wiley.

Winton, E. C., Clark, D. M., & Edelmann, R. J. (1995). Social anxiety, fear of negative evaluation and detection of emotion in others. *Behaviour Research and Therapy, 33,* 193–196.

Yuen, P. K. (1994). *Social anxiety and the allocation of attention: Evaluation using facial stimuli in a dot-probe paradigm.*. Unpublished research project, Department of Experimental Psychology, University of Oxford, UK.

CHAPTER FIVE

The Self-Presentation Model of Social Phobia

MARK R. LEARY
ROBIN M. KOWALSKI

The central question for any theory of social phobia is, *What are people afraid of* when they experience anxiety in interpersonal settings? What is so threatening about social encounters that many people feel nervous when interacting with others, avoid social interactions when possible, and leave particularly difficult social situations prematurely? Furthermore, why do people differ in how socially anxious they tend to be? Why are some people at ease in most encounters, whereas others are so distressed about social interactions that they may be classified as social phobics?

The self-presentation theory of social anxiety was offered to address these questions in reference to people's interpersonal goals (Schlenker & Leary, 1982). At the time the self-presentation approach was proposed, the prevailing theories of social anxiety focused primarily on the role of social skills deficits (Curran, 1977; Twentyman & McFall, 1975) or on people's negative self-evaluations (Cacioppo, Glass, & Merluzzi, 1979; Clark & Arkowitz, 1975; Rehm & Marston, 1968). These approaches identified important specific causes of social anxiety, but in focusing on the anxious individual's dysfunctional behaviors or cognitions, they did not adequately address the question of *why* poor social skills or negative self-evaluations should make people nervous in social encounters.

Although the self-presentation theory emerged from the study of "normal" social anxiety in ordinary social interactions, we argue that it applies equally well to cases of social phobia as defined by the fourth edition of the *Diagnostic and Statistical Manual of Mental Disorders* (DSM-IV; American Psychiatric Association, 1994): "a marked and persistent fear of one or more social or performance situations in which the person is exposed to unfamiliar people or to possible scrutiny by others. The individual fears that he or she will act in a way (or show anxiety symptoms) that will be humiliating or embarrassing" (p. 411). As we explore in detail below, the self-presentation model parsimoniously accounts for individual differences in the degree to which people experience anxiety in social encounters. In our view, social phobia simply reflects a level of social anxiousness so extreme that the individual meets the DSM-IV criteria (Rapee, Sanderson, & Barlow, 1988). For example, comparisons of subclinically shy people with diagnosed social phobic individuals showed that social phobics display more extreme deficits than do shy individuals in daily functioning, a more serious course of the disorder, more extreme avoidant behaviors, stronger physiological reactions to social evaluation, and in some instances, a greater deficit in social skills (Turner, Beidel, & Larkin, 1986; Turner, Beidel, & Townsley, 1990). Yet no clear-cut evidence of qualitative differences between shy persons and social phobics was obtained. Thus, everything we say about the self-presentation underpinnings of social anxiety applies equally to social phobia.

This chapter reviews the self-presentation approach and its empirical support. Because the theory is described in detail elsewhere (Leary, 1983c; Leary & Kowalski, 1995; Schlenker & Leary, 1982, 1985), our coverage of the model itself will be brief. Rather, we will devote most of the chapter to research that has been conducted since the theory was proposed and to treatment recommendations that emerge from the model (most of which remain untested).

THE SELF-PRESENTATION APPROACH

According to the self-presentation theory of social anxiety (Schlenker & Leary, 1982), people experience social anxiety in a particular situation when two conditions co-occur: the person (1) is motivated to make particular impressions on other people but (2) doubts that he or she will be able to make the desired impressions successfully. If either of these conditions is not present—when people do not care how they are perceived by others, or if they are confident of making the desired impressions—social anxiety should not occur.

Some researchers have misinterpreted the theory as suggesting that social anxiety arises when people think they will make negative or unfavorable impressions on others. This interpretation is incorrect for two reasons. First, in some instances, people want to make negative, socially undesirable impressions on others. For example, they may want to appear intimidating to induce compliance, helpless to obtain support, or incompetent to avoid certain onerous responsibilities (Jones & Pittman, 1982; Kowalski & Leary, 1990; Leary & Miller, 1986). In cases such as these, people may become anxious when they think they will not make *undesirable* impressions.

Second, people may feel socially anxious even when they know they are making good impressions if they do not think they are being perceived *favorably enough* to accomplish their goals. A job applicant in an interview, a political candidate in a debate, or an adolescent on a first date may each think others view them positively, yet feel anxious because they do not think they are being viewed as positively as they would like (positively enough to get the job, to win the election, or to get a second date). When asked to rate how they think others perceive them, people who score relatively high in social anxiety usually give positive ratings (i.e., ratings above the neutral point of the scale; see Leary, 1986b; Leary, Kowalski, & Campbell, 1988). So it is not true that people must think they are regarded unfavorably in order for them to feel socially anxious.

For these reasons, we refer to making "particular" or "desired" impressions, rather than to making "positive," "favorable," or "socially desirable" impressions. A person's assessment of his or her self-presentation effectiveness can be made only relative to the impressions he or she desires to make; whether those impressions are positive or negative, as judged by others or by social norms, is irrelevant. Admittedly, in most instances the impressions people want others to form of them are positive, socially desirable ones, but this need not always be the case.

If we accept the premise that social anxiety arises from people's self-presentation concerns, we must address the broader question of why people experience anxiety when they feel incapable of making the kinds of impressions they desire. The impressions people make on others are a central determinant of their outcomes in social life (Goffman, 1959; Leary, 1995; Leary & Kowalski, 1990; Schlenker, 1980). Consider for a moment two people. Person A generally makes a "good" impression wherever she goes; others view her as friendly, competent, socially skilled, and interesting. Person B, in contrast, tends to leave others with a "bad" impression—that he is aloof, incompetent, socially unskilled, and boring. The importance of making certain, usually desirable impressions is obvious if we compare how these two individuals fare in life in terms of their friendships, romantic prospects, career opportunities, and even the quality of their daily interactions. Put simply, social interactions are mediated by the impressions that interactants form of one another.

Most people recognize that the impressions they make on others are important. In light of this, it is neither surprising nor irrational that people should often be concerned about making the "right" impression—whatever that may be in a particular situation. People can obviously be too concerned with what others think of them, or they may be concerned about the impressions they make when such concerns are simply not appropriate, but in principle, impression motivation is natural and understandably pervasive.

In fact, far from indicating vanity or neuroticism, occasional feelings of social discomfort, including social anxiety and embarrassment, may serve important functions. Baumeister and Tice (1990) persuasively argued that anxiety is a natural consequence of concerns about the nature of one's social bonds. Because humans find it difficult, if not impossible, to survive in isolation, mechanisms evolved that promote social inclusion by motivating people to develop and sustain supportive relationships. According to Baumeister and Tice, one of these mechanisms is an affective system that causes anxiety and other dysphoric reactions when one's relations with important others are in jeopardy. These reactions not only alert the individual to threats to his or her social relationships, but they influence the individual to stop ongoing behavior (so as not to dig him- or herself into a deeper interpersonal hole) and motivate remedial behavior to restore normal social relations and reduce the anxiety (Leary, 1990; Trower & Gilbert, 1989). Just as physical pain serves to warn us about threats to our physical well-being and motivates behaviors that reduce the pain, dysphoric social emotions—including social anxiety—may serve to warn us about threats to our social well-being (which, in a natural state, have direct implications for physical well-being as well) (Miller & Leary, 1992).

The degree to which people are included and accepted versus excluded and rejected by others is determined, in large part, by how others regard them. Those who are seen as incompetent, immoral, or socially undesirable, for example, risk exclusion relative to those whom others see as competent, upstanding, and socially desirable. Thus, people may be predisposed to experience anxiety when they fear they will fail to make desired impressions because self-presentation failures are associated with social exclusion. Such fears may be anticipatory, as in the case of social anxiety that occurs because of the possibility that one will make an undesired impression, or reactive, as in the case of embarrassment experienced after one's public image has already been damaged (Miller & Leary, 1992).

The self-presentation approach suggests that, although all social anxiety arises from self-presentation worries of one kind or another, people may be concerned about others' impressions of them for a variety of specific reasons. For example, some socially anxious people may be excessively concerned with obtaining social approval from others (i.e., their motivation to make particular impressions may be exceptionally high), whereas others may be anxious because they evaluate themselves negatively (and, thus, doubt that they will make the impressions they desire on others). Still others may recognize that they lack important social skills needed to suitably impress others (thereby accounting for the relationship between social skills deficits and social anxiety) or may have developed a conditioned negative emotional response to certain social situations as the result of having experienced the aversive consequences of previous self-presentation failures. Thus, the etiology of social anxiety can be understood in terms of characteristics that predispose people to experience excessive self-presentation concerns.

The self-presentation theory can parsimoniously incorporate other explanations of social anxiety, such as approaches based on unrealistic needs for approval, negative self-evaluations, social skills deficits, and classical conditioning (see Leary, 1983c, for a review). The causes of social anxiety specified by other perspectives can be regarded as particular factors that lead some people to be highly motivated to make particular impressions on others or to doubt that they will successfully make those impressions. As we will see, this facet of the theory has implications for the treatment of socially anxious clients: Although all socially anxious people have a high degree of concern over others' impressions of them, different clients may be concerned for different reasons.

When the self-presentation approach to social anxiety was first proposed (Leary, 1980, 1983c; Schlenker & Leary, 1982), little direct support for the model existed. During the last decade, however, we and others have accumulated increasing evidence that social anxiety can be traced to people's concerns with others' impressions of them. Below we review two general bodies of data that deal with the relationship between self-presentation and social anxiety: The first involves the effects of self-presentation concerns on anxiety in particular social settings (state social anxiety), and the second focuses on the relationship between self-presentation concerns and the general tendency to experience social anxiety (trait social anxiety). We then discuss the behavioral manifestations of social anxiety—withdrawal, reticence, and interpersonal avoidance—within the self-presentation perspective, and conclude with a discussion of treatment implications.

SELF-PRESENTATION CONCERNS
AND STATE SOCIAL ANXIETY

Considerable evidence supports the central premise of the self-presentation approach—that social anxiety emerges from people's self-presentation concerns with how they are being perceived and evaluated by others. In the initial study that tested the self-presentation model of social anxiety (Leary, 1980), subjects who were told how to make a desired impression on another person reported feeling less anxious than subjects who were not told how to make a desired impression. In everyday interactions, uncertainty about the impressions one should make or about how to effectively make those impressions causes people to feel socially anxious. This explains why encounters involving strangers, ambiguity, or novel roles often evoke considerable anxiety.

Leary (1980) also found that subjects who thought they possessed a trait that was associated with making good impressions were more relaxed and less shy than subjects who doubted that they possessed this trait. Furthermore, subjects' responses to the question "How good an impression do you think you made on the other subject?" correlated .42 with self-reported relaxation in a dyadic conversation. In another, role-playing study, subjects' beliefs regarding their ability to make desired impressions in a particular situation correlated −.49 with how anxious they expected to feel (Maddux, Norton, & Leary, 1988).

For ethical reasons, we have hesitated to experimentally induce social anxiety by leading subjects to think they made undesired impressions on another person. However, one experiment (Leary, 1986b) attempted to *decrease* state social anxiety by lowering subjects' self-presentation concerns. The reasoning behind this study was that, to the extent that social anxiety emerges from people's self-presentation concerns, anxiety should be lower when a person's self-presentation difficulties can be attributed to situational impediments. A person interacting under very difficult circumstances need not be as concerned about the impressions he or she makes both because others would have difficulty forming clear-cut impressions to begin with and because a failure to make a desired impression could easily be attributed to the difficult situation.

Subjects identified as either low or high in trait social anxiety interacted in the presence of moderately loud, distracting noise. Some subjects were told that the noise was expected to have little effect on their ability to interact and form accurate impressions of one another, whereas other subjects were told that they would find the noise quite distracting, and that it would be difficult for them to interact and get to know one another. (In reality, the noise was equally loud in both situations.) As predicted, subjects who were told that the noise would be distracting had lower pulse rates (indicating lower anxious arousal) than did those who were told that the noise was expected to have little effect. In addition, the supposedly loud noise was particularly comforting for subjects high in trait social anxiety. The self-presentation interpretation of these findings is that the presence of a situational impediment that ostensibly interfered with interpersonal behavior released subjects from the negative implications of a mediocre or substandard self-presentation performance.

Social anxiety increases with the salience of interpersonal evaluation because explicit evaluation raises the possibility that one will not be perceived and judged as desired. Furthermore, the more difficult a person believes it will be to make a particular desired impression on someone, the more anxious he or she should feel and behave.

DePaulo, Epstein, and LeMay (1990) had women high and low in social anxiety tell four stories to a confederate. Subjects were instructed to tell two stories that would make them appear independent (one true and one false) and two that would make them appear dependent (one true and one false). Before telling the stories, subjects were presented with information that described the confederate as either very wary or very trusting, a manipulation designed to affect subjects' efficacy in making desired impressions. To manipulate self-presentation motivation, subjects were also told that the confederate either would or would not inform them of the impression she formed after each story. The researchers found that socially anxious women who anticipated evaluation told shorter and less personally revealing stories than did either socially anxious individuals who did not anticipate evaluation or non-socially anxious subjects. The researchers suggested that socially anxious subjects faced with interpersonal evaluation adopted a protective self-presentation style to avoid making a negative impression.

In a study of the cognitions associated with social anxiety, Mahone, Bruch, and Heimberg (1993) found that anxiety during a laboratory conversation was best predicted by the percent of the subject's thoughts that were self-deprecating and by the percent of the subject's thoughts that focused on the positive attributes of the conversational partner. These findings suggest that the self-presentation concerns that precipitate anxiety can emerge both from self-perceived personal shortcomings (deficiencies that undermine the person's confidence in making a particular impression) and from the belief that other people in an interaction have high standards for evaluating others (because they possess highly desirable attributes themselves). Thus, people who are more physically attractive, socially skilled, knowledgeable, or gifted in some other domain are more likely to engender social anxiety in those with whom they interact than are people who do not possess socially desirable characteristics (Leary, 1983c; Leary & Kowalski, 1995; Mahone et al., 1993).

In brief, research has supported the notion that state social anxiety is associated with self-presentation concerns. Individuals who anticipate interpersonal evaluation experience greater anxiety, particularly if they have a tendency to be socially anxious, than do individuals who do not expect evaluation. In addition, manipulations designed to raise or lower self-presentation worries are associated with concomitant changes in self-reported anxiety and physiological arousal, and self-reported anxiety correlates with the degree to which people are worried about others' impressions in a particular context.

SELF-PRESENTATION CONCERNS
AND TRAIT SOCIAL ANXIETY

As we have seen, the self-presentation approach proposes that people experience social anxiety when they are motivated to make certain impressions but doubt that they will be able to do so. A corollary of this proposition is that individual differences in trait social anxiety are based, to a degree, on differences in variables related to impression motivation and efficacy. That is, if the self-presentation approach is accurate, we should find that dispositionally socially anxious people, including those who can be classified as social phobic, are more motivated to make impressions on other people and less likely to think they will do so than are less anxious persons. Two lines of research clearly support this view.

Dispositional Correlates

The first body of evidence comes from studies that have examined dispositional correlates of social anxiousness or social phobia. First, compared to individuals low in trait social anxiety, socially anxious people score higher on measures that reflect a high degree of self-presentation motivation: (1) public self-consciousness (e.g., they are more aware of others' impressions of them) (Buss, 1980; Leary, 1983a; Reno & Kenny, 1992), (2) self-monitoring (e.g., they more regularly monitor and control others' impressions of them) (Glass & Arnkoff, 1989; Leary & Kowalski, 1993), and (3) fear of negative evaluation (e.g., they are more concerned about being perceived unfavorably) (Leary, 1983b; Leary & Kowalski, 1993).

Second, trait social anxiety is correlated with doubts about one's ability to make desired impressions on others. Most important, trait social anxiety correlates moderately with trait self-esteem (e.g., Clark & Arkowitz, 1975; Leary, 1983b; Leary & Kowalski, 1993; Leary & Meadows, 1991). From the standpoint of the self-presentation approach, the relationship between self-esteem and social anxiety is indirect, being mediated by people's beliefs about how others perceive them. Because persons with low self-esteem assume that others regard them less favorably than do persons with high self-esteem (partly because they present themselves less positively to others; Baumeister, Tice, & Hutton, 1989), they experience greater social anxiety when they are motivated to manage their impressions.

Thus, in contrast to cognitive explanations that trace social anxiety to negative self-beliefs per se, the self-presentation model stresses the primacy of people's expectancies about *others'* impressions. Evidence in support of this distinction is provided by Wallace and Alden (1991). Male subjects classified as low or high in social anxiety rated their ability to meet or exceed three standards of performance in an upcoming interaction: their own personal standards, the performance of the average subject, and the experimenter's standards. Men low in anxiety felt confident that they could meet, if not exceed, the expectations of not only themselves but also others, including the experimenter. In contrast, men high in social anxiety thought they could meet their own personal standards but expected to fall short of the experimenter's standards. Significantly, the anxious and nonanxious men did not differ in their perceptions of the experimenter's standard for performance. Although this study did not explicitly assess standards for *self-presentation* performance, it highlights the fact that trait social anxiety is more closely related to people's concerns about meeting others' standards than to concerns about meeting their own standards. This is consistent with the tenets of self-discrepancy theory, which proposes that "agitation-based" emotions, such as anxiety, occur when there is a discrepancy between the attributes that people think they possess and the attributes that they think others believe they ought to possess (e.g., Higgins, Bond, Klein, & Strauman, 1986).

Some dispositional characteristics may contribute jointly to the motivational and the efficacy components of the self-presentation model. For example, individuals who are publicly self-conscious are focused on the aspects of themselves that are observable to others and thus, should be more concerned with the impressions that others are forming and more motivated to control those impressions (Buss, 1980; Fenigstein, 1979). At the same time, however, preoccupation with the self may lead to negative self-thoughts (Burgio, Merluzzi, & Pryor, 1986) and decrease the amount of attention publicly self-conscious individuals devote to their interaction partners. As a result, they may be more likely to doubt their ability to effectively manage their impressions (Hope, Gansler, & Heimberg, 1989; Hope & Heimberg, 1988).

Some studies have shown an inverse relationship between one's perceived level of physical attractiveness and trait social anxiety or shyness (Phillips, 1991; Pilkonis, 1977; but see Cheek & Buss, 1981). From the self-presentation perspective, anxiety is associated with low perceived attractiveness because people recognize that attractive people tend to make better impressions than do less attractive people (Berscheid & Walster, 1974; Feingold, 1992). Thus, some people may be chronically anxious because they worry about how others are judging their appearance. For example, people with physique anxiety are frequently distressed when they think their bodies are being scrutinized by other people (Hart, Leary, & Rejeski, 1989).

A more extreme case is body dysmorphism—a phenomenon in which individuals experience intense anxiety because of an imagined flaw in their appearance, even though they actually appear perfectly normal (Phillips, 1991). Because of their obsessive concern over the imagined defect, such individuals are highly vigilant of the reactions of others, worrying that others are continually noticing and commenting on their supposed physical defect. The consequence of this is that dysmorphic individuals frequently experience extreme social anxiety and embarrassment.

Impression-Relevant Cognitions of Socially Anxious People

The second body of evidence relevant to the self-presentation explanation of trait social anxiety or phobia comes from findings regarding the cognitions of persons low and high in social anxiety before, during, and after laboratory conversations. First, subjects high in trait social anxiety report thinking more about the impressions they are making on others in laboratory conversations than do subjects low in social anxiety (Leary, 1986b).

Second, relative to subjects low in social anxiety, socially anxious people consistently think that they are making less favorable impressions on other people (DePaulo et al., 1990; Lake & Arkin, 1985; Leary & Kowalski, 1993; Melchior & Cheek, 1990; Smith & Sarason, 1975). For example, in one study, high and low socially anxious subjects indicated their perception of an interaction partner's impression of them (Pozo, Carver, Wellens, & Scheier, 1991). The interaction partner was actually a videotape in which facial expressions were varied to indicate acceptance, rejection, or neutrality. Relative to individuals low in social anxiety, those high in social anxiety felt that the interaction partner was less accepting of them (see also Curran, Wallander, & Fischetti, 1980).

In another study (Clark & Arkowitz, 1975), high and low socially anxious men engaged in two tape-recorded interactions with female confederates. Following the interactions, the men listened to the tapes and rated their level of social skill, social anxiety, and the positivity of the woman's response during the interaction. They also rated additional tapes (purportedly by other participants) in which a male confederate played the role of a socially anxious or nonanxious individual. Two judges also coded the tapes along the same dimensions as did the subjects. Relative to men low in social anxiety, socially anxious men perceived themselves to be less socially skilled. The socially anxious men also devalued their performance relative to the judges' ratings.

Similar findings have been reported in socially anxious subjects' self-reports of everyday social interactions. In one study, socially anxious and nonanxious individuals used a diary format to record their interpersonal interactions over a 2-week period (Dodge, Heimberg, Nyman, & O'Brien,

1987). Relative to non-socially anxious individuals, those high in social anxiety evaluated their interpersonal performance more negatively and were less satisfied with the interactions that occurred. In part, these effects are exacerbated by the fact that socially anxious people tend to remember more negative information about themselves than do less anxious people (Breck & Smith, 1983; O'Banion & Arkowitz, 1977).

Based on Bandura's (1977) distinction between self-efficacy and outcome expectancies, Maddux et al. (1988) reasoned that socially anxious people are not only more likely to doubt that they can make the impressions they would like to make (self-presentation self-efficacy expectancy) but may also believe that making the "right" impression is less likely to lead to the outcomes they desire (self-presentation outcome expectancy). In support of this, trait social anxiety correlated negatively both with self-presentation self-efficacy expectancies ($r = -.65$) and with outcome expectancies ($r = -.32$).

In many cases, however, people's perceived self-presentation difficulties are more imagined than real. Although judges often rate people high in social anxiety less positively than they rate those who are low (e.g., Bellack & Hersen, 1979; Curran, 1977), socially anxious individuals tend to overestimate others' negative reactions to them. For example, one study showed that socially anxious subjects assumed they had made a worse impression on another person than did less anxious subjects even if the other person had only glanced at them (Leary, Kowalski, & Campbell, 1988). Socially anxious people also overestimate the degree to which their nervousness is apparent to other people (Bruch, Gorsky, Collins, & Berger, 1989).

For several years, we assumed that socially anxious people often experience self-presentation doubts because they believe that they make less-desired impressions than most other people do. However, a study we conducted (Leary, Kowalski, & Campbell, 1988, Experiment 2) casts doubt on this assumption. Subjects classified as low or high in trait social anxiety rated how they thought another person in an imaginary encounter would perceive either them or other people. Consistent with other research, high socially anxious subjects thought they would make a less positive impression than did low socially anxious subjects, even after very short interactions.

More interesting, however, was the fact that highly anxious subjects did *not* assume that they would make worse impressions than they thought others would make. However, subjects low in social anxiety thought that they would make *better* impressions than would most other people. Put differently, subjects who scored low in social anxiety indicated that they would make better impressions than would most other people, but highly anxious subjects thought that they made the same sorts of impressions as did others. These effects were obtained across three different self-presentation dimensions, reflecting effectance (e.g., intelligent, competent), socio-emotionality (e.g., friendly, socially skilled), and social attractiveness (e.g., interesting, popular).

This finding offers an intriguing twist on the relationship between self-presentation concerns and social anxiety. Individual differences in social anxiety may occur not so much because socially anxious people think they make worse impressions than others do, but rather, because relative to people low in anxiety, socially anxious people may think they *and everyone else* make less favorable impressions. Thus, these data suggest that perceived self-presentation deficiencies do not create a tendency to experience social anxiety as much as the belief that one makes better impressions than other people lowers anxiety. One remaining question is whether social phobics resemble the high socially anxious subjects in this study or whether they actually believe that they make poorer impressions than do most other people. Research is needed to examine the self-presentation motives and confidence of social phobics.

The self-presentation concerns of socially anxious people can become exacerbated if they come to believe that they appear excessively nervous during a particular encounter. Because appearing anxious, tense, or flustered is valued negatively in our society, people usually try to conceal evidence of their social discomfort. If they feel unable to do so (because their hands tremble or their voice cracks, for example), they may become increasingly anxious. Unfortunately, socially anxious people do overestimate the extent to which others can detect that they feel anxious, so that these concerns are often unfounded (Bruch et al., 1989).

SOCIAL ANXIETY AND INTERPERSONAL BEHAVIOR

Any useful theory of social anxiety must explain not only the subjective experience of fear that accompanies certain kinds of social encounters but also the reticent, withdrawn, and socially avoidant behavior that tends to accompany episodes of social anxiety and that characterizes the interpersonal style of many social phobics. From the standpoint of the self-presentation model, the behavior of socially anxious or social phobic people reflects attempts to manage one's impressions under less than ideal circumstances (Leary, 1986a; Leary, Knight, & Johnson, 1987). Because the impressions people make have such important implications for their well-being, people are unlikely to completely abandon their efforts to manage their impressions even when they believe they will not make the impressions they desire. Yet because they do not think they will make desired impressions, socially anxious people must modify the self-presentation tactics they use.

Specifically, when socially anxious, people appear to adopt a "protective" as opposed to an "acquisitive" self-presentation style (Leary, 1983c; Shepperd & Arkin, 1990). According to Arkin (1981), whereas acquisitive self-presentation involves efforts to gain social approval, protective self-presentation involves attempts to avoid losses in approval. After people conclude that they are unlikely to make the impressions they desire, they may retreat to safe, protective tactics.

Evidence for this comes from a study by Greenberg, Pyszczynski, and Stine (1985) in which high and low socially anxious individuals interacted with a person of the other sex with whom they either did or did not expect to have future interactions. Individuals low in social anxiety who anticipated future interactions attempted to convey a very favorable image to the other individual. Socially anxious individuals, on the other hand, did not manage their impressions so as to make a particularly positive impression on the other person. Because socially anxious individuals have a low expectancy of sustaining a positive image in the eyes of others over time, they adopt a protective self-presentation strategy aimed toward minimizing social losses.

The reticence and withdrawal of socially anxious people can also be viewed as protective self-presentation. When people doubt that they will make the impressions they desire, the safest tactic is often to disaffiliate, either by remaining quietly present or by leaving the situation altogether. Such tactics allow people to avoid further damage to their social images.

In addition, when people who doubt their ability to make desired impressions remain in a social encounter, they tend to engage in relatively safe interpersonal behaviors—behaviors that allow them to remain at least minimally engaged but that allow them to protect their social image. For example, socially anxious people tend to be innocuously sociable (Leary, 1983c)—smiling and nodding frequently and using a high number of acknowledgments to indicate that they are attentive to the conversation (i.e., "uh-huh"). They also tend to ask more questions (a low-risk tactic that conveys friendly interest while keeping attention off oneself) while making fewer statements of fact (Leary, Knight, & Johnson, 1987). Such behaviors are useful ways of remaining engaged in an interaction without risking damage to one's image, and they help to keep the spotlight on other interactants and off oneself. Indeed, one study showed that instructing subjects to "find out as much as you can" about another person significantly lowered social anxiety and awkwardness, presumably because such a tactic focused attention on the other person and reduced the questioner's self-presentation concerns (Leary, Kowalski, & Bergen, 1988).

Evidence of protective self-presentation can also be seen in the attributions of socially anxious people. Unlike non-socially anxious individuals, who exhibit the self-serving bias by taking credit for success while denying responsibility for failure, socially anxious individuals show a tendency to reverse the self-serving bias (Arkin, Appelman, & Burger, 1980; Hope et al., 1989; Teglasi & Fagin, 1984). Although other interpretations are possible, these findings are consistent with the idea that socially anxious people are careful not to present overly self-aggrandizing images of themselves that might lead to scoffing, criticism, or rejection (Arkin et al., 1980).

Although some have interpreted these behavioral manifestations of social anxiety as reflecting deficits in social skills, others have suggested that these "protective" behaviors actually require considerable interpersonal ability. For example, Trower and Gilbert (1989), operating from a psychobiological model, suggested that socially anxious individuals adopt submissive behaviors in response to an appraisal process informing them that important relationships are in jeopardy. However, rather than reflecting a social skills deficit, these behaviors are intentionally enacted to avoid negative evaluations by other people.

TREATMENT IMPLICATIONS

As later chapters in this book describe, a variety of psychotherapeutic models have been successful in reducing social anxiety and phobia. A number of specific treatments have been examined, but most have reflected some variation of systematic desensitization (Arkowitz, Hinton, Perl, & Himadi, 1978), social skills training (for a review, see Curran, 1977), or cognitive-behavioral therapy (Lucock & Salkovskis, 1988; Mitchell, 1988; Heimberg & Juster, Chapter 12, this volume).

In identifying concerns with others' impressions as the precipitating factor in social phobia, the self-presentation approach sheds a new light on the treatment of social anxiety. Specifically, although all social anxiety is self-presentationally mediated, "a variety of specific attributes may predispose people to be highly motivated to control the impressions they make on others and/or to harbor doubts that they can do so" (Leary, 1987, p. 128).

Put differently, not all social phobic clients are anxious for precisely the same set of reasons (Leary, 1987; Schneier, 1991). As noted earlier, some people are socially anxious because they are excessively high in need for approval and thus walk through life trying to convey the impressions they think will stave off unfavorable evaluations. In contrast, other socially anxious people lack important social skills, which leads them to doubt that they will make desired impressions in social encounters. Yet other socially anxious people have generally low self-esteem, assuming that others share their less than flattering self-views. Still other people are social phobic because they hold excessively high and rigid standards for evaluating their social performances; failing to meet these high standards leads to anxiety. And, of course, in severe cases, a socially anxious person may manifest several of these predisposing factors. Even when this is the case, however, some factors may contribute more to the person's distress than others.

Although each of these people's anxiety can be traced to interpersonal, self-presentation concerns, their specific difficulties differ. To the extent this is so, treatments are most likely to be effective when they are matched to the characteristics that underlie a particular client's problems (Leary, 1987, 1988; Leary & Kowalski, 1995). Thus, counselors and therapists should try to determine the precise source of a particular client's self-presentation concerns and use this information in treatment planning.

SUMMARY

Research during the past 15 years generally supports the self-presentation model as a parsimonious, overarching explanation that offers insights into the causes and treatment of social insecurities. Although most research conducted to explicitly test the model has involved subclinical social anxiety in normal (i.e., undergraduate) samples, we have every reason to believe that the differences between social anxiety and social phobia are largely a matter of degree. From this perspective, social phobics are people who are extraordinarily motivated to make desired impressions on others, particularly doubtful of their ability to be perceived and evaluated as they desire, and in general, excessively concerned about others' impressions.

Although the definition of social phobia provided by the DSM-IV acknowledges the central role of social scrutiny and potential embarrassment, little research involving social phobics has adopted a self-presentation perspective. A more explicit emphasis on the impression-relevant concerns of social phobics may enhance our understanding and treatment of this problem. Thus, research is needed that examines the self-presentation model in clinical populations and in nonclinical populations other than college undergraduates.

Research is also needed to test the usefulness of matching treatment approaches to the factors that underlie a particular client's social anxiety. Rather than continuing the tradition of pitting one treatment model against another, we should begin to explore the possibility that treatment efficacy depends on the source of a particular client's anxiety.

REFERENCES

American Psychiatric Association. (1994). *Diagnostic and statistical manual of mental disorders* (4th ed.). Washington, DC: Author.

Arkin, R. M. (1981). Self-presentation styles. In J. T. Tedeschi (Ed.), *Impression management theory and social psychological research* (pp. 311–333). New York: Academic Press.

Arkin, R. M., Appelman, A. J., & Burger, J. M. (1980). Social anxiety, self-presentation, and the self-serving bias in causal attribution. *Journal of Personality and Social Psychology, 38*, 23–35.

Arkowitz, H., Hinton, R., Perl, J., & Himadi, W. (1978). Treatment strategies for dating anxiety in college men based on real-life practice. *Counseling Psychologist, 7*, 41–46.

Bandura, A. (1977). Self-efficacy: Toward a unifying theory of behavioral change. *Psychological Review, 84*, 191–215.

Baumeister, R. F., & Tice, D. M. (1990). Anxiety and social exclusion. *Journal of Social and Clinical Psychology, 9*, 165–195.

Baumeister, R. F., Tice, D. M., & Hutton, D. G. (1989). Self-presentational motivations and personality differences in self-esteem. *Journal of Personality, 57*, 547–579.

Bellack, A. S., & Hersen, M. (Eds.). (1979). *Research and practice in social skills training.* New York: Plenum Press.

Berscheid, E., & Walster, E. (1974). Physical attractiveness. In L. Berkowitz (Ed.), *Advances in experimental social psychology* (Vol. 7, pp. 157–215). San Diego, CA: Academic Press.

Breck, B. E., & Smith, S. H. (1983). Selective recall of self-descriptive traits by socially anxious and nonanxious females. *Social Behavior and Personality, 11*, 71–76.

Bruch, M. A., Gorsky, J. M., Collins, T. M., & Berger, P. A. (1989). Shyness and sociability revisited: A multicomponent analysis. *Journal of Personality and Social Psychology, 57*, 904–915.

Burgio, K. L., Merluzzi, T. V., & Pryor, J. B. (1986). Effects of performance expectancy and self-focused attention on social interaction. *Journal of Personality and Social Psychology, 50*, 1216–1221.

Buss, A. H. (1980). *Self-consciousness and social anxiety.* San Francisco: Freeman.

Cacioppo, J. T., Glass, C. R., & Merluzzi, T. V. (1979). Self-statements and self-evaluations: A cognitive-response analysis of heterosocial anxiety. *Cognitive Therapy and Research, 3*, 249–262.

Cheek, J. M., & Buss, A. H. (1981). Shyness and sociability. *Journal of Personality and Social Psychology, 41*, 330–339.

Clark, J. V., & Arkowitz, H. (1975). Social anxiety and self-evaluation of interpersonal performance. *Psychological Reports, 36*, 211–221.

Curran, J. P. (1977). Skills training as an approach to the treatment of heterosexual–social anxiety: A review. *Psychological Bulletin, 84*, 140–157.

Curran, J. P., Wallander, J. L., & Fischetti, M. (1980). The importance of behavioral and cognitive factors in heterosexual-social anxiety. *Journal of Personality, 48*, 285–292.

DePaulo, B. M., Epstein, J. A., & LeMay, C. S. (1990). Responses of the socially anxious to the prospect of interpersonal evaluation. *Journal of Personality, 58*, 623–640.

Dodge, C. S., Heimberg, R. G., Nyman, D., & O'Brien, G. T. (1987). Daily heterosocial interactions of high and low socially anxious college students: A diary study. *Behavior Therapy, 18*, 90–96.

Feingold, A. (1992). Good-looking people are not what we think. *Psychological Bulletin, 111*, 304–341.

Fenigstein, A. (1979). Self-consciousness, self-attention, and social interaction. *Journal of Personality and Social Psychology, 37,* 75–86.

Glass, C. R., & Arnkoff, D. B. (1989). Behavioral assessment of social anxiety and social phobia. *Clinical Psychology Review, 9,* 75–90.

Goffman, E. (1959). *The presentation of self in everyday life.* Garden City, NY: Doubleday/Anchor.

Greenberg, J., Pyszczynski, T., & Stine, P. (1985). Social anxiety and anticipation of future interaction as determinants of the favorability of self-presentation. *Journal of Research in Personality, 19,* 1–11.

Hart, E. A., Leary, M. R., & Rejeski, W. J. (1989). The measurement of social physique anxiety. *Journal of Sport and Exercise Psychology, 11,* 94–104.

Higgins, E. T., Bond, R. N., Klein, R., & Strauman, T. (1986). Self-discrepancies and emotional vulnerability: How magnitude, accessibility, and type of discrepancy influence affect. *Journal of Personality and Social Psychology, 51,* 5–15.

Hope, D. A., Gansler, D. A., & Heimberg, R. G. (1989). Attentional focus and causal attributions in social phobia: Implications from social psychology. *Clinical Psychology Review, 9,* 49–60.

Hope, D. A., & Heimberg, R. G. (1988). Public and private self-consciousness and social phobia. *Journal of Personality Assessment, 52,* 626–639.

Jones, E. E., & Pittman, T. (1982). Toward a general theory of strategic self-presentation. In J. Suls (Ed.), *Psychological perspectives on the self* (Vol. 1, pp. 231–262). Hillsdale, NJ: Erlbaum.

Kowalski, R. M., & Leary, M. R. (1990). Strategic self-presentation and the avoidance of aversive events: Antecedents and consequences of self-enhancement and self-depreciation. *Journal of Experimental Social Psychology, 26,* 322–336.

Lake, E. A., & Arkin, R. M. (1985). Reactions to objective and subjective interpersonal evaluation: The influence of social anxiety. *Journal of Social and Clinical Psychology, 3,* 143–160.

Leary, M. R. (1980). *The social psychology of shyness: Testing a self-presentational model.* Unpublished doctoral dissertation, University of Florida, Gainesville.

Leary, M. R. (1983a). A brief version of the Fear of Negative Evaluation Scale. *Personality and Social Psychology Bulletin, 9,* 371–376.

Leary, M. R. (1983b). Social anxiousness: The construct and its measurement. *Journal of Personality Assessment, 47,* 66–75.

Leary, M. R. (1983c). *Understanding social anxiety: Social, personality, and clinical perspectives.* Bevery Hills, CA: Sage.

Leary, M. R. (1986a). Affective and behavioral components of shyness: Implications for theory, measurement, and research. In W. H. Jones, J. M. Cheek, & S. R. Briggs (Eds.), *Shyness: Perspectives on research and treatment* (pp. 27–38). New York: Plenum Press.

Leary, M. R. (1986b). The impact of interactional impediments on social anxiety and self-presentation. *Journal of Experimental Social Psychology, 22,* 122–135.

Leary, M. R. (1987). A self-presentational model for the treatment of social anxieties. In J. E. Maddux, C. D. Stoltenberg, & R. Rosenwein (Eds.), *Social processes in clinical and counseling psychology* (pp. 126–138). New York: Springer-Verlag.

Leary, M. R. (1988). A comprehensive approach to the treatment of social anxieties: The self-presentation model. *Phobia Practice Research Journal, 1,* 48–57.

Leary, M. R. (1990). Responses to social exclusion: Social anxiety, jealousy, loneliness, depression, and low self-esteem. *Journal of Social and Clinical Psychology*, *9*, 221–229.

Leary, M. R. (1995). *Self-presentation: Impression management and interpersonal behavior*. Milwaukee, WI: Brown & Benchmark.

Leary, M. R., Knight, P. D., & Johnson, K. A. (1987). Social anxiety and dyadic conversation: A verbal response analysis. *Journal of Social and Clinical Psychology*, *5*, 34–50.

Leary, M. R., & Kowalski, R. M. (1990). Impression management: A literature review and two-component model. *Psychological Bulletin*, *107*, 34–47.

Leary, M. R., & Kowalski, R. M. (1993). Psychometric properties of the Interaction Anxiousness Scale. *Journal of Personality Assessment*, *61*, 136–146.

Leary, M. R., & Kowalski, R. M. (1995). *Social anxiety*. New York: Guilford Press.

Leary, M. R., Kowalski, R. M., & Bergen, D. J. (1988). Interpersonal information acquisition and confidence in first encounters. *Personality and Social Psychology Bulletin*, *14*, 68–77.

Leary, M. R., Kowalski, R. M., & Campbell, C. (1988). Self-presentational concerns and social anxiety: The role of generalized impression expectancies. *Journal of Research in Personality*, *22*, 308–321.

Leary, M. R., & Meadows, S. (1991). Predictors, elicitors, and concomitants of social blushing. *Journal of Personality and Social Psychology*, *60*, 254–262.

Leary, M. R., & Miller, R. S. (1986). *Social psychology and dysfunctional behavior*. New York: Springer-Verlag.

Lucock, M. P., & Salkovskis, P. M. (1988). Cognitive factors in social anxiety and its treatment. *Behaviour Research and Therapy*, *26*, 297–302.

Maddux, J. E., Norton, L. W., & Leary, M. R. (1988). Cognitive components of social anxiety: An investigation of the integration of self-presentation theory and self-efficacy theory. *Journal of Social and Clinical Psychology*, *6*, 180–190.

Mahone, E. M., Bruch, M. A., & Heimberg, R. G. (1993). Focus of attention and social anxiety: The role of negative self-thoughts and perceived positive attributes of the other. *Cognitive Therapy and Research*, *17*, 209–224.

Melchior, L. A., & Cheek, J. M. (1990). Shyness and anxious self-preoccupation during a social interaction. In M. Booth-Butterfield (Ed.), *Communication, cognition, and anxiety* (pp. 117)130). San Rafael, CA: Select Press.

Miller, R. S., & Leary, M. R. (1992). Social sources and interactive functions of emotion: The case of embarrassment. In M. Clark (Ed.), *Emotion and social behavior* (pp. 202–221). Beverly Hills, CA: Sage.

Mitchell, C. E. (1988). Some psychotherapeutic techniques useful in the treatment of social phobias. *Journal of College Student Psychotherapy*, *3*, 73–82.

O'Banion, K., & Arkowitz, H. (1977). Social anxiety and selective memory for affective information about the self. *Social Behavior and Personality*, *5*, 321–328.

Phillips, K. A. (1991). Body dysmorphic disorder: The distress of imagined ugliness. *American Journal of Psychiatry*, *148*, 1138–1149.

Pilkonis, P. A. (1977). The behavioral consequences of shyness. *Journal of Personality*, *45*, 596–611.

Pozo, C., Carver, C. S., Wellens, A. R., & Scheier, M. F. (1991). Social anxiety and social perception: Construing others' reactions to the self. *Personality and Social Psychology Bulletin*, *17*, 355–362.

Rapee, R. M., Sanderson, W. C., & Barlow, D. H. (1988). Social phobic features across the DSM-III-R anxiety disorders. *Journal of Psychopathology and Behavioral Assessment, 10*, 287–299.

Rehm, L. P., & Marston, A. R. (1968). Reduction of social anxiety through modification of self-reinforcement. *Journal of Consulting and Clinical Psychology, 32*, 565–574.

Reno, R. R., & Kenny, D. A. (1992). Effects of self-consciousness and social anxiety on self-disclosure among unacquainted individuals: An application of the social relations model. *Journal of Personality, 60*, 79–94.

Schlenker, B. R. (1980). *Impression management: The self-concept, social identity, and interpersonal relations.* Monterey, CA: Brooks/Cole.

Schlenker, B. R., & Leary, M. R. (1982). Social anxiety and self-presentation: A conceptualization and model. *Psychological Bulletin, 92*, 641–669.

Schlenker, B. R., & Leary, M. R. (1985). Social anxiety and communication about the self. *Journal of Language and Social Psychology, 4*, 171–192.

Schneier, F. R. (1991). Social phobia. *Psychiatric Annals, 21*, 349–353.

Shepperd, J. A., & Arkin, R. M. (1990). Shyness and self-presentation. In W. R. Crozier (Ed.), *Shyness and embarrassment* (pp. 286–314). New York: Cambridge University Press.

Smith, R. E., & Sarason, I. G. (1975). Social anxiety and the evaluation of negative interpersonal feedback. *Journal of Consulting and Clinical Psychology, 43*, 429.

Teglasi, H., & Fagin, S. S. (1984). Social anxiety and self–other biases in causal attribution. *Journal of Research in Personality, 18*, 64–80.

Trower, P., & Gilbert, P. (1989). New theoretical conceptions of social anxiety and social phobia. *Clinical Psychology Review, 9*, 19–35.

Turner, S. M., Beidel, D. C., & Larkin, K. T. (1986). Situational determinants of social anxiety in clinic and non-clinic samples: Physiological and cognitive correlates. *Journal of Consulting and Clinical Psychology, 54*, 523–527.

Turner, S. M., Beidel, D. C., & Townsley, R. M. (1990). Social phobia: Relationship to shyness. *Behaviour Research and Therapy, 28*, 497–505.

Twentyman, C. T., & McFall, R. M. (1975). Behavioral training of social skills in shy males. *Journal of Consulting and Clinical Psychology, 43*, 384–395.

Wallace, S. T., & Alden, L. E. (1991). A comparison of social standards and perceived ability in anxious and nonanxious men. *Cognitive Therapy and Research, 15*, 237–254.

CHAPTER SIX

Neurobiology of Social Phobia

P. V. NICKELL
THOMAS W. UHDE

Social phobia is the clinically significant fear of being "exposed to unfamiliar people or to possible scrutiny by others" or that one may "act in a way . . . that will be humiliating or embarrassing" (American Psychiatric Association, 1994, p. 416). Investigating the neurobiological correlates of normal and pathological degrees of social anxiety is important for several reasons. First, such information is useful in delineating the boundaries between social phobia and normal degrees of social discomfort, other anxiety disorders, and phenomenologically related conditions. For example, there is some debate among academicians regarding the relationship between social phobia and avoidant personality disorder (C. S. Holt, Heimberg, & Hope, 1992). If these syndromes were found to have common biological abnormalities, one might contend that social phobia and avoidant personality disorder simply represented different clinical variants of a single diathesis rather than distinct disorders. In contrast, consistently different biological abnormalities across the two syndromes would support the concept of two separate and distinct conditions. On the other hand, if neither social phobia nor avoidant personality disorder were associated with alterations in biological function, one might reach quite different conclusions regarding the neuropsychopathology of these phenomenologically related syndromes. In short, the neurobiological study of social phobia provides a methodology for investigating the validity of current diagnostic classifications (e.g., the fourth edition of the *Diagnostic and Statistical Manual of Mental Disorders* [DSM-IV]; American Psychiatric Association, 1994).

Second, an improved understanding of the neurobiological underpinnings of social phobia may lead to novel treatment approaches. Although many therapeutic advances in biological psychiatry have been discovered through serendipity (West & Dally, 1959), an improved understanding of the neurobiological basis of social phobia should lead to the development of new drugs with relatively specific mechanisms of action and improved side-effect profiles (Nickell & Uhde, in press).

Third, an understanding of possible biological predispositions or risk factors for the development of a given syndrome may lead to successful secondary prevention techniques. Rosenbaum, Biederman, Hirshfeld, Bolduc, and Chaloff (1991) have suggested such interventions for children at risk to develop social phobia.

This chapter will provide an update on social phobia in the following areas: behavioral pharmacology, genetics, sleep physiology, and neuroendocrinology.

BEHAVIORAL PHARMACOLOGY

Drug Therapy

By investigating the range of therapeutic responses to different pharmacological agents with known mechanisms of action, one can gain insights into the pathophysiology of the condition being treated. Similar responses across phenomenologically distinct syndromes denote a possible overlap in underlying pathophysiology, whereas different response patterns suggest (but do not confirm) a divergence in neurobiology. Defining the cellular and molecular actions of a compound known to be active in a given syndrome can yield further insights into the disordered functioning of the organism. Although pharmacological treatments are discussed in depth elsewhere in this book (see Potts & Davidson, Chapter 14, and Liebowitz & Marshall, Chapter 15, this volume), a brief review for the drug therapies for social phobia is presented here as a tool for examining a possible role for one or more neurotransmitter—receptor systems in the neurobiology of social phobia.

Several different medications have been reported to be effective in social phobia. Those studied under double-blind conditions include phenelzine, moclobemide, alprazolam, atenolol, clonazepam, and brofaromine. Our group conducted a 12-week study comparing cognitive-behavioral group therapy with the monoamine oxidase inhibitor (MAOI) phenelzine (Nardil), alprazolam (Xanax), and pill placebo, administered under double-blind conditions (Gelernter et al., 1991). Clinician ratings showed significantly greater improvement with phenelzine and alprazolam than with the placebo, with phenelzine having some advantage over alprazolam. At follow-up 2 months after drug discontinuation, the phenelzine-treated group remained improved compared with placebo, whereas the alprazolam-treated group did not.

Liebowitz et al. (1992) treated 74 patients in a double-blind, randomized trial of phenelzine, the cardioselective beta blocker atenolol (Tenormin), and placebo. Phenelzine was significantly superior to both atenolol and placebo after 8 weeks and superior to placebo after 16 weeks. Atenolol was not different from placebo at either assessment.

Versiani et al. (1992) recently compared the reversible MAOI moclobemide to phenelzine and placebo in a double-blind trial (moclobemide is not available in the United States). Both active drugs were found to be statistically and clinically superior to placebo at 8 and 16 weeks, with phenelzine somewhat more effective but moclobemide better tolerated. A double-blind trial of the reversible MAOI brofaromine (no longer produced) supported its efficacy in the treatment of social phobia (van Vliet, den Boer, & Westenberg, 1992). Davidson et al.'s (1993) double-blind, placebo-controlled trial of clonazepam (Klonopin) showed it to be more effective than placebo. Counter to these positive findings, however, Clark and Agras (1991) conducted a placebo-controlled trial of the novel anxiolytic buspirone (BuSpar). Buspirone is a relatively selective serotonin agonist at the serotonin 1A receptor. There was no difference between buspirone and placebo. However, Schneier et al. (1993), in an open label trial, did find buspirone to be moderately effective. (See Potts & Davidson, Chapter 14, this volume, for a more detailed review of these studies.)

Open label studies have suggested efficacy for additional compounds, including the irreversible MAOI tranylcypromine (Parnate) (Versiani, Mundim, Nardi, & Liebowitz, 1988) and the selective serotonin reuptake inhibitor fluoxetine (Prozac) (Black, Uhde, & Tancer, 1992; Schneier, Chin, Hollander, & Liebowitz, 1992; Sternbach, 1990; Van Ameringen, Mancini, & Steiner, 1993). Goldstein (1987) reported the successful treatment of a single patient with social phobia who responded to the central alpha-2 agonist clonidine (Catapres). Similarly, Emmanuel, Lydiard, and Ballenger (1991) reported the successful treatment of a single patient with social phobia with the antidepressant bupropion (Wellbutrin). Benca, Matuzas, and Al-Sadir (1986) reported using imipramine (Tofranil) to successfully treat two patients with social phobia and echocardiographically defined mitral valve prolapse. This report is at odds, however, with a study by Tancer and Uhde (unpublished observations, 1989) in which only 1 of 10 social phobics responded to maximally tolerated doses of imipramine (mean dose 111 ± 45 mg per day).

A review of drug studies in children with elective mutism (renamed "selective mutism" in DSM-IV) is relevant to this chapter because this enigmatic syndrome is almost always associated with disabling amounts of social anxiety. In fact, 97% of 30 children with elective mutism were recently found to suffer from concomitant social phobia (Black & Uhde, 1995). This finding, among other observations, led Black and Uhde to conclude that elective mutism may be a childhood variant of social phobia rather than a distinct syndrome. Black and Uhde (1994) tested 15 children in a double-blind controlled study with either placebo ($n = 9$) or fluoxetine ($n = 6$; 0.6 mg per kg per day) and found that while the children in both groups demonstrated improvement on many different types of rating scales (teacher-rated, parent-rated, and physician-rated scales), the fluoxetine-treated children were significantly more improved than placebo-treated children only on the parent-rated scales of "mutism change" and "global improvement." For reasons discussed elsewhere (Black & Uhde, 1995), the authors believe that parents of children with elective mutism may be better able than teachers or physicians to identify early and more subtle signs of improvement. For example, the earliest signs of improvement might be the observed willingness of the child to talk for the first time with another child in the neighborhood or to talk more often and comfortably with a member of the child's extended family. These changes might be evident to the parents early in the course of pharmacotherapy, whereas more profound changes might not occur in the school (i.e., the more threatening environment) until later in the course of therapy. This pattern of symptom resolution in children with elective mutism is not dissimilar to the gradual elimination of selective avoidance behaviors seen in adults with either panic disorder or social phobia who are successfully treated with either drug or cognitive-behavioral therapies. Nonetheless, most of the children treated with fluoxetine were only partial responders. That is, although there was a clinically relevant degree of improvement associated with fluoxetine therapy, most of the children remained symptomatic. This preliminary study indicates that serotonergic reuptake inhibitors may have a role in the treatment of elective mutism. These findings further suggest that additional studies should be conducted to investigate the relationship between elective mutism and social phobia. In an initial attempt to examine the familial relationship between elective mutism and social phobia, Black and Uhde (1995) found that social phobia was evident in 70% of the first-degree relatives of probands with elective mutism.

The above brief review suggests that several medications effective in the treatment of panic disorder (e.g., phenelzine, alprazolam, clonazepam, and fluoxetine) may also be effective in the treatment of social phobia. On the other hand, imipramine, still considered by many clinical investigators to be the "gold standard" in treating panic disorder, may have minimal efficacy in the treatment of most patients with social phobia. It would appear, therefore, that social phobia and panic disorder represent partially overlapping anxiety conditions in terms of their pharmacological responses to psychotropic medications. On the other hand, the divergence of response to imipramine suggests that social phobia and panic disorder do not represent identical neurobiological diatheses with different clinical presentations and should be further investigated.

Do these drug treatment findings provide any clues regarding the neurobiological basis of social phobia? Given the array of drug therapies that are effective in the treatment of social phobia, it would appear that there is no *single* neurotransmitter system implicated in the neurobiology (or mediation of therapeutic responses) of social phobia. The MAOIs seem to increase levels of serotonin, dopamine, and norepinephrine; fluoxetine blocks the reuptake of serotonin from the synaptic cleft; and the benzodiazepines facilitate gamma-aminobutyric-acid-mediated neurotransmission. Yet representatives from each class have been shown to be efficacious in the treatment of social phobia.

With the possible exception of obsessive–compulsive disorder (which has been strongly linked to serotonergic system dysfunction), social phobia appears to be similar to other anxiety disorders insofar as several different classes of drugs are known to be effective. Any number of conclusions might be drawn from these observations, including the possibility that social phobias, as currently diagnosed, represent a heterogeneous group of neurobiological conditions. Likewise, it is possible that none of these drugs target the final common pathway in the pathogenesis of social phobia. Of particular interest, however, are the data supporting the effectiveness of MAOIs in the treatment of most patients with social phobia. These observations, combined with other lines of evidence indicating an unusually high rate of social phobia in patients with Parkinson's disease (Stein, Heuser, Juncos, & Uhde, 1990), suggest that dopaminergic neurotransmitter–receptor system function may be involved in pathologic social anxiety, a hypothesis first elaborated by Liebowitz, Campeas, and Hollander (1987) and discussed in greater depth later in this chapter.

Challenge Paradigms

The provocation of anxiety symptoms by administration of selective anxiogenic compounds is a research strategy that has achieved considerable popularity in recent years. Chemical models have been widely used in the study of panic disorder (Uhde & Tancer, 1989) and, to a lesser degree, social phobia. The basic idea underlying this line of investigation is that patients with a truly distinct and homogeneous anxiety syndrome should demonstrate qualitatively and/or quantitatively different biochemical, physiologic, and behavioral responses to anxiogenic probes compared to subjects with different neuropsychiatric syndromes and normal controls. For example, our laboratory reported that panic disorder patients have a lower threshold for caffeine-induced panic attacks and greater caffeine-induced increases in blood lactate and cortisol than do normal controls (Uhde, 1990). The use of chemical challenge paradigms, however, is based on the tacit assumption that the physiology underlying the chemically induced anxiety state has some relevance to that of the native (i.e., "naturally occurring") anxiety state under study, an assumption that may or may not be accurate. This section will review the literature on biological challenge paradigms in social phobia—including sodium lactate, epinephrine, and caffeine—and orthostatic challenges, and will briefly comment on behavioral challenges.

As an outgrowth of their work with panic disorder patients, Liebowitz et al. (1985a) performed single-blind lactate infusions in 15 subjects with social phobia, 9 with agoraphobia with panic attacks, and 20 with panic disorder. The clinician judging whether a panic attack had occurred was blind to the patient's diagnosis. One of the 15 (6.7%) social phobic patients, 4 of the 9 (44%) agoraphobic patients, and 10 of the 20 (50%) panic disorder patients suffered a panic attack. These findings of increased lactate-induced panic attacks in anxiety disorder subjects who have naturally occurring (i.e., spontaneous) panic attacks supports the current diagnostic distinction between social phobia and panic disorder.

Stressful social or performance situations often are associated with high levels of plasma catecholamines (Ward et al., 1983). In light of this fact and the knowledge that compounds that block beta adrenoreceptors (e.g., propranolol) often reduce performance anxiety in normal subjects (Liebowitz, Gorman, Fyer, & Klein, 1985b), Papp et al. (1988) studied the effects of intravenously administered epinephrine in 11 social phobic patients. Despite increases in mean plasma epinephrine levels from 113 to 928 pg per ml, only one subject experienced "observable" anxiety, which he described as typical but of shorter duration than his naturally occurring, socially provoked anxiety. His epinephrine level rose from 25 pg per ml at baseline to 1,198 pg per ml. These findings were interpreted to suggest that a significant increase in plasma epinephrine alone is insufficient to cause pathological degrees of social anxiety. Indeed, there remains the very real possibility that physiological arousal in a social phobic individual outside of a social context has no real psychological meaning and thus may not be reported as distressing.

Our laboratory also investigated the caffeine model of anxiety in a small group of social phobic patients. As noted above, we had earlier reported that panic disorder patients were more easily aroused by caffeine than were normal controls (Uhde, 1990). Moreover, patients who panicked in response to caffeine had significantly greater lactate increases than did patients who did not panic. In a separate study, we studied 11 subjects in each of three groups: social phobic, panic disorder, and normal controls.

We found that social phobic patients' cortisol, but not lactate, levels increased similarly to caffeine-induced increments found in the patients with panic disorder (Tancer, Stein, & Uhde, 1995). Taken together, these findings suggest that increases in lactate levels after caffeine are linked to panic attacks. Although the pathophysiological meaning of this observation is not clear, our data, along with the work of Papp et al. (1988), further support the current diagnostic distinction between social phobia and panic disorder.

Many of the symptoms of pathologic degrees of anxiety, such as sweating, tremor, and tachycardia, appear to be mediated by a relative hyperfunctioning of the sympathetic nervous system. One way to indirectly assess the integrity of this system is to measure physiological and biochemical changes with changes in posture (i.e., from lying to sitting, or from sitting to standing), a technique known as the "orthostatic challenge paradigm." In short, a postural change is accompanied by a greater or lesser tendency for blood to pool in the lower extremity venous system. The sympathetic nervous system reacts to this threat to blood pressure by increasing its output, which constricts vascular musculature and increases heart rate. Stein, Tancer, and Uhde (1992) used this technique to compare patients with social phobia and panic disorder with age-matched normal controls, measuring heart rate, blood pressure, and plasma norepinephrine. The social phobic subjects had supine and upright plasma norepinephrine levels that were significantly higher than those of the patients with panic disorder or normal control subjects. The three groups did not differ in supine heart rate or blood pressure, or in systolic blood pressure or mean arterial pressure change to orthostatic challenge. While the challenge produced greater increases in heart rate in the panic patients than in either of the other groups, the patients with social phobia did not differ from the panic disorder patients or the normal controls. Although there were some potential methodological weaknesses in the study (e.g., perhaps the experimental paradigm represented a "performance" situation for the patients with social phobia and was thus singularly anxiogenic for them), the data suggested that subjects with panic disorder and social phobia may display different abnormalities in the autonomic nervous system. That is, the panic patients' increase in heart rate without a parallel increase in norepinephrine could reflect a decrease in parasympathetic outflow, thereby altering the balance in sympathetic/parasympathetic activity without a change in sympathetic outflow. Indeed, Yeragani et al. (1990), using an indirect measurement of parasympathetic nervous tone, noted increased tone in panic patients. On the other hand, our finding of increased norepinephrine in social phobic patients suggests exaggerated sympathetic tone in this patient group. Our findings need to be replicated, but at this time, they suggest a discrete defect in the sympathetic limb of the autonomic nervous system.

A challenge paradigm commonly used in psychological studies, but that has received relatively little attention in the biological literature, is the exposure of the subject to experimentally designed phobic stimuli (Heimberg, Becker, Goldfinger, & Vermilyea, 1985; P. E. Holt, & Andrews, 1989; Mersch, Emmelkamp, Bögels, & van der Sleen, 1989). Although this topic is covered in some depth in other chapters of this volume (see Heimberg & Juster, Chapter 12, and McNeil, Ries, & Turk, Chapter 10, this volume), a brief comment here is warranted. Social phobia is phenomenologically distinct from panic disorder (Uhde, Tancer, Black, & Brown, 1991) in a variety of areas, but most fundamentally in the situationally cued nature of anxiety in social phobia and the (at least initially) spontaneous nature of anxiety attacks in panic disorder. Thus, while chemical challenge paradigms have an intrinsic value in studying panic disorder by inducing phenomena (i.e., panic attacks) in the laboratory that do not usually occur in observable settings, the same may not be as true for social phobia. A promising area of future research will be the expanded use of provocative "social anxiety" challenges (e.g., social interactions) to study the neurobiology of social phobia. For example, Levin et al. (1993) noted physiological differences (in heart rate) between both normal controls and generalized social phobic patients and between those with discrete and generalized forms of social phobia. Combining behavioral challenges with psychophysiological and neuroendocrinological assessments could potentially yield new and enlightening data.

In summary, the literature on challenge studies in social phobic patients is relatively small. Most studies to date have not differentiated social phobics from normal controls. A positive finding, however, is increased supine and upright norepinephrine levels in response to orthostatic challenge.

GENETICS

It has long been suspected that many anxiety syndromes cluster in families. This is now known to be true for social phobia. While a full chapter is devoted to the topic elsewhere in this text (see Chapman, Mannuzza, & Fyer, Chapter 2, this volume), some comment is warranted in a chapter on neurobiology.

Torgersen (1979) published a study of monozygotic and dizygotic twins. Monozygotic twins have identical genetic material, while dizygotic twins have no more genetic homogeneity than do other pairs of siblings. Assuming that the environment affects both types of twins equally, a higher concordance rate for a given syndrome in monozygotic twins than in dizygotic twins suggests a genetic contribution to the development of the disorder. Torgersen personally interviewed 99 same-sex twin pairs, of which 49 were dizygotic and 50 were monozygotic, and concluded that "genetic factors" play a role in the development of several phobias, including social phobia. However, the fact that this study was conducted before the implementation of the diagnostic criteria of the third edition of the *Diagnostic and Statistical Manual of Mental Disorders* (DSM-III; American Psychiatric Association, 1980) makes interpretation of the data somewhat difficult.

Reich and Yates (1988) used the family history technique to study the relatives of patients with panic disorder or social phobia and of normal control subjects. They found that social phobics had significantly more relatives with social phobia than did panic disorder patients, and there was a trend for probands with social phobia to have a greater proportion of relatives with social phobia compared with the relatives of normal controls.

In a recent paper by Fyer, Mannuzza, Chapman, Liebowitz, and Klein (1993), the investigators interviewed 30 probands with social phobia but without comorbid anxiety disorders and 83 of their first-degree relatives and 77 never mentally ill subjects and 231 of their first-degree relatives. The relatives of social phobic probands had a significantly increased risk of social phobia (16%) compared with the relatives of the never mentally ill controls (5%), an increased risk that was not evident for other anxiety disorders.

An intriguing and different approach to the study of genetic contributions to anxiety disorders is found in the work of Kagan, Rosenbaum, and colleagues. Kagan's group at the Harvard Infant Study Laboratory found approximately 10–15% of infants to be predisposed toward being irritable in infancy, more fearful than their peers in preschool years, and more cautious and introverted at school age (Kagan, Reznick, & Snidman, 1987). They hypothesized that these inhibited children had an inborn low arousal threshold in the amygdala and hypothalamus and that this low threshold manifested itself as increased sympathetic activation. Indeed, they noted in inhibited children high resting heart rate, low heart rate variability, and magnified acceleration of heart rate to mild stress (Kagan, Reznick, & Snidman, 1988). Building on these findings, Rosenbaum and coworkers (Rosenbaum, Biederman, Hirshfeld, Bolduc, & Chaloff, 1991; Rosenbaum, Biederman, Hirshfeld, Bolduc, Faraone, et al., 1991) postulated that the "behavioral inhibition" shown by these children in infancy is a risk factor for the later development of pathological anxiety conditions and that children of patients with anxiety disorders would have a higher prevalence of behavioral inhibition than control groups. To investigate this hypothesis, they initially studied children at risk to develop anxiety disorders by virtue of having a parent with panic disorder. Included in the study were children of parents with panic disorder alone and with both panic disorder and major depression and a control group of children of parents with neither panic disorder nor major depression. The rates of behavioral inhibition in children of parents with panic disorder, with or without depression (70% and 85%, respectively), were significantly higher than the rate for children of parents with major depression alone (50%) or the control group of children of parents without panic disorder or major depression (15%) (Rosenbaum et al., 1988).

In the next phase, children from the initial sample selected at birth to take part in the longitudinal studies of Kagan and coworkers on behavioral inhibition were studied. Using family study methodology, the first-degree relatives of the inhibited and uninhibited children were examined and compared to the relatives of a control group of children from the outpatient pediatric clinic of Massachusetts General Hospital. When compared with parents of uninhibited and control children, parents of inhibited children had significantly greater risks for more than two anxiety disorders, anxiety disorders from childhood continuing into adulthood, social phobia, and childhood avoidant and overanxious disorders (Rosenbaum, Biederman, Hirshfeld, Bolduc, Faraone, et al., 1991). The parallels between the presentation of these children and patients with social phobia is intriguing. It is tempting to speculate on how aversion to novel situations could spawn clinically significant social anxiety. The heightened physiological arousal of these children could leave them more vulnerable to being conditioned, in a negative sense, by adverse social interactions. Additional replication and longitudinal studies are necessary to define whether behavioral inhibition in childhood conveys an increased risk of developing an anxiety disorder as an adult, but these data provide intriguing support for this hypothesis.

To review, the available data support a genetic contribution to social phobia. A twin study conducted before DSM-III diagnostic criteria were adopted suggested greater concordance in monozygotic than dizygotic twins. Two family studies noted a greater risk for social phobia in first-degree relatives of probands with social phobia than with other anxiety disorders. Lastly, novel longitudinal investigations focusing on behaviorally inhibited children suggest the possibility of inborn risk factors for the later development of anxiety disorders, especially social phobia and panic disorder.

SLEEP PHYSIOLOGY

Disturbance of the normal sleep–wake cycle is an element common to many psychiatric syndromes, including thought disorders, substance-use disorders, depression, and panic disorder. Different syndromes, however, appear to be associated with different patterns of sleep disruption, as can be demonstrated by polysomnography. As part of the process of attempting to unravel the pathophysiology of these syndromes, much attention has been paid to the formal study of the sleep of patients, with some intriguing findings. For example, the shortened time of onset to the first rapid-eye-movement (REM) period in depression is one of the most robust biological markers in psychiatry (Reynolds & Kupfer, 1987). Patients with panic disorder and social phobia do not have shortened REM latencies (Uhde, 1994). Sleep panic attacks, however, are a frequently encountered phenomenon in panic disorder patients, occurring in perhaps 60% of patients (Mellman, 1989; Mellman & Uhde, 1989, 1990; Uhde, 1994). These attacks typically occur early in the sleep cycle, emerging from late stage 2 or early stage 3 sleep. Patients report no dream recall associated with a sleep panic attack, a finding consistent with their onset during non-REM sleep. Dreading the occurrence of sleep panic attacks, some patients develop a conditioned fear of sleeping (Uhde, 1994). This leads to sleep deprivation, which has been shown to worsen symptoms of anxiety and increase the frequency of panic attacks (Roy-Byrne, Uhde, & Post, 1986b).

Social phobic patients, on the other hand, typically do not complain of insomnia or sleep panic attacks and do not develop avoidance of sleep. A recent polysomnographic study found no evidence of disturbed sleep efficiency, architecture, or REM latency (Brown, Black, & Uhde, 1994; Uhde, 1994). Thus, studying the sleep of patients with panic disorder and social phobia, while yielding no distinct insights into the pathophysiology or neurobiology of social phobia, does further support the classification of these two syndromes as separate and distinct entities.

NEUROENDOCRINOLOGY

In parallel with the relative paucity of treatment studies in social phobia, there are few studies exploring the neuroendocrine correlates of pathological social anxiety. A small number of studies have examined the functional status of the hypothalamic–pituitary–thyroid and hypothalamic–pituitary–adrenal axes and growth hormone responses to noradrenergic system stimulation.

Abnormalities in thyroid function have been hypothesized in a variety of neuropsychiatric syndromes (Loosen & Prange, 1982), including panic disorder (Fishman, Sheehan, & Carr, 1985; Katerndahl & Vande Creek, 1983). Moreover, many clinicians believe that thyroid disease is commonly associated with anxiety disorders. Because of this view, we investigated hypothalamic–pituitary–thyroid axis function in patients with social phobia versus normal control subjects (Tancer, Stein, Gelernter, & Uhde, 1990). Consistent with most prior studies of panic disorder, we found no significant differences between 26 patients with social phobia and 26 age- and sex-matched controls in blood levels of standard measures of thyroid function, that is, triiodothyronine (T_3), total and free thyroxine (T_4), and thyroid-stimulating hormone (TSH). Likewise, there were no significant differences between the two groups in the proportion of subjects with positive antithyroid antibodies, which can be associated with hypothyroidism.

The integrity of one limb of the hypothalamic–pituitary–thyroid axis can be assessed using the so-called TRH stimulation test. In this procedure, the hypothalamic hormone thyrotropin-releasing hormone (TRH) is infused into the patient, and the magnitude of the release of TSH from the pituitary is measured. Hypothyroidism is reflected by an exaggerated TSH response to TRH, and some investigators maintain that major depression is often associated with a blunted response (M. S. Gold et al., 1981). In a subgroup of Tancer, Stein, Gelernter, and Uhde's (1990) subjects on whom this test was performed, (22 normal controls, 13 patients with social phobia), there were also no significant differences in the maximal TSH response to TRH or the proportion of social phobic patients and normal controls having maximal TSH response outside the normal range (95% confidence interval). Loosen and Prange (1982), in their studies of patients with major depression, described the use of an operational cutoff. In a sample of never mentally ill controls, the lowest change in TSH was 5.6 μU per ml. Loosen and Prange then arbitrarily defined a blunted TSH response to TRH as being 5.0 μU per ml or less. When we applied this operational cutoff, significantly more of the patients than normal controls had blunted responses.

In a related study (Tancer, Stein, & Uhde, 1990), we examined the effects of TRH on blood pressure and heart rate in 10 patients with social phobia, 10 patients with panic disorder, and 10 age- and sex-matched controls. Twenty-nine subjects had been free of medication for at least 2 weeks, and the 30th had had a single 50-mg dose of the beta blocker atenolol 1 week prior to the study. With the subject supine, a single dose of 500 μg of TRH was infused intravenously over 1 minute. Heart rate and blood pressure were checked at 1, 6, and 11 minutes postinfusion. The patients with social phobia had significantly greater rises in systolic blood pressure and mean arterial pressure at 1 minute after the infusion compared with both the patients with panic disorder and normal control subjects. Supportive of Stein et al's. (1992) data from the orthostatic challenge paradigm, these data suggest possible autonomic hyperactivity in social phobic patients.

The hypothalamic–pituitary–adrenal axis has been studied in both affective (P. W. Gold, Goodwin, & Chrousos, 1988) and anxiety disorders (Roy-Byrne, Bierer, & Uhde, 1985; Roy-Byrne, Uhde, & Post, 1986a; Stein & Uhde, 1988). In preliminary work, social phobic patients seem to have normal function of at least some limbs of the hypothalamic–pituitary–adrenal axis. Uhde and coworkers (Uhde, Tancer, Gelernter, & Vittone, 1994) found normal levels of free cortisol in a 24-hour urine collection, normal morning cortisol levels, and appropriate suppression of post-dexamethasone cortisol levels in social phobic patients. Potts, Davidson, Krishnan, Doraiswamy, and Ritchie (1991) conducted a similar study, measuring urinary free cortisol in 10 patients with social phobia and 15 age- and sex-matched normal controls. Their results were consistent with those of Uhde et al. (1994) insofar as there were no differences between the two groups on either levels of urinary free cortisol or in the ratio of free cortisol to creatinine. Despite these negative studies, Potts et al. (1991) caution that more sensitive probes of the hypothalamic–pituitary–adrenal axis (e.g., corticotropin-releasing factor infusions or glucocorticoid receptor assays) may be necessary to show any altered patterns in neuroendocrine system function in patients with social phobia.

The response of growth hormone secretion to clonidine challenge is a putative reflection of the integrity of noradrenergic systems that impinge upon the hypothalamus (Uhde et al., 1992). Noradrenergic systems have been hypothesized by many research teams to be involved in the genesis and maintenance of pathological anxiety syndromes (Redmond & Huang, 1979). Patients with panic disorder have been shown to have blunted growth hormone responses to clonidine (Uhde et al., 1992). Tancer, Stein, and Uhde (1993) have presented preliminary evidence of a similarly blunted response in subjects with social phobia compared with normal controls when using *intravenously* administered clonidine. Of interest, there are inconsistent between-group differences reported with *orally* administered clonidine (Tancer, 1993), complicating comparison of data from studies using oral versus intravenous methods of administration.

Tancer et al. (1995), in one of the most comprehensive assessments of the neuroendocrinology of social phobic patients, performed what they called the "quadruple challenge" on 21 patients and 22 age- and sex-matched controls. Each subject received, in randomized double-blind fashion, levodopa, fenfluramine, oral clonidine, and placebo. The three active probes are believed to stimulate the dopaminergic, serotonergic, and noradrenergic systems, respectively. Measures of dopaminergic function were chosen a priori and were prolactin response and change in rate of eyeblink. Prolactin secretion is inhibited by dopamine, and the rate of eyeblink is considered to be a good indicator of dopamine activity. Prolactin release was markedly inhibited to the same degree in both groups. Similarly, eyeblink rate increased in both groups by an identical amount. These findings suggest normal dopaminergic functioning in patients with social phobia, although it is possible that there is a "floor effect" in the prolactin response to levodopa.

Fenfluramine has been used to study the serotonin system. This compound stimulates serotonin secretion and blocks its reuptake (Rowland & Carlton, 1986). Serotonin in turn stimulates prolactin release (Lowy & Meltzer, 1988) and cortisol secretion (Charney et al., 1988). In the Tancer et al. (1995) study, prolactin response to fenfluramine was also not different between the patient and control groups. Cortisol secretion, however, was significantly greater in the social phobic patients at several timepoints.

Growth hormone response to oral clonidine did not differ between the two groups, in contrast to the earlier study by Tancer et al. (1993). As noted above, though, the meaning of different findings from parenteral and oral clonidine challenges is not clear.

Table 6.1 shows social phobics' endocrine responses to various biological tests.

An interesting but preliminary line of evidence suggests a role for central dopamine in the symptoms of social phobia. King (1986) has postulated that the temperament of extraversion could be correlated with increased central dopamine release. As social incentives are important reinforcers, he hypothesized that central levels of dopamine release might be correlated with measures of social activity such as extraversion. Supportive of this hypothesis, the timid NC 100 strain of mice has markedly decreased dopaminergic activity in the nucleus accumbens but normal serotonergic and noradrenergic functioning (Tancer, 1993). Elevated dopamine

TABLE 6.1. Neuroendocrine Function in Social Phobia

Biological test	Response
Dexamethasone suppression test	5–10% nonsuppressors
Clonidine challenge	
Growth hormone	Normal/blunted
TRH infusion	
TSH response	Normal
Heart rate	Normal
Mean arterial pressure	Enhanced
Systolic blood pressure	Enhanced
Thyroid function studies	
T_4	Normal
T_3	Normal
Free T_4	Normal
Antithyroid antibodies	Normal
Urinary free cortisol (24 hr)	Normal

Note. TRH, thyrotropin-releasing hormone; TSH, thyroid-stimulating hormone; T_3, triiodothyronine; T_4, thyroxine.

release in rodents is associated with increased motor responsiveness to incentives such as food or sex (King et al., 1986). King et al. (1986) studied 16 depressed inpatients, measuring their degree of self-reported extraversion and cerebrospinal fluid levels of dopamine. Log cerebrospinal fluid dopamine was significantly correlated with extraversion scores on the Eysenck Personality Inventory (Eysenck & Eysenck, 1968). As King et al. point out, however, this study needs to be replicated in a normal control group, who should have a stable value for extraversion-scale scores.

Liebowitz et al. (1987) expanded upon the hypothesis of King, noting the efficacy of MAOIs in patients with social phobia. They further commented on the differential efficacy in social phobia of the MAOIs versus the tricyclic antidepressants, the former possessing adrenergic, serotonergic, and dopaminergic activity, the latter having neither significant dopamine activity nor, apparently, efficacy in social phobia. The preliminary findings of Tancer et al. (1995) described above, however, argue against a major role for dopaminergic transmission in the symptoms of social phobia.

A case report by Emmanuel et al. (1991) is consistent with King et al.'s (1986) hypothesis. As noted above, they reported the successful treatment of a social phobic patient with bupropion, an antidepressant with dopamine agonist properties. Although additional treatment studies supporting this hypothesis are not yet available, Emmanuel et al. also postulated that the dopamine agonist activity of bupropion explains the differential treatment efficacy of this agent versus the tricyclic antidepressants.

Further evidence supporting this hypothesis comes from a paper by Stein et al. (1990), in which they report the results of semistructured interviews in patients with Parkinson's disease. Of those studied, 38% had a clinically significant current anxiety disorder. Twenty-one percent had panic disorder or panic disorder with agoraphobia, and 17% met criteria for social phobia. An additional 12% of the subjects had clinically significant social anxiety, but it was judged to be secondary to self-consciousness about their Parkinsonian symptoms and thus not considered to be social phobic per the criteria of the revised third edition of the *Diagnostic and Statistical Manual of Mental Disorders* (DSM-III-R; American Psychiatric Association, 1987). There were no significant differences between the groups with and without current anxiety disorders in the cumulative exposure to L-dopa therapy, the current dose of L-dopa, or degree of motor disability. These findings suggested a higher rate of anxiety disorders, especially social phobia, in the Parkinsonian patients than in other populations of chronically physically ill patients.

Further studies exploring the neuroendocrine characteristics of patients with social phobia are clearly needed. Such investigations should further clarify the overlap and divergence of social phobia and panic disorder and could lead to novel treatment approaches for pathological social anxiety.

CONCLUSION

Although research into the pathophysiology and treatment of social phobia has increased rapidly in recent years, we still have little knowledge about the neurobiology of this syndrome, especially when compared to other more extensively studied conditions, such as panic disorder or major depression. Available data support the current classification of social phobia as a distinct syndrome of abnormally excessive social anxiety that is substantially different from panic disorder in relation to the aforementioned array of neurobiological "tests." There is preliminary evidence that decreased function of central dopaminergic neuronal systems may be involved in the neurobiology of excessive social anxiety, although current strategies for testing the functional status of central dopaminergic systems in humans are quite limited.

Social phobia may be linked to patterns of behavioral inhibition in approximately 15% of children. However, the field has not yet fully determined whether features of behavioral inhibition in childhood are reliable predictors of social phobia or other anxiety or affective disturbances in adults. The work of Kagan, Rosenbaum, and coworkers (e.g., Rosenbaum et al., 1988) is a provocative line of investigation that promises to provide us with an improved understanding of the nature versus nurture contributions to the acquisition of positive social skills and the development of social phobia.

While the neurobiology of social phobia appears to be largely different from that of panic disorder, a question with more far-reaching implications is whether the neurobiology of social phobia is *qualitatively* different from that of shyness or other forms of social anxiety experienced by all humans from time to time in their lifetimes. We have a paucity of information on the neurobiology of social phobia; however, what available data have been collected across different laboratories suggest that tests of biological function in patients with social phobia are more typically similar to, rather than different from, those of normal control subjects. If this is true, then the development of both cognitive-behavioral and drug *strategies* that diminish or block experimentally induced social anxiety in *normal control subjects* might represent an extremely valuable line of investigation for developing new treatments for social phobia. While this "continuum" view of social anxiety to social phobia might appear to be self-evident in some scientific circles, it is, in truth, a different theoretical construct from the widely held "disease model" of panic and obsessive–compulsive disorders.

Further testing is required to establish the validity of a continuum model of social anxiety. If proven to be correct, it will have far-reaching implications for the methodological approaches to the study and treatment of social phobia and related conditions.

REFERENCES

American Psychiatric Association. (1980). *Diagnostic and statistical manual of mental disorders*, (3rd ed.). Washington, DC: Author.

American Psychiatric Association. (1987). *Diagnostic and statistical manual of mental disorders* (3rd ed., rev.). Washington, DC: Author.

American Psychiatric Association. (1994). *Diagnostic and statistical manual of mental disorders* (4th ed.). Washington, DC: Author.

Benca, R., Matuzas, W., & Al-Sadir, F. (1986). Social phobia, MVP, and response to imipramine. *Journal of Clinical Psychopharmacology, 6,* 50–51.

Black, B., & Uhde, T. W. (1994). Treatment of elective mutism with fluoxetine: A double-blind, placebo-controlled study. *Journal of the American Academy of Child and Adolescent Psychiatry, 33,* 1000–1006.

Black, B., & Uhde, T. W. (1995). Psychiatric characteristics of children with selective mutism: A pilot study. *Journal of the American Academy of Child and Adolescent Psychiatry, 34,* 847–856.

Black, B., Uhde, T. W., & Tancer, M. E. (1992). Fluoxetine for the treatment of social phobia. *Journal of Clinical Psychopharmacology, 12,* 293–295.

Brown, T. M., Black, B., & Uhde, T. W. (1994). Sleep architecture in social phobia. *Biological Psychiatry, 35,* 420–421.

Charney, D. S., Goodman, W. K., Price, L. H., Woods, S. W., Rassmussen, S. A., & Heninger, G. R. (1988). Serotonin function in obsessive–compulsive disorder. *Archives of General Psychiatry, 45,* 177–185.

Clark, D. B., & Agras, W. S. (1991). The assessment and treatment of performance anxiety in musicians. *American Journal of Psychiatry, 148,* 598–605.

Davidson, J. R. T., Potts, N., Richichi, E., Krishnan, R., Ford, S. M., Smith, R., & Wilson, W. H. (1993). Treatment of social phobia with clonazepam and placebo. *Journal of Clinical Psychopharmacology, 13,* 423–428.

Emmanuel, N. P., Lydiard, R. B., & Ballenger, J. C. (1991). Treatment of social phobia with bupropion. *Journal of Clinical Psychopharmacology, 11,* 276– 277.

Eysenck, H. J., & Eysenck, S. B. G . (1968). *Manual for the Eysenck Personality Inventory (EPI)*. San Diego, CA: Educational and Instructional Testing Service.

Fishman, S. M., Sheehan, S. W., & Carr, D. B. (1985). Thyroid indices in panic disorder. *Journal of Clinical Psychiatry, 46,* 432–433.

Fyer, A. J., Mannuzza, S., Chapman, T. F., Liebowitz, M. R., & Klein, D. F. (1993). A direct interview family study of social phobia. *Archives of General Psychiatry, 50,* 286–293.

Gelernter, C. S., Uhde, T. W., Cimbolic, P., Arnkoff, D. B., Vittone, B. J., Tancer, M. E., & Bartko, J. J. (1991). Cognitive-behavioral and pharmacological treatments for social phobia: A controlled study. *Archives of General Psychiatry, 48,* 938–945.

Gold, M. S., Pottash, A. L. C., Extein, I., Martin, D. M., Howard, E., Mueller, E. A., & Sweeney, D. R. (1981). The TRH test in the diagnosis of major and minor depression. *Psychoneuroendocrinology, 6,* 159–169.

Gold, P. W., Goodwin, F. K., & Chrousos, G. P. (1988). Clinical and biochemical manifestations of depression: Relation to the neurobiology of stress. *New England Journal of Medicine, 319,* 348–353.

Goldstein, S. (1987). Treatment of social phobia with clonidine. *Biological Psychiatry, 22,* 369–372.

Heimberg, R. G., Becker, R. E., Goldfinger, K., & Vermilyea, J. A. (1985). Treatment of social phobia by exposure, cognitive restructuring, and homework assignments. *Journal of Nervous and Mental Disease, 173,* 236–245.

Holt, C. S., Heimberg, R. G., & Hope, D. A. (1992). Avoidant personality disorder and the generalized subtype of social phobia. *Journal of Abnormal Psychology, 101,* 318–325.

Holt, P. E., & Andrews, G. (1989). Provocation of panic: Three elements of the panic reaction in four anxiety disorders. *Behaviour Research and Therapy, 27,* 253–261.

Kagan, J., Reznick, J. S., & Snidman, N. (1987). The physiology and psychology of behavioral inhibition in children. *Child Development, 58,* 1459–1473.

Kagan, J., Reznick, J. S., & Snidman, N. (1988). Biological bases of childhood shyness. *Science, 240,* 167–171.

Katerndahl, D. A., & Vande Creek, L. (1983). Hyperthyroidism and panic attacks. *Psychosomatics, 24,* 491–496.

King, R. (1986). Motivational diversity and mesolimbic dopamine: A hypothesis concerning temperament. In R. Plutchik & H. Kellerman (Eds.), *Emotions: Theory, research, and experience: Biological foundations of emotions* (Vol. 3, pp. 363–380). Orlando, FL: Academic Press.

King, R. J., Mefford, I. N., Wang, C., Murchison, A., Caligari, E. J., & Berger, P. A. (1986). CSF dopamine levels correlate with extraversion in depressed patients. *Psychiatry Research, 19,* 305–310.

Levin, A. P., Saoud, J. B., Strauman, T., Gorman, J. D., Fyer, A. J., Crawford, R., & Liebowitz, M. R. (1993). Responses of "generalized" and "discrete" social phobics during public speaking. *Journal of Anxiety Disorders, 7,* 207–221.

Liebowitz, M. R., Campeas, R., & Hollander, E. (1987). MAOIs: Impact on social behavior [Letter to the editor]. *Psychiatry Research, 22,* 89–90.

Liebowitz, M. R., Fyer, A. J., Gorman, J. M., Dillon, D., Davies, S., Stein, J. M., Cohen, B. S., & Klein, D. F. (1985a). Specificity of lactate infusions in social phobia versus panic disorder. *American Journal of Psychiatry, 142,* 947–950.

Liebowitz, M. R., Gorman, J. M., Fyer, A. J., & Klein, D. F. (1985b). Social phobia: Review of a neglected anxiety disorder. *Archives of General Psychiatry, 42,* 729–736.

Liebowitz, M. R., Schneier, F., Campeas, R., Hollander, E., Hatterer, F., Fyer, A., Gorman, F., Papp, L., Davies, S., Gully, R., & Klein, D. F. (1992). Phenelzine vs. atenolol in social phobia: A placebo-controlled comparison. *Archives of General Psychiatry, 49,* 290–300.

Loosen, P. T., & Prange, A. J. J. (1982). Serum thyrotropin response to thyrotropin-releasing hormone in psychiatric patients: A review. *American Journal of Psychiatry, 139,* 405–416.

Lowy, M. T., & Meltzer, H. (1988). Stimulation of serum cortisol and prolactin secretions in humans by MK-212, a centrally active serotonin agonist. *Biological Psychiatry, 23,* 818–828.

Mellman, T. A. (1989). Sleep panic attacks: New clinical findings and theoretical implications. *American Journal of Psychiatry, 146,* 1204–1207.

Mellman, T. A., & Uhde, T. W. (1989). Electroencephalographic sleep in panic disorder. *Archives of General Psychiatry, 46,* 178–184.

Mellman, T. A., & Uhde, T. W. (1990). Patients with frequent sleep panic: Clinical findings and response to medication treatment. *Journal of Clinical Psychiatry, 51,* 513–516.

Mersch, P. P. A., Emmelkamp, P. M. G., Bögels, S. M., & van der Sleen, J. (1989). Social phobia: Individual response patterns and the effects of behavioral and cognitive interventions. *Behaviour Research and Therapy, 27,* 421–434.

Nickell, P. V., & Uhde, T. W. (in press). Theoretical basis for developing and evaluating anxiolytics. In N. Cutler, J. J. Sramek, & P. K. Narang (Eds.), *Pharmacodynamics: Perspectives in clinical pharmacology.* New York: Wiley-Liss.

Papp, L. A., Gorman, J. M., Liebowitz, M. R., Fyer, A. J., Cohen, B., & Klein, D. F. (1988). Epinephrine infusions in patients with social phobia. *American Journal of Psychiatry, 145,* 733–736.

Potts, N. L. S., Davidson, J. R. T., Krishnan, R. R., Doraiswamy, P. M., & Ritchie, J. C. (1991). Levels of urinary free cortisol in social phobia. *Journal of Clinical Psychiatry, 52,* 41–42.

Redmond, D. E. J., & Huang, Y. H. (1979). New evidence for a locus ceruleus–norepinephrine connection with anxiety. *Life Sciences, 25,* 2149–2162.

Reich, J., & Yates, W. (1988). Family history of psychiatric disorders in social phobia. *Comprehensive Psychiatry, 29,* 72–75.

Reynolds, C. F., & Kupfer, D. J. (1987). Sleep research in affective illness: State of the art circa 1987. *Sleep, 10,* 199–215.

Rosenbaum, J. F., Biederman, J., Gersten, M., Hirshfeld, D. R., Meminger, S. R., Herman, J. B., Kagan, J., Reznick, J. S., & Snidman, N. (1988). Behavioral inhibition in children of parents with panic disorder and agoraphobia: A controlled study. *Archives of General Psychiatry, 45,* 463–470.

Rosenbaum, J. F., Biederman, J., Hirshfeld, D. R., Bolduc, E. A., & Chaloff, J. (1991). Behavioral inhibition in children: A possible precursor to panic disorder or social phobia. *Journal of Clinical Psychiatry, 52*(11, Suppl.), 5–9.

Rosenbaum, J. F., Biederman, J., Hirshfeld, K. R., Bolduc, E. A., Faraone, S. V., Kagan, F., Snidman, N., & Reznick, J. S. (1991). Further evidence of an association between behavioral inhibition and anxiety disorders: Results from a family study of children from a non-clinical sample. *Journal of Psychiatric Research, 25,* 49–65.

Rowland, N. E., & Carlton, J. (1986). Neurobiology of an anorectic drug: Fenfluramine. *Progress in Neurobiology, 27,* 13–62.

Roy-Byrne, P. P., Bierer, L., & Uhde, T. W. (1985). The dexamethasone suppression test in panic disorder: Comparison with normal controls. *Biological Psychiatry, 20,* 1237–1240.

Roy-Byrne, P. P., Uhde, T. W., & Post, R. M. (1986a). The corticotropin-releasing hormone stimulation test in patients with panic disorder. *American Journal of Psychiatry, 143,* 896–899.

Roy-Byrne, P. P., Uhde, T. W., & Post, R. M. (1986b). Effects of one night's sleep deprivation on mood and behavior in panic disorder. *Archives of General Psychiatry, 43,* 895–899.

Schneier, F. R., Chin, S. J., Hollander, E., & Liebowitz, M. R. (1992). Fluoxetine in social phobia. *Journal of Clinical Psychopharmacology, 12,* 62–63.

Schneier, F. R., Saoud, J. B., Campeas, R., Fallon, B. A., Hollander, E., Coplan, J., & Liebowitz, M. R. (1993). Buspirone in social phobia. *Journal of Clinical Psychopharmacology, 13,* 251–256.

Stein, M. B., Heuser, I. J., Juncos, J. L., & Uhde, T. W. (1990). Anxiety disorders in patients with Parkinson's disease. *American Journal of Psychiatry, 147,* 217–220.

Stein, M. B., Tancer, M. E., & Uhde, T. W. (1992). Heart rate and plasma norepinephrine responsivity to orthostatic challenge in anxiety disorders. *Archives of General Psychiatry, 49,* 311–317.

Stein, M. B., & Uhde, T. W. (1988). Cortisol response to clonidine in panic disorder: Comparison with depressed patients and normal controls. *Biological Psychiatry, 24,* 322–330.

Sternbach, H. (1990). Fluoxetine treatment of social phobia. *Journal of Clinical Psychopharmacology, 10,* 230–231.

Tancer, M. E. (1993). Neurobiology of social phobia. *Journal of Clinical Psychiatry, 54*(12, Suppl.), 26–30.

Tancer, M. E., Mailman, R. B., Stein, M. B., Mason, G. A., Carson, S. W., & Golden, R. N. (1995). Neuroendocrine responsivity to monoaminergic system probes in generalized social phobia. *Anxiety, 1,* 216–223.

Tancer, M. E., Stein, M. B., Gelernter, C. S., & Uhde, T. W. (1990). The hypothalamic–pituitary–thyroid axis in social phobia. *American Journal of Psychiatry, 147,* 929–933.

Tancer, M. E., Stein, M. B., & Uhde, T. W. (1990). Effects of thyrotropin-releasing hormone on blood pressure and heart rate in phobic and panic patients: A pilot study. *Biological Psychiatry, 27,* 781–783.

Tancer, M. E., Stein, M. B., & Uhde, T. W. (1993). Growth hormone response to clonidine in patients with social phobia. *Biological Psychiatry, 34,* 591–595.

Tancer, M. E., Stein, M. B., & Uhde, T. W. (1995). Lactic acid response to caffeine in panic disorder: Comparison with social phobics and normal controls. *Anxiety, 1,* 138–140.

Torgersen, S. (1979). The nature and origin of common phobic fears. *British Journal of Psychiatry, 134,* 343–351.

Uhde, T. W. (1990). Caffeine provocation of panic: A focus on biological mechanisms. In J. C. Ballenger (Ed.), *Neurobiology of panic disorder* (pp. 219–242). New York: Wiley-Liss.

Uhde, T. W. (1994). The anxiety disorders. In M. H. Kryger, T. Roth, & W. Dement (Eds.), *Principles and practice of sleep medicine* (pp. 871–898). Philadelphia: Saunders.

Uhde, T. W., & Tancer, M. E. (1989). Chemical models of panic: A review and critique. In T. Tyrer (Ed.), *Psychopharmacology of anxiety* (pp. 109–131). New York: Oxford Medical Publications.

Uhde, T. W., Tancer, M. E., Black, B., & Brown, T. M. (1991). Phenomenology and neurobiology of social phobia: Comparison with panic disorder. *Journal of Clinical Psychiatry, 52,* 31–39.

Uhde, T. W., Tancer, M. E., Gelernter, C. S ., & Vittone, B. J. (1994). Normal urinary free cortisol and postdexamethasone cortisol in social phobia: Comparison to normal volunteers. *Journal of Affective Disorders, 30,* 155–161.

Uhde, T. W., Tancer, M. E., Rubinow, D. R., Roscow, D. B., Boulenger, J.-P., Vittone, B., Gurguis, G., Geraci, M., Black, B., & Post, R. M. (1992). Evidence for hypothalamo-growth hormone dysfunction in panic disorder: Profile of growth hormone (GH) responses to clonidine, yohimbine, caffeine, glucose, GRF and TRH in panic disorder patients versus healthy volunteers. *Neuropsychopharmacology, 6,* 101–118.

Van Ameringen, M., Mancini, C., & Steiner, D. L. (1993). Fluoxetine efficacy in social phobia. *Journal of Clinical Psychiatry, 54,* 27–32.

van Vliet, I. M., den Boer, J. A., & Westenberg, H. G. M. (1992). Psychopharmacological treatment of social phobia: Clinical and biochemical effects of brofaromine, a selective MAO-A inhibitor. *European Neuropsychopharmacology, 2,* 21–29.

Versiani, M., Mundim, F. D., Nardi, A. E., & Liebowitz, M. R. (1988). Tranylcypromine in social phobia. *Journal of Clinical Psychopharmacology, 8,* 279–283.

Versiani, M., Nardi, A. E., Mundim, F. D., Alves, A. B., Nick, E., & Liebowitz, M. R. (1992). Pharmacotherapy of social phobia: A controlled study with moclobemide and phenelzine. *British Journal of Psychiatry, 161,* 353–360.

Ward, M. M., Mefford, I. N., Parker, S. D., Chesney, M. A., Taylor, C. B., Keegan, D. L., & Barchas, J. D. (1983). Epinephrine and norepinephrine responses in continuously collected human plasma to a series of stressors. *Psychosomatic Medicine, 45,* 471–486.

West, E. D., & Dally, P. J. (1959). Effect of iproniazid in depressive syndrome. *British Medical Journal, 1,* 1491–1494.

Yeragani, V. K., Balon, R., Pohl, R., Ramesh, C., Glitz, D., Weinberg, P., & Merlos, B. (1990). Decreased R-R variance in panic disorder patients. *Acta Psychiatrica Scandinavica, 81,* 554–559.

CHAPTER SEVEN

Conditioning and Ethological Models of Social Phobia

SUSAN MINEKA
RICHARD ZINBARG

In the years since 1969, when social phobia was first identified a distinct type of phobia (cf. Marks, 1969; Marks & Gelder, 1966), significant progress has been made in understanding the origins, maintenance, and treatment of this interesting disorder. Theories regarding the origins of social phobia range from neurobiological (e.g., Liebowitz, Gorman, Fyer, & Klein, 1985; Sheehan, 1983) and evolutionary–genetic (Öhman, 1986; Öhman, Dimberg, & Öst, 1985) to behavioral (e.g., Barlow, 1988; Marks, 1987) and cognitive (e.g., Beck & Emery, 1985). In this chapter we review research and theories that to some extent span these different levels of analysis. That is, although our focus is on theories originally inspired by the behavioral tradition, these theories have been integrated with ethological and behavior genetic approaches from the more biological tradition. In addition, the behavioral theories are also integrated with more cognitive theories ranging from theories emphasizing the importance of perceptions of control versus helplessness to theories emphasizing the role of automatic information processing in helping to account for the irrationality of social phobia. We discuss both animal and human research from these traditions that we consider to be useful in understanding the origins and maintenance of social phobia.

First let us consider how contemporary understanding of social phobia has been enhanced by considering it in an adaptive/ functional framework. In 1985, Öhman, Dimberg, and Öst proposed that Mayr's (1974) behavior classification system from evolutionary biology could provide a useful framework for understanding different classes of human fears and phobias.

Mayr's framework distinguishes between noncommunicative behavior, interspecific communicative behavior (as between predator and prey), and intraspecific communicative behavior (as between two members of the same species). As noted by Öhman et al. (1985), the fears occuring in each of these three systems correspond quite well to three of the major categories of phobias identified by Marks (1969) and Torgersen (1979)—miscellaneous specific phobias (for inanimate objects and aspects of nature), animal phobias, and social phobias.

Öhman et al. (1985; Öhman, 1986) used this framework and other current ideas from evolutionary biology to compare and contrast what is known about animal fears and phobias with what is known about social fears and phobias. For example, they note that animal fears (i.e., corresponding to interspecific fears of potential predators) evolved to help organisms develop efficient responses to deal with threatening predators. Therefore, animal fears should involve rapid and strong activation of the fight-or-flight response of the sympathetic nervous system, preparing the animal for fighting or fleeing from the potential predator. They summarize a good deal of psychophysiological research consistent with this characterization of the fear responses of animal phobics. Moreover, they also note that animal fears and phobias should be most likely to originate early in development because the young of a species are most vulnerable to predation; this is consistent with what is known about the average age of onset of animal phobias. By contrast, they argue that social fears (i.e., corresponding to intraspecific fears) evolved as a by-product of dominance hierarchies, which are a common way in which social life is coordinated in social living animals such as primates. Agonistic or combative encounters between members of a social group help to establish such dominance hierarchies, and a defeated animal typically displays fear and submissive behavior, although the fear less often involves total escape from the situation than a short dash to get out of the immediate reach of the attacker. They summarize a good deal of psychophysiological research consistent with the notion that the fear response seen in social phobics is "much more loosely and conditionally concocted, with a less prominent and reflexive role for active avoidance behavior" (1985, p. 141). Moreover, they also note that the typical age of onset for social phobias (adolescence and young adulthood) coincides with the time when dominance conflicts become prominent.

Our review first focuses on conditioning models. We also highlight experiential, evolutionary, and temperamental variables that are likely to affect the outcome of traumatic conditioning experiences in causing social phobia. We then discuss the relevance of the now very large literature on the importance of perceived uncontrollability over important life events. This literature helps illuminate certain important features of the origins and maintenance of social phobia.

CONDITIONING MODELS

One prominent theory regarding the origins of social phobia is that it may develop in the same way as do many specific phobias, that is, as a consequence of one or more traumatic conditioning experiences (e.g., Barlow, 1988; Öst & Hugdahl, 1981). The primary difference in whether someone would develop a social or a specific phobia would be in the nature of the conditioned stimuli (CSs) that acquire the capacity to elicit fear—social situations such as public speaking or eating in public versus discrete stimuli such as snakes or airplanes. In addition, although there is little evidence on this, it might be expected that the unconditioned stimuli (UCSs) might also tend to differ for social versus specific phobias. In the case of social phobia, one would expect most of the UCSs that would be effective in conditioning fear to involve some kind of perceived social defeat or humiliating experience or being the target of anger or criticism (i.e., a trauma involving intraspecific social interactions), whereas with specific phobias one would more often expect perceived physical danger to be effective in conditioning fear (i.e., traumas such as being bitten by a snake or surviving a near-fatal plane crash).

Direct Traumatic Conditioning

What evidence do we have that social phobias can originate in this way? At least two studies have now documented that a large proportion of social phobics can recall direct traumatic conditioning experiences as being involved in the origins of their phobia. In the first, Öst and Hugdahl (1981) studied 41 small animal phobics, 34 social phobics, and 35 claustrophobics who had presented for treatment in Sweden. All subjects completed a questionnaire inquiring about the origins of their phobia. Öst and Hugdahl found that 58.1% of their social phobic sample recalled direct traumatic conditioning experiences as having been involved in the origin of their phobia (vs. 47.5% for small animal phobics and 68.6% for claustrophobics).

A more recent study by Townsley (1992) examined a sample of 67 patients diagnosed with social phobia according to the criteria of the revised third edition of the *Diagnostic and Statistical Manual of Mental Disorders* (DSM-III-R; American Psychiatric Association, 1987) and compared them to a normal control sample consisting of 25 control subjects who did not meet criteria for any current or past DSM-III-R disorders. The social phobic sample was further subdivided into those with specific social phobia (i.e., those with fears of one or more discrete social situations, $n = 17$) and those with generalized social phobia (i.e., those with significant fears of most social situations, $n = 50$), in order to determine whether different factors might be involved in the origins of specific versus generalized sub-types. All subjects were interviewed regarding the course and nature of social phobia symptoms, as well as about a variety of possible etiological variables, including their recollections of traumatic experiences in social situations. For the traumatic experience to qualify as having had causal significance, the social phobics also had to report that the recalled episode was associated either with the onset of their fears or with a dramatic increase in the intensity of their fears. Comparing the patient sample as a whole with the control group, there was a significant difference in the proportion who recalled traumatic conditioning experiences (44% vs. 20%). When the results were analyzed separating the two subgroups of social phobics, an interesting pattern emerged. A greater percentage of specific social phobics recalled traumatic conditioning experiences (56%) than did controls (20%), with the generalized subtype being intermediate and not differing significantly from either of the other two groups (40%). The 56% for the specific subtype group is nearly identical to that reported by Öst and Hugdahl (1981), leading us to speculate that their sample may have consisted primarily of specific social phobics (this distinction did not exist when their study was conducted).

Observational or Vicarious Conditioning

In recent years increasing attention has also been paid to the role that observational or vicarious conditioning experiences might play in the origins of fears and phobias. That is, simply observing someone else behaving fearfully in the presence of some object or situation may be sufficient to cause the conditioning of a fear or phobia. As is the case with human research on direct conditioning, human research on observational conditioning of fear has involved conditioning of only very mild and transient fears (e.g., Hygge & Öhman, 1983). Thus, for humans there is only anecdotal evidence that strong and persistent fear, like that involved in clinical phobias, can develop through vicarious conditioning. Nevertheless, at least with regard to conditioning of predator fears, strong empirical evidence that robust conditioning of phobic-like fears can indeed occur through observation alone comes from the work of Mineka and Cook on the observational conditioning of snake fear in rhesus monkeys (e.g., Cook & Mineka, 1991; Mineka, 1987; Mineka & Cook, 1988). In these studies, laboratory-reared monkeys, who were not initially afraid of snakes, underwent a discriminative observational conditioning procedure in which they watched wild-reared monkeys behaving with high levels of fear on trials when a snake was present and nonfearfully on other trials when a neutral stimulus was present. After only 4–8 minutes of exposure to the wild-reared models behaving fearfully with snake stimuli, the laboratory-reared observer monkeys acquired an intense fear of snakes (Mineka & Cook, 1993). In other studies involving a total of 24 minutes of exposure to the wild-reared models behaving fearfully, it was shown that the fear did not diminish in intensity over a 3-month follow-up interval (see Mineka, 1987; Mineka & Cook, 1988, for reviews).

Although this work on observational conditioning of snake fear was never actually extended to the learning of social fears, it does seem likely that such learning could indeed occur. For example, in the context of living in a large social group with its associated dominance hierarchies, the offspring of parents low in the dominance hierarchy would have substantial occasion to observe their parents behaving submissively after defeat in dominance conflicts and might be expected to learn to fear defeat and to acquire submissive behaviors. By contrast, the offspring of dominant parents would have very different opportunities for social learning and would not be expected to acquire social fear or submissive behaviors. In this regard, it is interesting to note that in at least some species dominance hierarchies are passed down from one generation to the next. For example, de Waal (1989) described this phenomenon in rhesus monkeys and noted that "rank positions of daughters depend on those of their mothers. We can predict with almost total certainty which position in the hierarchy a newborn female will occupy when she moves into adulthood" (p. 93). Although the mechanisms underlying such transmission are undoubtedly complex and are as yet not completely understood, de Waal argues that "genetics does not seem to play much of a role in the transmission of rank. . . . The status tradition is primarily a *social* institution. Juvenile members of high-ranking lineages behave dominantly only when their relatives are nearby; their rank depends on the presence of supporters rather than on some inborn predisposition" (pp. 93–94). Moreover, he also notes that in all three instances in which infants were adopted by nonbiological parents, their rank was what was predicted for the biological offspring of their adoptive parents, rather than what was predicted based on their own biological parents. Although this evidence is only indirect, it does support the idea that vicarious learning of social behaviors relating to dominance and submissiveness can indeed occur. It should be noted, however, that de Waal himself later acknowledged that definitive studies ruling out a genetic contribution have not yet been conducted. Moreover, our review below of the behavioral inhibition literature leads us to suspect that it is quite likely that genetic factors may well interact with direct or social learning factors.

The relevance of these ideas to understanding social phobias in humans is also quite speculative at this point, but it is interesting to note that Öst and Hugdahl (1981) found that 13% of their social phobic subjects reported recalling the onset of their social phobia as having occurred through vicarious learning experiences of some sort. This is somewhat lower than the percentage of animal phobics who recalled vicarious experiences (27.5%), but nevertheless strongly suggestive that observational conditioning of social phobia can indeed occur in humans. Unfortunately, Townsley (1992) did not question her subjects about observational conditioning experiences, and so there is no independent replication of these findings as there is for direct conditioning.

Several points regarding these studies involving retrospective recall of direct traumatic or observational conditioning experiences are noteworthy. First, although reliance on retrospective recall is always problematic, the convergence between the results of the two studies regarding estimates of direct traumatic conditioning experiences is encouraging. Second, at first glance one might find the results from the normal control group of the Townsley study to be troubling, given that 20% of these subjects also recalled traumatic conditioning experiences but did not develop social phobia. Some have argued that such results tend to undermine a conditioning account of the origins of phobias (e.g., Rachman, 1978, 1990) because if traumatic experiences really play a causal role in the origins of phobias and given all the traumatic conditioning experiences that people may undergo in a lifetime, more people should have phobias. However, as we have argued elsewhere (Mineka, 1985a, 1985b, 1987; Mineka & Zinbarg, 1991), this argument rests on an overly simplistic view of the conditioning theory of the origins of fears and phobias. In particular, this view involves a mistaken belief that conditioning experiences occur in a vacuum, whereas it is well documented in contemporary conditioning research that there are a multitude of experiential and temperamental variables occuring prior to, during, and following a conditioning experience that affect the amount of fear that is experienced, conditioned, and maintained into the future (see Mineka, 1985a, 1985b; Mineka & Zinbarg, 1991).

Experiential Variables Affecting the Amount of Conditioning That Occurs

One example of an experiential variable occuring prior to a conditioning event that can have powerful effects on the amount of fear that gets conditioned involves prior experience with the conditioned stimulus. Although there is no direct evidence on this for social fears, one can reason by analogy from research on the acquisition of snake fear. For example, Mineka and Cook (1986) demonstrated that rhesus monkeys first exposed to a nonfearful model behaving nonfearfully with snakes were later immunized against the effects of exposure to a fearful model behaving fearfully with snakes.

Simple prior exposure to snakes also had a small effect, although it was not significant in that study. Related results have been found in studies of human children. For example, Poser and King (1975) took children who were not afraid of snakes and exposed them to a film of a model interacting nonfearfully with snakes. Later, these children approached a snake more closely than did children who had simply seen a film of a snake with no model. Moreover, Melamed and colleagues showed that children who watched a film of a similar-aged peer undergoing a dental restorative treatment later showed less fear and distress during their own dental work than did children who saw a demonstration film that lacked a peer model (Melamed, Yurcheson, Fleece, Hutcherson, & Hawes, 1978). By analogy, then, for the acquisition of social fear, one would expect, for example, that someone who had a reasonable amount of public speaking experience, and especially someone who had observed peers handle public speaking with confidence, might be less likely to develop a fear of public speaking after having a traumatic experience while speaking than would someone without such prior experience (direct or observational).

There are also a multitude of variables occurring following a conditioning experience that help to shape the outcome of that experience. For example, with Rescorla's well-known inflation effect (1974), it was shown that a mild conditioned fear response (CR) can become an intense fear if the organism is later exposed to a more intense UCS than was originally involved in the conditioning experience, even though the CS is never paired with the more intense UCS. Thus, the CR becomes inflated in the direction that would have been expected if the more intense UCS had been involved in the conditioning experience in the first place. Thus, by analogy, if a person had a mildly traumatic conditioning experience with social stimuli and acquired a mild level of fear, later exposure to a more intense social trauma, even though it is not paired with the same social stimuli, might result in an inflated fear CR to the social stimuli.

Mineka (1992) has also discussed a number of findings about generalization of conditioned fears that are relevant in this context. For example, Riccio, Richardson, and Ebner (1984) discussed evidence showing that generalization gradients around an excitatory CS (CS +) flatten with the passage of time following conditioning, and the flattening is caused by larger CRs being exhibited to the generalization test stimuli, rather than by smaller CRs being exhibited to the original CS +. By contrast, Hendersen (1978) and Thomas (1979) have shown that with the passage of time, inhibitory fear CS − s, or safety signals, are forgotten; that is, they lose their inhibitory properties. This combination of increasing generalization of excitatory fear CRs, combined with the fragility of inhibitory fear CRs, may help to account for the common clinical observation of increasing generalization of fears with the passage of time (see Mineka, 1992, for further discussion).

In summary, from the standpoint of contemporary knowledge about conditioning theory, it is not problematic, or even surprising, that not all individuals who undergo a traumatic or a vicarious conditioning experience acquire clinically significant levels of fear (e.g., Townsley's 20% of normal controls reporting traumatic conditioning and no current social anxiety). Moreover, it is also not surprising that there will be wide individual differences in how much fear is maintained over time based on experiential variables occurring following conditioning, with some showing exacerbations of fear (as with the inflation effect) or generalization of the range of situations that elicit the fear.

Preparedness and Conditioning Models

An additional important perspective on conditioning models was added with the introduction of the preparedness theory of fears and phobias (e.g., Öhman, 1986; Öhman, Dimberg, & Öst, 1985; Seligman, 1971). When Seligman introduced the preparedness concept, he was attempting to help to account for the nonrandom distribution of fears and phobias seen clinically, as well as to account for important characteristics of phobias that are often not shared by fears conditioned in the laboratory. These characteristics of phobias include rapid acquisition, high resistance to extinction, and their apparent irrationality. The basic idea is that human and nonhuman primates have an evolutionarily based predisposition to acquire fears and phobias to objects or situations that may once have posed a threat to our early evolutionary ancestors because individuals who easily acquired fears of dangerous objects or situations might have had a selective advantage in the struggle for existence.

Much of the empirical research testing various aspects of this theory has involved comparing characteristics of conditioning of electrodermal or heart rate responses to prepared or fear-relevant CSs with conditioning to unprepared or fear-irrelevant CSs. In a typical paradigm used by Öhman and his colleagues, one group of subjects has a fear-relevant CS + (such as a slide of a snake or a spider) paired with mild electric shock as a UCS, and another fear-relevant inhibitory CS (CS −) paired with the absence of shock. A second group of subjects receives fear-irrelevant CSs (such as flowers or mushrooms) as both CS + and CS −. What is typically found is that the group conditioned with fear-relevant CSs shows superior conditioning relative to what is seen in the group conditioned with fear-irrelevant CSs, where the superior conditioning is usually indexed by superior resistance to extinction (although Cook, Hodes, & Lang, 1986, also reported significant differences in acquisition using heart rate as their measure).

One important question left unanswered by the human research on this topic is whether the differences in conditionability seen in the human subjects used in these studies really derive from phylogenetic factors, as proposed by preparedness theory, as opposed to ontogenetic factors, as has been claimed by some (e.g., Delprato, 1980). The problem stems from the fact that human subjects all come to these experiments with prior ontogenetically based experiences with the CSs used in the experiments. Thus, differences seen in conditioning could derive simply from the fact that the subjects have prior negative associations to the stimuli used as fear-relevant CSs.

In part to address these limitations of human research on this topic, Cook and Mineka (1989, 1990, 1991) compared conditioning to fear-relevant and fear-irrelevant stimuli in laboratory-reared rhesus monkeys who had had no prior exposure to any of the stimuli used during conditioning. These experiments were an extension of the vicarious conditioning experiments described earlier, except that these experiments used videotapes of wild-reared models responding fearfully to different objects rather than live models. An initial demonstration of the viability of the videotape technique for conditioning fear (Cook & Mineka, 1990, Experiment 1) allowed the construction of spliced videotapes in which model monkeys would appear to be reacting fearfully to fear-relevant or fear-irrelevant stimuli. In one experiment, one group of laboratory-reared monkeys watched videotapes of wild-reared models behaving fearfully with toy snakes and nonfearfully with flowers, and a second group watched models behaving fearfully with the flowers and nonfearfully with the toy snakes (Cook & Mineka, 1990, Experiment 2). Note that the fear performances exhibited by the models were identical; it was only the stimuli toward which the fear was directed that differed. Monkeys in the first group did indeed acquire a fear of toy (and real) snakes, but monkeys in the second group did not acquire a fear of flowers (or snakes). In another experiment, parallel results were found when a toy crocodile was used as the fear-relevant stimulus and a toy rabbit was used as the fear-irrelevant stimulus (Cook & Mineka, 1989). Because the monkeys used in these experiments had no prior experiences with any of these stimuli, the results strongly implicate phylogenetic rather than ontogenetic factors as the source of the differences in conditionability (see Cook & Mineka, 1991, for a detailed discussion).

In 1978, Öhman and Dimberg reported the first extension of the preparedness theory of phobias to the understanding of social fears and phobias. As noted at the outset, Öhman and Dimberg believe that social fears evolved as a by-product of dominance hierarchies, which in turn evolved as a means of establishing order in the social life of many group-living animals. Dominance hierarchies develop and change as a function of agonistic encounters, many of which involve highly ritualized displays of threat on the part of the dominant animal and of fear and submissiveness on the part of the defeated animal (see Öhman et al., 1985, for an excellent summary). Because these ritualized displays have a strong facial component (threat or anger facial expressions on the part of the dominant animal and fear grimaces on the part of the submissive animal), Öhman and Dimberg (1978) predicted that superior conditioning would occur when slides of angry facial expressions were used as CSs, relative to what would be seen with happy or neutral faces. Thus, their experimental design was parallel to that used in their experiments with other kinds of fear-relevant and fear-irrelevant stimuli. As predicted, results indicated that superior conditioning occurred when angry faces were used as CSs relative to what was seen when happy or neutral faces were used as CSs.

In further extensions of this work, Öhman and Dimberg reasoned that fear should only be exhibited when the gaze is directed at the target subject. This is consistent with observations that staring promotes escape behavior in humans, and that a common component of submissive behavior is averting one's eyes from the aggressor (Öhman et al., 1985). Moreover, they reasoned that because facial expressions change frequently and may be directed at multiple group members at different points in time, it would be most adaptive for an individual to learn which group members are most dangerous and to respond with fear only when an angry facial expression is directed at the individual. Consistent with these ideas were the results of an experiment by Dimberg and Öhman (1983) in which subjects only showed the superior resistance to extinction characteristic of prepared conditioning when the angry facial expression was directed at the subject—not when it was averted by about 30% to the side. In a second experiment, they also showed that it was the direction of the gaze during extinction trials that was critical; subjects conditioned with an angry face looking away during acquisition showed enhanced resistance to extinction if the face was directed at them during extinction. This suggests that subjects learn that a particular person may be dangerous, but they only exhibit the "fear" when the angry gaze is directed at them.

In yet another experiment, Dimberg (1986) tested for generalization of the conditioned response to another angry face. Subjects were conditioned with the angry face of person A as a CS+ (and a happy face as a CS−), and then tested in extinction with the angry face of person B. In this situation the response extinguished immediately, leading Öhman et al. (1985) to conclude that "the expression per se did not carry any effect at all, which strongly suggests that the effect was carried by the person" (p. 158). However, in our view this conclusion may be premature for several reasons. First, the UCS used in these experiments—mild electric shocks—may not have maximal "belongingness" with prepared social stimuli as would be needed to produce the strongest conditioning effects (cf. Hamm, Veitl, & Lang, 1989). Instead, we would expect that UCSs more relevant to social fears, such as angry voices or some aspect of social humiliation or defeat, would be more likely to produce generalized fears. In addition, it may well be that to get conditioned responsiveness to angry facial expressions per se, one would need to have aversive conditioning experiences with multiple different angry faces. For example, if five different angry faces were used in acquisition, one might expect to see generalization to a sixth angry face in extinction. Indeed, this may be more analogous to what goes on in the acquisition of true social phobia, which is not a simple acquired fear of one particular individual; that is, by its very definition, even specific social phobia involves fears of many different individuals. Thus, although this work on conditioning to prepared facial stimuli provides important insights into the kinds of stimuli that are likely to become the sources of fear, it has some limitations at this point as a model of the origins of true social phobia because of the high degree of specificity to the individual used as the CS +. Whether this limitation reflects weaknesses in the design of the experiments conducted to date (namely, the nature of the UCS used and the use of only one face as a CS + during conditioning) or something more inherently problematic about the model is unclear at present.

Importantly, Öhman and colleagues (Öhman, 1986; Öhman, Dimberg, & Esteves, 1989) have also demonstrated that following conditioning with prepared CSs (such as angry faces), it is possible to elicit the CR even with subliminally presented CSs in extinction. That is, following conditioning, one can elicit a CR with very brief (approximately 30 msec) CSs presented in such a fashion so as to prevent access to conscious awareness. This "preattentive" activation of conditioned responses is seen only with prepared CSs—not with unprepared CSs such as happy faces. They argue that such results may help in part to account for the irrational quality of social phobia, in that the emotional reaction can be activated without conscious awareness of the threat cue.

In summary, the work of Öhman and colleagues on preparedness and social fears and phobias suggests that there is an evolutionarily based predisposition to acquire fears of angry, critical, or rejecting faces (Öhman et al., 1985; Öhman, 1986). Barlow (1988) further argues that for most individuals, such social fears will be mild or transient, with full-blown social phobia only developing in individuals who are vulnerable for biological and/or psychological reasons to develop what he calls anxious apprehension about future situations in which this social anxiety may be elicited. The biological sources of vulnerability undoubtedly include the temperamental variables discussed below. Moreover, the psychological vulnerabilities undoubtedly include the experiential variables occurring prior to, during, and following a conditioning experience discussed earlier. Finally, other important aspects of psychological vulnerability seem to stem from the individual's sense of control (or lack thereof) over his or her environment, as will also be discussed below.

Temperamental Variables Affecting Conditioning

The idea that temperament contributes to individual differences in conditioning traces back to the origins of the modern study of conditioning (see Mineka & Zinbarg, 1991). In his initial studies of conditioning, Pavlov (1927) recognized at least four distinct temperamental types of dogs, including the "sanguine," "melancholic," "phlegmatic," and "choleric," that were said to differ in the ease with which they acquired and extinguished conditioned responses.

The temperamental construct that is most relevant for the study of anxiety—behavioral inhibition—is also one of the most widely researched in the field of temperament (e.g., Biederman et al., 1990; Gray, 1982; Kagan, Reznick, & Snidman, 1988). Although there is some debate as to whether behavioral inhibition is best thought of in dimensional (Gray, 1982) or typological (Kagan, 1989; Kagan & Snidman, 1991) terms, there is growing consensus about the psychological and physiological correlates of behavioral inhibition. The behavioral inhibition system is responsible for inhibiting behavior in response to novelty and to signals for either punishment or frustration. Behavioral inhibition system functioning has been related to the experience of negative affects, including anxiety and fear, and to the personality traits of introversion (Gray, 1982; Kagan, 1989), anxiety (Gray, 1982), negative affectivity (Tellegen, 1985), and impulsivity versus constraint (Fowles, 1987, 1992). Although much of the research on behavioral inhibition has been done with human subjects (see Bruch & Cheek, Chapter 8, this volume), we will confine ourselves here to a primary focus on animal research contributions to the literature on behavioral inhibition.

Scott and Fuller (1965) reported what is perhaps the most extensive study of the genetic origins of behavioral inhibition. Their sample consisted of 470 puppies from five different breeds studied longitudinally from birth and tested on a wide battery of tests of problem solving, emotional reactivity, and psychophysiology. The emotional reactivity measures included reactions to novel objects or situations, mildly frightening environmental stimuli, interactions with humans and one measure of the dog's relationships with other dogs. On the basis of factor analyses of this battery of measures, Scott and Fuller concluded that "the only verified general trait is an emotional one" (p. 375). They named this factor "timidity or fear" and noted that it was defined primarily by fear of novel objects but also involved fear of humans. In addition, there were large differences on markers of this timidity factor between different breeds of dogs with evidence for a substantial genetic contribution to this trait.

Evidence for the existence of a behavioral inhibition factor has been replicated in several other species. Of even greater significance for the topic of this chapter is the fact that many of these studies included more extensive measures of relationships among conspecifics (members of the same species) and explicitly demonstrated that behavioral inhibition is related to reactivity to conspecific stressors as well as to nonsocial stressors. That is, these results suggest that behavioral inhibition acts as a predispositional factor to the development of social anxiety in addition to other forms of anxiety. For example, evidence from subhuman primates comes from a study reported by Chamove, Eysenck, and Harlow (1972). Chamove et al. found a major factor among measures of group behavior in rhesus monkeys that was loaded on most highly by nonsocial fear, but also was defined by high loadings on measures of social fear and withdrawal (see Stevenson-Hinde & Zunz, 1978, for very similar results).

In cats, Adamec (1975) examined aggressiveness versus submissiveness in response to various social and nonsocial stressors. In comparison to rat-killing cats, non-rat-killing cats showed less exploration of a novel room, as well as greater withdrawal and shelter-seeking tendencies to a human and to sounds of cat threat howls and catfight noises. These results suggest significant covariation among the fears labeled by Öhman et al. (1985) as "noncommunicative" (novel room), "interspecific communicative" (rats, people), and "intraspecific communicative" (other cats).

A good deal of the evidence regarding behavioral inhibition and its relationship to agonistic interactions among conspecifics comes from studies of rats. Hall (1941) reviewed evidence revealing moderate to large positive intercorrelations among measures of timidity and fearfulness displayed by rats in response to a wide variety of nonsocial stressors. Hall and Klein (1942) went on to demonstrate that rats bred for timidity and fearfulness in such nonsocial situations were also significantly more socially submissive than were rats bred for fearlessness in nonsocial situations. The timid rats not only initiated fewer attacks, but they also were more than twice as likely not to resist when attacked in comparison to the nonfearful rats. Billingslea (1940) reported similar results—that is, rats bred for timidity in nonsocial situations were also less likely to fight with conspecifics for access to food. Interestingly, Hall (1941) also cites evidence indicating that individual differences in timidity in nonsocial situations are negatively correlated with copulation frequency. Although there may be several possible explanations of this finding, it is consistent with the notion that the timid animals are not as bold with the opposite sex as are their fearless comrades. Social anxiety in humans has also been found to be negatively correlated with sexual experience (Leary & Dobbins, 1983). Furthermore, at least in men, sexual dysfunction has been conceptualized as a form of social phobia, given that evaluation anxiety tends to be associated with a higher incidence of premature ejaculation and temporary impotence (Barlow, 1986, 1988; Heimberg & Barlow, 1988).

In summarizing the animal literature presented above, behaviorally inhibited animals are more likely to be socially anxious, submissive, and acquiescent to others and appear to be more timid in their heterosexual interactions than other animals. These characteristics seem to parallel some of the more common features of socially phobic people, who are often submissive, fearful of asserting themselves, and fearful of dating and talking with the opposite sex (e.g., Hope & Heimberg, 1990; Scholing & Emmelkamp, 1990; Trower, Gilbert, & Sherling, 1990). Thus, our reading of the animal literature on behavioral inhibition suggests the following two hypotheses: (1) There is significant overlap between social anxiety and other forms of anxiety, and (2) behavioral inhibition may be a temperamental risk factor common to all the anxiety disorders, including social phobia.

Zinbarg and Barlow (1992) recently reported evidence consistent with these two hypotheses. First, a higher-order factor analysis was performed on 23 subscales from eight inventories tapping various forms of anxiety, including panic, social anxiety, worry, tension, agoraphobia, obsessions, compulsions, and specific fears. This analysis revealed a second-order general factor that was loaded on by each of the 23 measures and, on average, accounted for almost one-third of the variance in each of these scales. Next, a discriminant function analysis was performed to compare six patient groups representing all of the principal DSM-III-R anxiety disorder diagnoses (except posttraumatic stress disorder) and a no-mental-disorder control group. Each of the six anxiety disordered groups obtained significantly higher scores than did the no-mental-disorder control group on a discriminant function corresponding to the second-order general factor described above; there were no significant differences among the patient groups. Although other interpretations are plausible, these results are consistent with the notion that the second-order general factor was tapping a common predispositional core to all the anxiety disorders, including social phobia. Stronger tests of this hypothesis will obviously require longitudinal designs to rule out the possibility that the second-order general factor was a consequence rather than a cause of having an anxiety disorder.

Indirect evidence that behavioral inhibition is a risk factor for the development of anxiety disorders also comes from human studies of individual differences in conditionability. Numerous studies have found that introverts learn to inhibit a response to avoid punishment more rapidly than do extraverts (see Gray, 1982 for a review). Zinbarg and Revelle (1989) and Zinbarg (1994) have found similar results using the Trait

Anxiety Scale from the State–Trait Anxiety Inventory (STAI; Spielberger, Gorsuch, & Luschene, 1970) and the Impulsivity versus Constraint subscale from the Eysenck Personality Inventory (Eysenck & Eysenck, 1975). That is, individuals scoring high on the STAI and high on constraint show the most rapid acquisition of an avoidance response. When we added a measure of expectancies to our standard approach–avoidance paradigm, we found a significant correlation between STAI scores and the rate of acquiring expectancies for punishment. Because the STAI correlates almost as highly with measures of depression as it does with other measures of anxiety, it is probably best thought of as a measure of negative affectivity (Clark, 1989). Given that introversion, negative affectivity, and constraint have all been hypothesized to relate to behavioral inhibition system functioning, these results support the notion that behavioral inhibition is related to the ease of acquisition of aversive associations and avoidance responses. Although this work on personality and the acquisition of aversive associations has not yet been extended to observational conditioning paradigms, we expect that a similar relationship will hold. Therefore, we suggest that of all individuals who undergo a traumatic or vicarious conditioning experience, those who are high on the trait of behavioral inhibition are likely to acquire significantly higher levels of fear and avoidance.

Finally, given the evidence for an inherited basis to behavioral inhibition, we would expect to find a genetic contribution to the etiology of social phobia (see Chapman, Mannuzza, & Fyer, Chapter 2, this volume). Specifically, we would predict that what would be inherited would be a predisposition that is common to most, if not all, of the anxiety disorders. Although more and better data on this issue are needed, Barlow's (1988) conclusion based on a review of the available evidence is consistent with our prediction: "What seems to be inherited is a 'vulnerability' to develop an anxiety disorder, rather than a specific clinical syndrome itself" (p. 176).

ROLE OF PERCEIVED UNCONTROLLABILITY IN SOCIAL ANXIETY

Uncontrollability Moderates Levels of Fear Conditioning and Causes Increased Submissiveness

Animal models of phobias suggest that perceptions of controllability are a potent moderator of the intensity of learned fear. Along these lines, several studies have found that a CS for inescapable shock produces greater fear than does a CS for escapable shock (e.g., Desiderato & Newman, 1971; Mineka, Cook, & Miller, 1984; Osborne, Mattingly, Redmon, & Osborne, 1975). Similarly, the finding that animals that can avoid or escape shocks show less contextual fear than do animals that receive inescapable shock has been replicated several times (e.g., Brennan & Riccio, 1975; Mineka et al., 1984; Mowrer & Viek, 1948).

The animal literature not only suggests a role of perceived uncontrollability in the onset of phobias in general, but it also contains evidence supporting the more specific suggestion that perceived uncontrollability plays an important role in the etiology and maintenance of social phobia. This hypothesis has been explored in two directions. The first of these lines of research has involved investigations of the effects of uncontrollable shock upon submissiveness. Numerous studies have demonstrated that prior exposure to inescapable shock reduces shock-elicited aggression (e.g., Anderson, Crowell, Wickoff, & Lupo, 1980; Payne, Anderson, & Murcurio, 1970; Powell & Creer, 1969). Maier, Anderson, and Lieberman (1972) demonstrated that this effect is caused by the inescapability of the shocks rather than by mere exposure to shock per se. In two of three studies, Powell, Francis, Francis, and Schneiderman (1972, Experiments 1 and 2) replicated this finding. Moreover, Rapaport and Maier (1978) obtained similar results using competition for limited access to food as a measure of dominance versus submissiveness. Thus, it seems that rats exposed to inescapable shock are subsequently more submissive and less assertive. This behavior may be seen as analogous to that of socially anxious individuals, who behave more submissively and less assertively than do others (see Trower et al., 1990, for a brief review).

Although Williams (1982) has questioned the validity of the shock-elicited fighting and food competition paradigms as measures of aggressiveness versus submissiveness, he found similar results using what he considers to be a superior measure, the colony-intruder test (Williams, 1982; Williams & Lierle, 1986). The colony-intruder test also may provide a better analogue to human social anxiety because it involves interactions between strangers, which are among the most common situations that evoke anxiety among the socially anxious (Scholing & Emmelkamp, 1990). In the colony-intruder paradigm, naive intruder rats are placed in an established colony of rats. Typically, the intruder is attacked, primarily by just the dominant male colony resident (e.g., Blanchard, Takahashi, & Blanchard, 1977; Williams, 1982). Williams (1982) conducted a phase of colony-intruder testing prior to shock training to identify the dominant male in each colony. The dominant residents of each colony were then randomly assigned to receive either escapable shock, inescapable yoked shock, or exposure to the shock chamber without shock, and the colony-intruder test was repeated. Inescapable shock markedly reduced all forms of aggression in the dominant rats and increased defensive behaviors among these animals; by contrast, there were no decreases in aggressive responses for dominant rats that had either escapable shock or no shock. Williams and

Lierle (1986) conducted a similar study, except that they examined the effects of shock controllability on animals that were later to be tested as the intruders in the colony-intruder test. They found that inescapable shock makes a colony intruder even more submissive, that is, that it spent more time engaged in either defensive rearing, lying on its back, and/or freezing than it otherwise would when confronting a dominant resident animal. By contrast, escapable shock did not potentiate submissiveness among the colony intruders.

Taken together, the evidence from the studies reported by Maier et al. (1972), Powell et al. (1972, Experiments 1 and 2), Rapaport and Maier (1978), Williams (1982), and Williams and Lierle (1986) provides strong support for the notion that inescapable shock leads to increased submissiveness and that this effect is caused by the uncontrollability of the shock rather than by the mere effects of shock per se. This evidence suggests that a perception of uncontrollability may play a role in the etiology and/or maintenance of the submissive, unassertive behavior characteristic of social phobics. An important limitation in generalizing from the animal studies cited above to social phobia in humans is that it is clear that inescapable electric shock is not involved in the etiology of social phobia. Fortunately, there is a second line of relevant animal research using a stressor that has more ecological validity for the study of social fears, and the conclusions drawn from this second line of work are highly similar.

Social Defeat as a Particularly Powerful Uncontrollable Stressor

This more ecologically valid line of animal research involves investigations of the effects of social defeat. To begin with, as might be expected, repeated defeat leads to an increase in submissive behavior and a lowering of position in a dominance hierarchy, whereas repeated victory leads to an increase in aggressiveness and a rise in position in a dominance hierarchy (e.g., Ginsburg & Allee, 1942; Kahn, 1951; Scott, 1948; Scott & Marston, 1953). Several points regarding the literature on the effects of social defeat on submissiveness are noteworthy. First, Scott and Marston (1953) seemed to be primarily measuring retaliatory behavior rather than the initiation of aggressive encounters. Thus, their results can be more directly interpreted as showing that repeated defeat leads to greater reluctance to actively defend oneself. Such timidity in retaliating when attacked would appear to offer a closer analogue to the lack of assertiveness associated with social phobia than does the strength of the tendency to initiate aggression.

A second notable feature of this literature is that is has been suggested that the defeated animals do not appear to learn to be submissive only to the specific animals by which they had formerly been defeated. For example, Ginsburg and Allee (1942) suggested that the submissiveness of defeated mice appeared to be in response to the "general deportment of an aggressive individual" (p. 492). Similarly, Uhrich (1938) concluded that "the subordinates do not recognize the dominant (as an individual) but merely flee from any mouse that happens to attack them or assumes a threatening attitude" (p. 402). To the extent that this generalization is valid, it suggests another parallel between the behavior of defeated, socially submissive animals and socially anxious people, because it is rare that socially anxious people are frightened only of a specific individual. Rather, socially anxious people are most often frightened by classes of people, such as strangers or people in authority. At least with respect to this feature, then, the animal social defeat literature appears to provide a better model of social phobia than do the studies of conditioning to facial stimuli discussed above (Öhman, 1986; Öhman et al., 1985).

Evidence suggesting that perceptions of control over socially stressful situations moderate the experience of social anxiety in animals also comes from a study of male tree shrews reported by Raab and Oswald (1980). The subjects in this study were introduced as intruders into the home cages of animals that had consistently attacked and defeated other intruders in pretesting. In one condition (inescapable visual presence), the defeated intruder was separated from the aggressive resident after combat by a wire mesh, but the cages were arranged in such a way that the intruder could not escape the visual presence of the victor. In a second condition (escapable visual presence), the cages were arranged such that the subordinate intruder could periodically escape behind blinds from the visual presence of the victor, even though the animals were not physically separated after combat. Intruders in the inescapable visual presence condition displayed greater weight loss and more evidence of physiological stress. These differences emerged despite the fact that the intruders in the escapable visual presence condition actually experienced four times as many aggressive encounters with the residents as did the intruders in the inescapable visual presence condition. In addition to suggesting a role of perceived uncontrollability in the onset of social anxiety, these results demonstrate that, even in animals, the mere act of being observed by an individual perceived to be more dominant than oneself can be very stressful.

Further evidence suggesting that perceptions of control may mediate the effects of social defeat comes from a growing body of literature documenting the effects of social defeat on a host of behaviors other than agonistic behavior. Of most relevance to our purposes are several studies from independent laboratories demonstrating that repeated social defeat produces many of the effects produced by inescapable shock. Perhaps the most well known of the effects of inescapable shock is the so-called learned helplessness escape deficit (e.g., Maier, Seligman, & Solomon, 1969; Overmier & Seligman, 1967; Seligman & Maier, 1967). Williams and Lierle (1988) compared the effects of a colony intruder's exposure to colonies that had either very aggressive (i.e., a dominant male) or nonaggressive residents. The authors reported that the intruders into the aggressive colonies were attacked and defeated on each of 25 days of such exposures, whereas the intruders into the nonaggressive colonies rarely encountered offensive postures from the residents and were never bitten. When tested on a shuttlebox measure of escape learning that is most sensitive to the effects of inescapable shock, the previously defeated animals showed no evidence of learning this escape response, whereas the nondefeated animals showed the expected learning curve. Thus, social defeat is associated with a similar impairment in the ability to associate one's actions with relief from aversive stimulation that is produced by inescapable shock.

In two interesting extensions of this work, S. F. Maier (personal communication, July 27, 1993) explicitly compared the effects of inescapable shock on the subsequent escape behavior of dominant and submissive animals. In the first study, dominance was determined by ratings of videotapes of the interactions of subjects living together in groups. In a second study, dominance was determined by pairwise competition for limited access to a food treat. In both studies, dominant animals showed significantly greater escape deficits subsequent to inescapable shock than did submissive animals. It is tempting to speculate that this effect may parallel the finding that the effects of loss of control are sometimes more deleterious than the effects of lack of control (e.g., Mineka & Kelly, 1989). That is, we interpret these findings as indicating that social dominance is ordinarily associated with perceptions of personal efficacy and control, which may be shattered by the experience of inescapable shock.

Another parallel between the effects of inescapable shock and social defeat is that both appear to lead to increases in conditioned fear. Williams and Scott (1989) assigned rats to be intruders for a single session in either aggressive or nonaggressive colonies and then tested the rats for fear in the presence of odors from either an aggressive colony or a nonaggressive colony. All the intruders in the aggressive colonies were defeated, meaning that they were each bitten at least five times and displayed a submissive on-the-back posture. On the other hand, none of the intruders in the nonaggressive colonies were defeated. The results of this experiment clearly showed that the rats that had been defeated and later tested for fear in the presence of the aggressive colony odors showed more freezing (a reliable index of fear; cf. Bolles & Collier, 1976; Mineka et al., 1984) than did the remaining three groups (i.e., defeated and tested with nonaggressive colony odors, undefeated and tested with aggressive colony odors, and undefeated and tested with nonaggressive colony odors). These results were replicated by Williams, Worland, and Smith (1990) and interpreted as suggesting that the aggressive colony odors became fear CSs for the defeated animals.

The hypothesis that aggressive colony odors become fear CSs during defeat sessions received further supporting evidence by Williams, Rogers, and Adler (1990). In this experiment, defeated animals tested in the presence of aggressive colony odors again showed higher levels of freezing than did nondefeated animals. However, additional groups of defeated animals given 2- or 12-hour exposure to aggressive-colony odors before prod-shock testing showed partial or complete reductions, respectively, of this effect. This type of extinction is exactly what one would predict if the freezing responses were indeed reflecting fear conditioned to the aggressive colony odors during the defeat session. Clearly, we are not suggesting that odors play a role in the acquisition or maintenance of social fears in humans. Rather, we would argue that odors may play an analogous role in rats to that played by facial expression in humans—communicating mood, including hostility, to conspecifics (e.g., Öhman et al., 1985). Thus, we would expect to find evidence demonstrating the preparedness of such odors in rats for the conditioning of social fear parallel to that found for facial expressions in humans.

Although the effects of inescapable shock on fear conditioning and escape learning may be well known, what may be less familiar to the reader is that there is a relationship between shock controllability and stress-induced analgesia. Recent reviews of this literature reveal that the analgesia produced by extensive inescapable shock is mediated by endogenous opioids to a greater extent than is the analgesia produced by escapable shock (Foa, Zinbarg, & Olasov-Rothbaum, 1992; Maier, 1986, 1989). There does not seem to be a clear analogy between stress-induced analgesia and any of the characteristics of social phobia as it is presently understood. We will devote a little attention to stress-induced opioid-mediated analgesia nonetheless, because there is evidence that the endogenous opioid system may mediate at least some of the effects of uncontrollable aversive stimuluation (e.g., Drugan & Maier, 1983; Maier, Coon, McDaniel, & Jackson, 1979; Maier, Sherman, Lewis, Terman, & Liebeskind, 1983). Just as extensive inescapable shock does, extensive exposure to attack from conspecifics results in opioid-mediated analgesia (Miczek, Thompson, & Shuster, 1982; Rodgers & Hendrie, 1983; Rodgers & Randall, 1985, 1986). Interestingly, it appears that this opioid-mediated analgesia is more highly correlated with the extent to which the animal being attacked assumes the characteristic postures of defeat, the upright submissive posture and the frozen crouch posture, than with the number of bites actually received (Miczek et al., 1982; Rodgers & Hendrie, 1983).

To briefly summarize the material covered thus far in this section, the evidence from two separate lines of research converge in demonstrating compelling parallels between the effects of social defeat and inescapable shock. First, the effects of inescapable shock parallel the effects of social defeat on measures of submissiveness. Second, the effects of social defeat parallel the effects of inescapable shock on several measures of nonsocial behavior, including escape learning, fear conditioning, and activation of endogenous opioid systems. These parallels strongly suggest the hypothesis that perceptions of control moderate the intensity of social fears.

Immunization Effects from Prolonged Exposure to Controllable Appetitive Events

Thus far the review of the literature on the effects of uncontrollability has stressed the deleterious consequences that stem from exposure to uncontrollable aversive events. However, there is also a smaller literature demonstrating that extensive experience with controlling appetitive events can also have beneficial consequences, serving at least partially to immunize the organism against the effects of various stressors. In one particularly relevant study, Mineka, Gunnar, and Champoux (1986) reared baby rhesus monkeys in controllable or uncontrollable environments. Across two replications, two groups of four master monkeys (who had extensive experience with control and mastery) lived in large cages that had various operant manipulanda, such as levers, chains, and keys, that could be operated in order to deliver food, water, and treats on various schedules of reinforcement. Two groups of four yoked monkeys (who had extensive experience with uncontrollability) lived in identical environments, except that their manipulanda were inoperative; that is, they received reinforcers only when a member of the master group successfully operated one of its manipulanda. The monkeys lived in these environments from approximately six weeks of age until approximately 11–12 months of age. Between 7 and 10 months of age, the monkeys were subjected to three fear tests, with a toy monster outside their home cage, and to three playroom tests, in which they were exposed to a large novel playroom environment. The master monkeys showed more rapid habituation to the fear-provoking toy monster than did the yoked groups, indicating superior ability to cope with transient stressful experiences. In the playroom tests, the master monkeys also habituated more rapidly to this novel scary situation, as evidenced by their emerging more quickly and spontaneously to play in the room with repeated tests; also, once in the playroom, they spent more time exploring the novel objects in the room and less time clinging to one another. Thus, with these two different measures, the master monkeys, who had extensive experience controlling important aspects of their environment, showed superior ability to cope with novel and threatening stimuli relative to yoked monkeys, who were reared in relatively uncontrollable environments.

Perhaps of greatest interest from the standpoint of social phobia, however, were the results of separation tests. Between 10 and 12 months of age, monkeys from the second replication were subjected to several different kinds of separations—ones in which they were individually housed, ones in which they were housed in pairs (with a familiar peer), and ones in which they were taken out of their own group one by one and placed in with the other group (intruder separations). Although the individual and pair separations did not reveal any interesting significant effects of rearing history, during the intruder separations, the master subjects coped better as intruders in the yoked group than vice versa. In particular, masters as intruders in the yoked group explored more and ate and drank more than did yoked monkeys as intruders in the master group. As hosts, the yoked group also showed more fear/submissive behavior toward the master intruders than vice versa. Thus, although these results are only suggestive in that they need to be replicated in independent groups of subjects, they do suggest that an early history of control over appetitive events can serve to immunize the organism against both inanimate stressors (such as a toy monster and a large novel playroom) and against social stressors (such as interacting with strangers during a time of stress, i.e., separation from one's peer group).

Summary

The evidence reviewed above suggests a strong role for perceived uncontrollability in the etiology and maintenance of social phobia. Exposure to uncontrollable stressors (both inescapable shock and social defeat) causes increased submissiveness and higher levels of fear conditioning, as well as all of the traditional learned helplessness effects. Moreover, there is some evidence that extensive experience with control over one's environment may immunize the organism against the effects of both nonsocial and social stressors.

Evidence for animal models of human psychopathology is always strengthened when parallel results can be found in humans. Although we are unaware of any studies that have directly manipulated controllability of stressors in humans and looked at the effects on social anxiety, there is some evidence that social phobia is associated with a diminished sense of control over social interactions. In particular, Cloitre, Heimberg, Liebowitz, and Gitow (1992) administered Levenson's (1973) Locus of Control scale to individuals with social phobia and with panic disorder and to no-mental-disorder control subjects. In comparison to the no-mental-disorder control subjects, both the social phobics and the individuals with panic disorder received significantly lower scores on a subscale reflecting belief in one's ability to influence events in one's life (e.g., "When I make plans, I am almost certain to make them work"). Further analyses indicated that, among social phobics, this diminished sense of personal control was primarily accounted for by beliefs that control over events occurring in their lives is primarily determined by "powerful others" (e.g., "If important people were to decide they didn't like me, I probably wouldn't make many friends"). As the samples were fairly small (14 subjects in each group), these results are in need of replication. Nevertheless, they suggest that social phobia is associated with diminished perceptions of the ability to influence the outcome of social interaction, as would be predicted by the above analysis of the animal uncontrollability and social defeat literature. (See Leung & Heimberg, 1994, for a replication of these results in an independent sample.)

CONCLUSIONS

In this chapter, we have reviewed research from a variety of different traditions that we believe helps to illuminate important factors involved in the origins and maintenance of social fears and phobias. Simple behavioral models that suggest the importance of direct or vicarious learning experiences in the origins of social fears and phobias need to be broadened to take into account the role of experiential variables, occurring prior to, during, and following a conditioning experience, that play a powerful role in determining the outcome of those direct or vicarious learning experiences. Moreover, these models also need to address the role of the preparedness of certain cues for social anxiety and to acknowledge the role of temperamental variables in putting certain individuals at higher risk than others. Finally, perceived uncontrollability over important life events—especially traumatic ones such as those described in the social defeat literature—may be related to a significant number of the symptoms of social phobia.

REFERENCES

Adamec, R. (1975). The behavioral bases of prolonged suppression of predatory attack in cats. *Aggressive Behavior, 1,* 297–314.

American Psychiatric Association. (1987). *Diagnostic and statistical manual of mental disorders* (3rd ed., rev.). Washington, DC: Author.

Anderson, D. C., Crowell, C. R., Wickoff, M. B., & Lupo, J. V. (1980). Activity during prior shock determines subsequent shock-elicited fighting in the rat. *Animal Learning and Behavior, 8,* 664–672.

Barlow, D. H. (1986). Causes of sexual dysfunction: The role of anxiety and cognitive interference. *Journal of Consulting and Clinical Psychology, 54,* 140–145.

Barlow, D. (1988). *Anxiety and its disorders: The nature and treatment of anxiety and panic.* New York: Guilford Press.

Beck, A., & Emery, G. (1985). *Anxiety disorders and phobias: A cognitive perspective.* New York: Basic Books.

Biederman, J., Rosenbaum, J., Hirshfeld, D., Faraone, S., Bolduc, E., Gersten, M., Meminger, S., Kagan, J., Snidman, N., & Reznick, J. S. (1990). Psychiatric correlates of behavioral inhibition in young children of parents with and without psychiatric disorders. *Archives of General Psychiatry, 47,* 21–26.

Billingslea, F. Y. (1940). The relationship between emotionality and various other salients of behavior in the rat. *Journal of Comparative Psychology, 31,* 69–77.

Blanchard, R. J., Takahashi, L. K., & Blanchard, D. C. (1977). The development of intruder attack in colonies of laboratory rats. *Animal Learning and Behavior, 5,* 365–369.

Bolles, R. C., & Collier, A. C. (1976). The effect of predictive cues on freezing in rats. *Animal Learning and Behavior, 4,* 6–8.

Brennan, J. F., & Riccio, D. C. (1975). Stimulus generalization of suppression in rats following aversively motivated instrumental or Pavlovian training. *Journal of Comparative and Physiological Psychology, 88,* 570–579.

Chamove, A. S., Eysenck, H. J., & Harlow, H. F. (1972). Personality in monkeys: Factor analyses of rhesus social behavior. *Quarterly Journal of Experimental Psychology, 24,* 496–504.

Clark, L. A. (1989). The anxiety and depressive disorders: Descriptive psychopathology and differential diagnosis. In P. Kendall & D. Watson (Eds.), *Anxiety and depression: Distinctive and overlapping features* (pp. 83–129). New York: Academic Press.

Cloitre, M., Heimberg, R. G., Liebowitz, M. R., & Gitow, A. (1992). Perceptions of control in panic disorder and social phobia. *Cognitive Therapy and Research, 16,* 569–577.

Cook, E. W., Hodes, R., & Lang, P. J. (1986). Preparedness and phobia: Effects of stimulus content on human visceral conditioning. *Journal of Abnormal Psychology, 95,* 195–207.

Cook, M., & Mineka, S. (1989). Observational conditioning of fear to fear-relevant versus fear-irrelevant stimuli in rhesus monkeys. *Journal of Abnormal Psychology, 98,* 448–459.

Cook, M., & Mineka, S. (1990). Selective associations in the observational conditioning of fear in rhesus monkeys. *Journal of Experimental Psychology: Animal Behavior Processes, 16,* 372–389.

Cook, M., & Mineka, S. (1991). Selective associations in the origins of phobic fears and their implications for behavior therapy. In P. Martin (Ed.), *Handbook of behavior therapy and psychological science: An integrative approach* (pp. 413–434). Elmsford, NY: Pergamon Press.

de Waal, F. (1989). *Peacemaking among primates.* Cambridge, MA: Harvard University Press.

Delprato, D. (1980). Hereditary determinants of fears and phobias. *Behavior Therapy, 11,* 79–103.

Desiderato, O., & Newman, A. (1971). Conditioned suppression produced in rats by tones paired with escapable or inescapable shock. *Journal of Comparative and Physiological Psychology, 77,* 427–431.

Dimberg, U. (1986). Facial expressions as excitatory and inhibitory stimuli for conditioned autonomic responses. *Biological Psychology, 22,* 37–57.

Dimberg, U., & Öhman, A. (1983). The effects of directional facial cues on electro-
    dermal conditioning to facial stimuli. *Psychophysiology, 20,* 160–167.
Drugan, R. C., & Maier, S. (1983). Analgesic and opioid involvement in the shock-
    elicited activity and escape deficit produced by inescapable shock. *Learning
    and Motivation, 14,* 30–47.
Eysenck, H. J., & Eysenck, S. B. G. (1975). *Manual of the Eysenck Personality Inventory*
    (2nd ed.). London: Hodder & Stoughton.
Foa, E., Zinbarg, R., & Olasov-Rothbaum, B. (1992). Uncontrollability and unpre-
    dictability in post-traumatic stress disorder: An animal model. *Psychological
    Bulletin, 112,* 218–238.
Fowles, D. (1987). Application of a behavioral theory of motivation to the concepts
    of anxiety and impulsivity. *Journal of Research in Personality, 21,* 417–435.
Fowles, D. C. (1992). Schizophrenia: Diathesis–stress revisited. *Annual Review of
    Psychology, 43,* 303–336.
Ginsburg, B., & Allee, W. C. (1942). Some effects of conditioning on social domi-
    nance and subordination in inbred strains of mice. *Physiological Zoology, 15,*
    485–506.
Gray, J. A. (1982). *The neuropsychology of anxiety: An enquiry into the functioning of
    the septo-hippocampal system.* Oxford, UK: Oxford University Press.
Hall, C. S. (1941). Temperament: A survey of animal studies. *Psychological Bulletin,
    38,* 909–943.
Hall, C. S., & Klein, S. J. (1942). Individual differences in aggressiveness in rats.
    Journal of Comparative Psychology, 33, 371–383.
Hamm, A., Veitl, D., & Lang, P. (1989) Fear conditioning, meaning, and belong-
    ingness: A selective association analysis. *Journal of Abnormal Psychology, 98,*
    395–406.
Heimberg, R. G., & Barlow, D. H. (1988). Psychosocial treatments for social phobia.
    Psychosomatics, 29, 27–37.
Hendersen, R. (1978). Forgetting of conditioned fear inhibition. *Learning and Moti-
    vation, 8,* 16–30.
Hope, D. A., & Heimberg, R. G. (1990). Dating anxiety. In H. Leitenberg (Ed.),
    Handbook of social and evaluation anxiety (pp. 217–246). New York: Plenum
    Press.
Hygge, S., & Öhman, A. (1978) Modeling processing in the acquisiton of fears:
    Vicarious electrodermal conditioning to fear-relevant stimuli. *Journal of Person-
    ality and Social Psychology, 36,* 271–279.
Kagan, J. (1989). The concept of behavioral inhibition to the unfamiliar. In J. S.
    Reznick (Ed.), *Perspectives on behavioral inhibition* (pp. 1–23). Chicago: Univer-
    sity of Chicago Press.
Kagan, J., Reznick, J. S., & Snidman, N. (1988). Biological bases of childhood
    shyness. *Science, 240,* 167–171.
Kagan, J., & Snidman, N. (1991) Temperamental factors in human development.
    American Psychologist, 46, 856–862.
Kahn, M. W. (1951). The effect of severe defeat at various age levels on the
    aggressive behavior of mice. *Journal of Genetic Psychology, 79,* 117–130.
Leary, M. R., & Dobbins, S. E. (1983). Social anxiety, sexual behavior and contra-
    ceptive use. *Journal of Personality and Social Psychology, 45,* 1347–1354.

Leung, A. W., & Heimberg, R. G. (1994). *Perceptions of control, homework compliance, and outcome of cognitive-behavioral treatment for social phobia.* Manuscript submitted for publication.

Levenson, H. (1973). Multidimensional locus of control in psychiatric patients. *Journal of Consulting and Clinical Psychology, 41,* 397–401.

Liebowitz, M., Gorman, J., Fyer, A., & Klein, D. (1985). Social phobia: Review of a neglected anxiety disorder. *Archives of General Psychiatry, 42,* 729–736.

Maier, S. F. (1986). Stressor controllability and stress-induced analgesia. *Annals of the New York Academy of Sciences, 467,* 55–71.

Maier, S. F. (1989). Determinants of the nature of environmentally induced hypoalgesia. *Behavioral Neuroscience, 103,* 131–143.

Maier, S. F., Anderson, C., & Lieberman, D. A. (1972). Influence of control of shock on subsequent shock-elicited aggression. *Journal of Comparative and Physiological Psychology, 81,* 94–100.

Maier, S. F., Coon, D. J., McDaniel, M. A., & Jackson, R. L. (1979). The time course of learned helplessness, inactivity, and nociceptive deficits in rats. *Learning and Motivation, 10,* 467–488.

Maier, S. F., Seligman, M. E. P., & Solomon, R. L. (1969). Pavlovian fear conditioning and learned helplessness: Effects on escape and avoidance behavior of a) the CS-US contingency and b) the independence of the US and voluntary responding. In B. A. Campbell & R. M. Church (Eds.), *Punishment* (pp. 299–342). New York: Appleton-Century-Crofts.

Maier, S. F., Sherman, J. E., Lewis, J. W., Terman, G. W., & Liebeskind, J. (1983). The opioid/nonopioid nature of stress-induced analgesia and learned helplessness. *Journal of Experimental Psychology: Animal Behavior Processes, 9,* 80–90.

Marks, I. (1969). *Fears and phobias.* New York: Academic Press.

Marks, I. (1987) *Fears, phobias and rituals: Panic, anxiety and their disorders.* New York: Oxford University Press.

Marks, I., & Gelder, M. (1966). Different ages of onset in varieties of phobias. *American Journal of Psychiatry, 123,* 218–221.

Mayr, E. (1974). Behavior programs and evolutionary strategies. *American Scientist, 62,* 650–659.

Melamed, B., Yurcheson, R., Fleece, E., Hutcherson, S., & Hawes, R. (1978). Effects of film modeling on the reduction of anxiety-related behaviors in individuals varying in the level of previous experience in the stress situation. *Journal of Consulting and Clinical Psychology, 46,* 1357–1367.

Miczek, K. A., Thompson, M. L., & Shuster, L. (1982). Opioid-like analgesia in defeated mice. *Science, 215,* 1520–1522.

Mineka, S. (1985a). The frightful complexity of the origins of fears. In F. R. Brush & J. B. Overmier (Eds.), *Affect, conditioning and cognition: Essays in the determinants of behavior* (pp. 55–73). Hillsdale, NJ: Erlbaum.

Mineka, S. (1985b). Animal models of anxiety-based disorders: Their usefulness and limitations. In J. Maser & A. Tuma (Eds.), *Anxiety and the anxiety disorders* (pp. 199–244). Hillsdale, NJ: Erlbaum.

Mineka, S. (1987). A primate model of phobic fears. In H. Eysenck & I. Martin (Eds.), *Theoretical foundations of behavior therapy* (pp. 87–111). New York: Plenum Press.

Mineka, S. (1992). Evolutionary memories, emotional processing and the emotional disorders. In D. Medin (Ed.), *The psychology of learning and motivation* (Vol. 28, pp. 161–206). New York: Academic Press.

Mineka, S., & Cook, M. (1986). Immunization against the observational conditioning of snake fear in rhesus monkeys. *Journal of Abnormal Psychology, 95,* 307–318.

Mineka, S., & Cook, M. (1988). Social learning and the acquisition of snake fear in monkeys. In T. Zentall & G. Galef (Eds.), *Comparative social learning* (pp. 51–73). Hillsdale, NJ: Erlbaum.

Mineka, S., & Cook, M. (1993). Mechanisms underlying observational conditioning of fear. *Journal of Experimental Psychology: General, 122,* 23–38.

Mineka, S., Cook, M., & Miller, S. (1984). Fear conditioned with escapable and inescapable shock: Effects of a feedback stimulus. *Journal of Experimental Psychology: Animal Behavior Processes, 10,* 307–323.

Mineka, S., Gunnar, M., & Champoux, M. (1986). Control and early socioemotional development: Infant rhesus monkeys reared in controllable versus uncontrollable environments. *Child Development, 57,* 1241–1256.

Mineka, S., & Kelly, K. (1989). The relationship between anxiety, lack of control, and loss of control. In A. Steptoe & A. Appels (Eds.), *Stress, personal control and health* (pp. 163–191). Chichester, UK: Wiley.

Mineka, S., & Zinbarg, R. (1991). Animal models of psychopathology. In C. Walker (Ed.), *Clinical psychology: Historical and research foundations.* (pp. 51–86). New York: Plenum Press.

Mowrer, H., & Viek, P. (1948). An experimental analogue of fear from a sense of helplessness. *Journal of Abnormal and Social Psychology, 43,* 193–200.

Öhman, A. (1986). Face the beast and fear the face: Animal and social fears as prototypes for evolutionary analyses of emotion. *Psychophysiology, 23,* 123–145.

Öhman, A., & Dimberg, U. (1978). Facial expressions as conditioned stimuli for electrodermal responses: A case of "preparedness"? *Journal of Personality and Social Psychology, 36,* 1251–1258.

Öhman, A., Dimberg, U., & Esteves, F. (1989). Preattentive activation of aversive emotions. In T. Archer & L.-G. Nilsson (Eds.), *Aversion, avoidance and anxiety: Perspectives on aversively motivated behavior* (pp. 169–199). Hillsdale, NJ: Erlbaum.

Öhman, A., Dimberg, U., & Öst, L.-G. (1985). Animal and social phobias: Biological constraints on the learned fear response. In S. Reiss & R. Bootzin (Eds.), *Theoretical issues in behavior therapy* (pp. 123–175). New York: Academic Press.

Osborne, F. H., Mattingly, B. A., Redmon, W. K., & Osborne, J. S. (1975). Factor affecting the measurement of classically conditioned fear in rats following exposure to escapable versus inescapable signalled shock. *Journal of Experimental Psychology: Animal Behavior Processes, 1,* 364–373.

Öst, L.-G., & Hugdahl, K. (1981). Acquisition of phobias and anxiety response patterns in clincal patients. *Behaviour Research and Therapy, 16,* 439–447.

Overmier, J. B., & Seligman, M. E. P. (1967). Effects of inescapable shock on subsequent escape and avoidance learning. *Journal of Comparative and Physiological Psychology, 63,* 28–33.

Pavlov, I. P. (1927). *Conditioned reflexes.* London: Oxford University Press.

Payne, R., Anderson, D. C., & Murcurio, J. (1970). Preshock-produced alterations in pain-elicited fighting. *Journal of Comparative and Physiological Psychology, 71*, 258–266.

Poser, E., & King, M. (1975). Strategies for the prevention of maladaptive fear responses. *Canadian Journal of Behavior Science, 7*, 279–294.

Powell, D. A., & Creer, T. L. (1969). The interaction of some environmental and developmental variables in shock-induced aggression. *Journal of Comparative and Physiological Psychology, 69*, 219–225.

Powell, D. A., Francis, M. J., Francis, J., & Schneiderman, N. (1972). Shock-induced aggression as a function of prior experience with avoidance, fighting, or unavoidable shock. *Journal of the Experimental Analysis of Behavior, 18*, 323–332.

Raab, A., & Oswald, R. (1980). Coping with social conflict: Impact on the activity of tyrosine hydroxylase in the limbic system and in the adrenals. *Physiology and Behavior, 24*, 387–394.

Rachman, S. (1978). *Fear and courage.* San Francisco: Freeman.

Rachman, S. (1990). *Fear and courage.* New York: Freeman.

Rapaport, P. M., & Maier, S. F. (1978). Inescapable shock and food-competition dominance in rats. *Animal Learning and Behavior, 6*, 160–165.

Rescorla, R. (1974). Effect of inflation of the unconditioned stimulus value following conditioning. *Journal of Comparative and Physiological Psychology, 86*, 101–106.

Riccio, D., Richardson, R., & Ebner, D. (1984). Memory retrieval deficits based upon altered contextual cues: A paradox. *Psychological Bulletin, 96*, 152–165.

Rodgers, R. J., & Hendrie, C. A. (1983). Social conflict activates status-dependent endogenous analgesic and hyperalgesic mechanisms in male mice. *Physiology and Behavior, 30*, 775–780.

Rodgers, R. J., & Randall, J. I. (1985). Social conflict analgesia: Studies on naloxone antagonism and morphine cross-tolerance. *Pharmacology, Biochemistry and Behavior, 23*, 883–888.

Rodgers, R. J., & Randdall, J. I. (1986). Extended attack from a resident conspecific is critical to the development of long-lasting analagesia in male intruder mice. *Physiology and Behavior, 38*, 427–430.

Scholing, A., & Emmelkamp, P. M. G. (1990). Social phobia: Nature and treatment. In H. Leitenberg (Ed.), *Handbook of social and evaluation anxiety* (pp. 217–246). New York: Plenum Press.

Scott, J. P. (1948). Studies on the early development of social behavior in puppies. *American Psychologist, 3*, 239–240.

Scott, J. P., & Fuller, J. L. (1965). *Genetics and the social behavior of the dog.* Chicago: University of Chicago Press.

Scott, J. P., & Marston, M. (1953). Nonadaptive behavior resulting from a series of defeats in fighting mice. *Journal of Abnormal and Social Psychology, 48*, 417–428.

Seligman, M. (1971). Phobias and preparedness. *Behavior Therapy, 2*, 307–320.

Seligman, M. E. P., & Maier, S. F. (1967). Failure to escape traumatic shock. *Journal of Experimental Psychology, 74*, 1–9.

Sheehan, D. (1983). *The anxiety disease.* New York: Charles Scribner's Sons.

Spielberger, C. D., Gorsuch, R., & Luschene, R. (1970). *The State–Trait Anxiety Inventory (STAI) Test Manual Form X.* Palo Alto, CA: Consulting Psychologists Press.

Stevenson-Hinde, J., & Zunz, M. (1978). Subjective assessment of individual rhesus monkeys. *Primates, 19,* 473–482.

Tellegen, A. (1985). Structures of mood and personality and their relevance to assessing anxiety, with an emphasis on self-report. In A. Tuma & J. Maser (Eds.), *Anxiety and the anxiety disorders* (pp. 681–706). Hillsdale, NJ: Erlbaum.

Thomas, D. (1979). Retention of conditioned inhibition in a bar-press suppression paradigm. *Learning and Motivation, 10,* 161–177.

Torgersen, S. (1979). The nature and origins of common phobic fears. *British Journal of Psychiatry, 134,* 343–351.

Townsley, R. (1992). Social phobia: Identification of possible etiological factors. Unpublished doctoral dissertation, University of Georgia, Athens.

Trower, P., Gilbert, P., & Sherling, G. (1990). Social anxiety, evolution, and self-presentation: An interdisciplinary perspective. In H. Leitenberg (Ed.), *Handbook of social and evaluation anxiety* (pp. 11–45). New York: Plenum Press.

Uhrich, J. (1938). The social hierarchy in albino mice. *Journal of Comparative Psychology, 25,* 373–413.

Williams, J. L. (1982). Influence of shock controllability by dominant rats on subsequent attack and defensive behaviors toward colony intruders. *Animal Learning and Behavior, 10,* 305–313.

Williams, J. L., & Lierle, D. M. (1986). Effects of stress controllability, immunization, and therapy on the subsequent defeat of colony intruders. *Animal Learning and Behavior, 14,* 305–314.

Williams, J. L., & Lierle, D. M. (1988). Effects of repeated defeat by a dominant conspecific on subsequent pain sensitivity, open-field activity, and escape learning. *Animal Learning and Behavior, 16,* 477–485.

Williams, J. L., Rogers, A. G., & Adler, A. P. (1990). Exposure to conspecific and predatory odors on defensive burying and freezing. *Animal Learning and Behavior, 18,* 453–461.

Williams, J. L., & Scott, D. K. (1989). Influence of conspecific and predatory stressors and the associated odors on defensive burying and freezing. *Animal Learning and Behavior, 17,* 383–393.

Williams, J. L., Worland, P., & Smith, M. G. (1990). Defeat-induced hypoalgesia in the rat: Effects of conditioned odors, naltrexone and extinction. *Journal of Experimental Psychology: Animal Behavior Processes, 16,* 345–357.

Zinbarg, R. (1994, March). *Individual differences in the acquisition of aversive associations and passive avoidance.* Poster presented at the Annual Meeting of the Anxiety Disorders Association of America, Santa Monica, CA.

Zinbarg, R., & Barlow, D. H. (1992, November). *The construct validity of the DSM-III-R anxiety disorders: Empirical evidence.* Presented at the 26th Annual Meeting of the Association for Advancement of Behavior Therapy, Boston.

Zinbarg, R., & Revelle, W. (1989). Personality and conditioning: A test of four models. *Journal of Personality and Social Psychology, 57,* 301–314.

CHAPTER EIGHT

Developmental Factors in Childhood and Adolescent Shyness

MONROE A. BRUCH
JONATHAN M. CHEEK

Specialization within psychology can inhibit interdisciplinary approaches to the study of human problems. Personality and developmental psychology, for instance, offer substantial research literatures that can contribute to clinical psychology's and psychiatry's understanding of disorders such as social phobia. Specifically, these fields provide information about the development and course of adaptive and maladaptive personality characteristics of normal individuals. Given this knowledge base, clinical researchers can then assess whether disordered persons show similar or different patterns in their personal and social development. Such comparisons may increase our knowledge about potential antecedent factors and processes that contribute to disordered behavior.

The purpose of this chapter is to discuss recent research in personality and developmental psychology that has focused on key individual and interpersonal variables that relate to child and adolescent shyness. Shyness is the normal personality characteristic that most closely parallels social phobia, in that they both share the antecedent of fear of negative evaluation. Although shyness and social phobia share cognitive and affective manifestations of fear of negative evaluation, it is not assumed that they are synonymous, because social phobia may involve a more pervasive pattern of avoidance and impairment in social and occupational functioning (Bruch, 1989). Nevertheless, research on the origins of childhood shyness has identified a number of reliable factors predictive of stable patterns of shyness over substantial time periods. Presumably these same developmental factors could exist for individuals who come to manifest symptoms of social phobia in adolescent and adult years.

In this chapter we will review selected research from four areas of the personality development literature that have provided insight about the origins and course of shyness. These four areas include research on temperament characteristics, family factors, socialization processes, and disturbance in self-esteem.

TEMPERAMENT AND SHYNESS

The idea that shyness is rooted in a biological predisposition is as old as the field of psychology. James (1890) quoted Darwin's discussion of shyness and included it in his list of basic human instincts. Baldwin (1894) also interpreted the emergence of bashfulness during the first year of life as an organic stage in the expression of instinctive emotion. Drawing on observations from his medical practice, Campbell (1896) argued that "no fact is more certain than that shyness runs in families" (p. 805). Recent work in behavior genetics tends to support these early speculations about the contribution of an inherited biological predisposition to the origins of shyness.

Plomin and Rowe (1979) conducted a study of 21 identical and 25 fraternal pairs of twins with an average age of 22 months. The twins were observed in their homes engaging in specific behaviors related to shyness, such as approaching, touching, smiling at, and playing with an adult stranger. Intraclass correlations were computed for the twin pairs, and significantly higher correlations for the identical than for the fraternal twins on several measures of social behavior indicated a heritable component in social responding to unfamiliar people. Studies of self-reported shyness among adolescent and adult samples of twins have yielded similar significant differences. For example, in a study of high school students, the intraclass correlations for scores on a shyness scale were .53 for identical twins and .24 for fraternal twins (Cheek & Zonderman, 1983). After reviewing 18 twin studies, one family study, and one adoption study, Plomin and Daniels (1986) concluded that heredity plays a more substantial role in shyness from infancy through adulthood than it does in other personality traits (e.g., activity level and gregariousness).

The research just reviewed indicates that shyness fulfills the two part criterion in the definition of a *temperament*: "inherited personality traits" and "present in early childhood" (Buss & Plomin, 1984, p. 84). There have, however, been some disagreements about the classification of shyness as a temperament. Buss and Plomin suggested that it might be better to consider shyness to be a derivative of the temperaments sociability and emotionality, especially because of the complicating factor of cognitive symptoms of shyness that first appear in later childhood and adulthood. Kagan and his colleagues have agreed that shyness has more complex connotations for adults and have, therefore, proposed the label "behavioral inhibition" for the temperamental qualities of wariness of unfamiliar people, timidity in situations that contain risk of harm, and cautiousness in situations that contain risk of failure (Kagan & Reznick, 1986; Kagan, Snidman, & Arcus, 1993).

Regardless of disagreements about terminology, Kagan and Reznick (1986) do agree with Plomin and Daniels (1986) that some children are born with a biological predisposition of increased vulnerability to developing shyness. Research in Kagan's laboratory has focused on measures of physiological reactivity that correlate with behavioral inhibition. For example, inhibited infants and young children tend to respond to novel stimuli and mild stress with high and stable heart rates, pupillary dilation, and tension in the skeletal muscles. These characteristics have been interpreted as being related to differential thresholds of excitability in the amygdala and its projections to parts of the nervous system (Kagan et al., 1993; for more details on biological models in humans and other animals, see Reznick, 1989). From a slightly different perspective, Rothbart and Mauro (1990) have suggested that temperamental individual differences in the flexibility and control of attention also play a role in the origins of shyness. Scholarly debate about terminology and specific mechanisms certainly will continue to be lively, but the basic idea that temperament makes a significant contribution to childhood shyness is now well established. In a parallel fashion, it is notable that there is increasing evidence for the heritability of social phobia. For instance, in a large sample of female twin pairs, Kendler, Neale, Kessler, Heath, and Eaves (1992) found that liability to social phobia was significantly correlated in twin pairs and was due more to genetic than to family-environment factors, consistent with an inherited phobia proneness model. Also, Fyer, Mannuzza, Chapman, Liebowitz, and Klein (1993), in a family study of social phobia, reported that relatives of uncomplicated social phobics, in contrast to relatives of nondisordered controls, showed a significantly increased risk (16% to 5%) for social phobia.

Later-Developing Shyness

Buss (1980, 1986) has proposed a distinction between early-developing, fearful shyness and later-developing, self-conscious shyness that is framed in the language of contemporary research on temperament and personality development. The fearful type of shyness typically emerges during the first year of life and is influenced by temperamental qualities of wariness, emotionality, and behavioral inhibition that includes the substantial genetic component discussed above. Buss's self-conscious type of shyness first appears around age 4 or 5, when the cognitive self has already begun to develop, and peaks between 14 and 17, as adolescents cope with cognitive egocentrism (the "imaginary audience" phenomenon) and identity issues (Adams, Abraham, & Markstrom, 1987; Cheek, Carpentieri, Smith, Rierdan, & Koff, 1986). In contrast to the somatic anxiety and behavioral inhibition that characterize early-developing shyness, later-developing shyness involves cognitive symptoms of psychic anxiety such as painful self-consciousness and self-preoccupation. This additional category of symptoms suggests a three-component definition of dispositional shyness: the tendency to feel tense, awkward, or worried during social interactions, especially with unfamiliar people (Cheek & Melchior, 1990).

Surveys employing retrospective reports of college students reveal four findings relevant to Buss's developmental conceptualization of shyness: (1) About 36% of currently shy respondents indicated that they had been shy since early childhood; (2) early-developing shyness is more enduring, with about 75% of those who said they were shy in early childhood reporting still being shy currently, but with only about 50% of those who were first shy during late childhood or early adolescence saying that they are currently shy; (3) the early-developing shy respondents also had developed cognitive symptoms of shyness upon entering adolescence, so that they differed from those with later-developing shyness by having more somatic anxiety symptoms but did not have fewer cognitive symptoms; and (4) early-developing shyness appears to be more of an adjustment problem, with males in that group reporting the most behavioral symptoms of shyness (Bruch, Giordano, & Pearl, 1986; Cheek et al., 1986; Shedlack, 1987). Also, it is interesting to note that epidemiological data on a sample of social phobics without comorbidity (Schneier, Johnson, Hornig, Liebowitz, & Weissman, 1992) showed a bimodal pattern for age at onset of social phobia. In the sample, the two largest groups reported onset either before 5 years of age (20 of 97, or 21%) or between the ages of 11 to 15 (25 of 97, or 26%).

The ongoing longitudinal study of childhood behavioral inhibition being conducted by Kagan and his colleagues is relevant to both types of shyness described by Buss. Kagan's construct is essentially equivalent to Buss's early-developing shyness (e.g., Kagan & Reznick, 1986), and the results from 21 months to 5 years support Buss's ideas about the physiological correlates and enduring quality of early-developing shyness. A more recent assessment occurred at age 7, which is after the time when later-developing shyness theoretically begins to emerge. At this point, about three-quarters of the children who were extremely shy when they were

21 months old were still shy, and about three-quarters of those not shy previously continued to be uninhibited (Kagan, Reznick, Snidman, Gibbons, & Johnson, 1988). The first finding suggests that beneficial socialization experiences can ameliorate the impact of a problematic temperament, for as James (1890) argued, in humans an instinct is only expressed in its pure form once and is thereafter subject to modification through interaction with the environment (see also Buss & Plomin, 1984).

Although Kagan et al. (1988) do not invoke it, Buss's theory may also help to explain their second finding, that one-quarter of the previously uninhibited children had become shy. This outcome is, in fact, absolutely necessary if his construct of later-developing shyness is valid. If no one became shy for the first time after age 5, then Buss's theory of a distinct type of shyness that primarily involves self-concept disturbances, rather than infant temperament, would be superfluous. Buss has suggested that the later-developing, self-conscious kind of shyness has no genetic component, but Cheek and Melchior (1990) speculated that research identifying separate genetic factors contributing to somatic and psychic anxiety symptoms might be applied eventually to a developmental model of shyness (cf. Kendler, Heath, Martin, & Eaves, 1987).

The early–late distinction implies that the ordering consistency assessed by test–retest stability for shyness should be high from infancy to age 5, more variable for assessments during middle childhood, depending on the exact age of each measurement, and then increasingly stable once again within adolescence and adulthood. The results from Kagan's project so far and from several other longitudinal studies generally support these expectations, although no one has yet analyzed longitudinal data specifically to test Buss's theory (for reviews see Cheek et al., 1986, and Moskowitz, Ledingham, & Schwartzman, 1985).

In a recent study in Kagan's laboratory of maternal behavior and infant temperament during the first year, Arcus (1991) found that mothers of temperamentally highly reactive infants who were direct in their limit setting and not overly responsive to fretting and crying appeared to be reducing the amount of behavioral inhibition subsequently displayed by their infants. As Plomin and Daniels (1986) have pointed out, however, findings of family-environmental influences on shyness do not necessarily undermine interpretations of the substantial genetic component found in early-developing shyness (within a studied population or group). In their study, the emotional expressiveness score from the Family Environment Scale (FES; Moos, 1986) had a much stronger negative correlation with infant shyness in nonadoptive families (i.e., biological parents were present) than in adoptive families. This is an important example of how genotype–environment correlations may influence the course of personality development (Scarr, 1987).

Two studies that traced the consequences of shyness from middle or late childhood into adulthood (average age about 35) found meaningful continuities in the trait and a coherent influence on the shy person's style of life but uncovered little psychopathology (Caspi, Elder, & Bem, 1988; Morris, Soroker, & Burruss, 1954). Gilmartin's (1987b) retrospective study of extremely shy adult men, however, demonstrates that early-developing shyness sometimes can have devastating consequences in terms of loneliness, under-employment, and unhappiness. In addition, it appears that the men in Gilmartin's study might fit Kagan's definition of behavioral inhibition as a qualitative category because they report somatic anxiety symptoms and other physical complaints, such as allergies, that date back to early childhood. Consequently, it would be important to test whether children who meet the criteria for behaviorally inhibited temperament, a group estimated to be about 15% of the population, are at greater risk for developing social phobia later in life than are children who are merely shy around strangers (Kagan et al., 1993).

The social phobic men in Gilmartin's (1987b) study reported that their childhood relationships with *both* their peers and their parents, especially their mothers, were simply terrible. In contrast, the typical pattern for shy children is poor relationships with peers but positive interactions at home, especially with their mothers (Stevenson-Hinde & Hinde, 1986). Thus, in spite of the strength of findings from temperament research, it appears that the home environment is also a decisive factor for developmental outcomes of shyness, even in extreme cases.

FAMILY FACTORS AND SHYNESS

The research on family antecedents to be reviewed consists of studies from the child development literature that focus on the relation between parental characteristics and childhood shyness. In addition, several studies from the clinical literature involving adult social phobics' retrospective reports of their parents' child-rearing attitudes will be reviewed. As previously mentioned, Plomin and Daniels (1986) were the first to provide evidence of a family-environment as well as genetic relation to infant shyness. Results from the FES indicated that families with higher cohesion, higher emotional expressiveness, and lower conflict and who placed emphases on intellectual and recreational orientations rated their infant children as less shy at 12 and 24 months of age. FES scores on the cohesion and expressiveness scales reflect qualities of open communication, while the intellectual and recreational scale scores reflect parental encouragement of social and cultural involvement. Consequently, the particular FES scores that correlated with infant shyness suggest that dimensions of parental support and social exposure may be associated with less likelihood of shyness in early childhood.

Engfer (1993) reports the results of a 6-year longitudinal study of antecedents of childhood shyness. Although based on only 39 German families, Engfer assessed maternal responsiveness to infant communication and maternal personality characteristics relative to childhood shyness as measured by an eight-item rating scale completed by a research assistant. Results showed that maternal responsiveness during the first 2.5 years was *inversely* correlated with shyness ratings at age 6.3 years for girls but not for boys. Maternal personality characteristics of nervousness, dysphoria, irritability, and shy inhibition were correlated with shyness ratings of girls at both 4 and 18 months. At 6.3 years, maternal personality characteristics were assessed with a reduced set of scales (i.e., dysphoria, irritability, and composure), and only dysphoria related to shyness. Engfer concludes that while boys' childhood shyness may be rather independent of maternal influence, girls' shyness appears to be meaningfully linked to maternal characteristics.

Recently, Rubin and his colleagues (Mills & Rubin, 1993; Rubin, LeMare, & Lollis, 1990) articulated a comprehensive, conceptual model of how parental characteristics contribute to the development of childhood shyness. In this model, he contends that children who are likely to become shy are those who are temperamentally fearful and inhibited in new situations *and* whose parents are unsupportive of this reaction because of their child-rearing attitudes. Presumably these factors have their greatest impact under conditions of family stress and/or limited resources for parental coping. The resultant relationship is one in which parents are, or are perceived to be, unavailable and unresponsive, leading to feelings of insecurity. In turn, it is assumed that this insecurity generalizes to other relationships and may produce a complementary belief that the self is unworthy and incompetent. If such a self-schema develops and is perpetuated by others' responses, the child is likely to manifest symptoms of shyness in various social situations.

Essentially Rubin suggests that childhood shyness is a joint product of characteristics of the child and conditions that influence parental support of the child. Recently, Mills and Rubin (1993) reported findings from a series of prospective studies that assessed the role of certain parental and situational conditions that presumably would reduce parental supportiveness. One variable consisted of parental beliefs and feelings about their child's social behavior including about how children learn socially competent behavior, strategies used for modifying unskilled social behavior, attributions about the causes of unskilled social behavior, and emotional responses toward unskilled social behaviors. The second variable consisted of external stressors that impair parental support as measured by socioeconomic status, and the third variable consisted of parental coping resources as measured by parental ratings of perceived social support.

Results are based on a sample of 122 mother–child dyads assessed initially when the child was aged 4, and a second time when the child was 6 for 45 out of 100 available dyads. The subsample of 45 dyads was demographically similar to the original sample. Generally the results of the study were consistent with Mills and Rubin's (1993) model. Mothers of shy children were more likely than were mothers of nonshy children to believe that social skills are best taught in a directive manner (i.e., being told exactly how to act) rather than some other manner (e.g., personal experience). Mothers of shy children also believed more strongly that unskilled behaviors should be responded to in a directive or coercive manner. Mothers of shy children were also more likely to feel angry, disappointed, guilty, and embarrassed by their child's unskilled behaviors and were more likely to attribute these unskilled behaviors to traits in their children rather than to mood or age-related factors. Furthermore, mothers of shy children were under more external stress (i.e., lower socioeconomic status), but the two groups of mothers did not differ in perceived social support. Although these results should be interpreted cautiously because mothers' beliefs may be a consequence as well as an antecedent of their child's shyness, differences in mothers' ratings were found when their children were aged 4 and 6 regardless of gender.

Unfortunately, results from a second study that employed a cohort of slightly older children were not highly consistent with the first study's findings. In fact, the results of the second study suggest that mothers of shy children were *underresponsive* rather than overreactive as was found in the first study. Mills and Rubin (1993) conclude that a longitudinal approach is needed to evaluate whether mothers reappraise their child's shyness as he or she grows older and whether such reappraisal leads to less facilitative interaction (e.g., mother comes to think of child's shyness as an unchangeable characteristic). In addition, they conclude that such reappraisal may be moderated by both the child's and the parent's gender, since there is evidence that fathers consider shyness more of a problem for boys than for girls (Bacon & Ashmore, 1985).

In contrast to the work by developmental investigators, clinical researchers have concentrated on adult phobics' retrospective report of their parent's child-rearing attitudes. Relative to social phobia, there are five published studies involving perceived parental child-rearing attitudes. Based on patients' anecdotal reports of their parents' behavior, Parker (1979), Arrindell, Emmelkamp, Monsma, and Brilman (1983), and Arrindell et al. (1989) assessed whether social phobics differed from agoraphobics and normal controls on child-rearing attitudes of affection and control. Parker found that social phobics relative to normal controls perceived both of their parents as controlling and expressing less affection, while agoraphobics differed from normals only in perceiving their mothers as less affectionate. Arrindell et al. (1983) reported a very similar pattern of findings in comparisons of social phobics to normals and agoraphobics to normals. In a comparison of social phobics to agoraphobics, Arrindell et al. (1989) found that social phobics reported significantly less affection from both parents than did agoraphobics.

Bruch, Heimberg, Berger, and Collins (1989) and Bruch and Heimberg (1994) compared social phobics to agoraphobics and to normal controls on a somewhat different set of parental child-rearing dimensions. Based in part on Buss's (1980) conception of family antecedents of shyness, Bruch and his colleagues assessed child-rearing dimensions of concern about the opinions of others, family sociability, and isolation of the child. According to Buss (1980), parental concern with others' opinions regarding appropriate behavior could sensitize a child to situations involving public scrutiny, while isolation (i.e., parental overprotection and control) and low family sociability may limit the child's access to socialization experiences that could reduce their fears.

In Bruch et al. (1989), generalized social phobics reported greater concern about the opinions of others, greater isolation, and lesser family sociability (i.e., visiting or inviting over friends and relatives) than did agoraphobics. Bruch and Heimberg (1994) extended the previous findings by comparing samples of generalized to nongeneralized social phobics and normal controls on the three previous child-rearing dimensions plus a fourth dimension of shame, a variable that is conceptually similar to affection–rejection (cf. Arrindell et al., 1983). Heimberg, Holt, Schneier, Spitzer, and Liebowitz (1993) define *nongeneralized* social phobics as those who fear various social and/or performance situations but are unimpaired in some area of social functioning. Bruch and Heimberg (1994) found that both generalized and nongeneralized social phobics differed from normal controls, but not each other, in reporting greater parental concern with the opinions of others and use of shame to discipline. However, generalized in contrast to nongeneralized social phobics and controls reported greater isolation and less family socializing.

The findings with adult social phobics show intriguing parallels to the results of the previously reviewed research on childhood shyness. For instance, Plomin and Daniels's (1986) finding that parents of shy children do not encourage an intellectual or recreational orientation is conceptually consistent with social phobics' perceptions of greater isolation and less family sociability. Also, Mills and Rubin's (1993) finding that mothers of shy children held stronger beliefs that social skills are best taught by directly telling their child how to act seems consistent with adult social phobics' report of parental concern with the importance of acting properly (i.e., concern about opinions of others). Finally, Mills and Rubin's (1993) evidence that mothers of shy children believe that unskilled behaviors should be dealt with in a directive or coercive manner appears consistent with adult subjects' report of parental control and use of shame to discipline.

SOCIALIZATION PROCESSES AND SHYNESS

Sex-Role Socialization and Gender Differences in Shyness

Despite the absence of gender differences on measures of shyness (Jones, Briggs, & Smith, 1986), shyness in boys may be associated with more negative feedback from parents and peers than shyness in girls. Bronson (1966) has argued, for example, that in terms of sex-role stereotypes in child development, it is more appropriate for girls than for boys to be seen as shy. Because the traditional male role requires that boys and men take the initiative rather than be passive in social relations, the correlates of shyness (e.g., nervousness, inhibition) are likely to be major impediments in males' social development. In fact, examination of common personality characteristics associated with shyness suggests that shyness is at odds with traditional role expectations for the American male. McCroskey, Daly, and Sorenson (1976) found that shyness was negatively correlated with self-control, adventurousness, dominance, emotional maturity, and self-confidence. Also, Buss (1984) states that it is the "relative absence of instrumental activity (traditional masculinity) that identifies shyness" (p. 39), while Cheek et al. (1986) note that the adjective "shy" is scored on the Femininity scale of the Bem (1981) Sex Role Inventory.

Presumably during childhood and adolescence, if a boy manifests symptoms of shyness in the presence of persons who hold traditional sex-role expectations, he is likely to experience negative feedback. Earlier we noted that Bacon and Ashmore (1985) and Mills and Rubin (1993) provide evidence that both fathers and mothers are more likely to admonish their sons than their daughters for shy and inhibited behavior, suggesting concerns about inappropriate sex-role behavior. Given the assumption that shy boys are less likely to manifest behaviors consistent with traditional sex-role expectations, they may experience more conflict from the sex-role socialization process. Specifically, a shy boy is likely to experience a discrepancy between societal expectations of how he should behave in various situations and his own expectations of how to behave. Although some discrepant behaviors are likely to be the consequence of anxiety and do not reflect how the person wants to behave, other discrepant behaviors may reflect the person's preferred response in a situation.

Similar to how the women's movement described negative consequences of socialized gender roles for women, O'Neil (1981) suggests that gender-role conflict in men stems from a socialized fear of femininity. Fear of femininity is defined as a negative affective reaction to anything associated with stereotypic feminine values, attitudes, and behaviors. Consequently, because deviance from traditional gender roles is likely to lead to negative consequences, O'Neil argues that fear of femininity (i.e., gender-role conflict) leads to restricted interest in and ability to engage in a wide range of human activities. In turn, such restricted behavior may lead to less effective social interaction and less relationship satisfaction.

Based on O'Neil's (1981) formulation, it seems possible that shy boys and young men could develop a greater fear of femininity if criticized for discrepant sex-role behaviors than do nonshy boys and young men. Furthermore, it can be argued that problems in later life may not necessarily arise directly from child or adolescent shyness but, rather, indirectly, as a result of how shyness impacts on developmental processes such as gender-role identity and self-concept. Recently, Berko (1993) tested the preceding notion in a sample of undergraduate men ($N = 199$). The criterion behavior he chose was intimate self-disclosure, an aspect of social relations relevant to shyness and gender-role conflict. Using a path-analytic methodology, Berko tested whether the predictor variables of shyness, self-esteem for physical abilities, masculinity, and femininity evidenced direct or indirect (via fear of femininity) relations with intimate self-disclosure. Self-confidence about physical abilities was selected because there is evidence that boys who dislike culturally masculine athletic and recreational activities (and thus, are likely to be low in physical self-esteem) report problematic shyness (Cheek & Melchior, 1990; Gilmartin, 1987b). Presumably, boys low in physical self-esteem would be likely to experience greater gender-role conflict (i.e., higher fear of femininity) and perhaps engage in less disclosure. Although shyness and physical self-esteem did not predict self-disclosure, shyness was positively related and physical self-esteem was negatively related to fear of femininity. In turn, fear of femininity and greater feminine gender identity were both predictive of intimate self-disclosure. Although Berko's results did not support the notion that shyness has either a direct or an indirect relation with intimate self-disclosure, limitations with the measure of self-disclosure may have attenuated his findings. Nevertheless, the negative relation between shyness and physical self-esteem and the pattern of relations of shyness and physical self-esteem with fear of femininity support the notion that shyness may complicate boys' sex-role socialization experiences.

Peer Relations and Shyness

In addition to gender-role socialization experiences, another important aspect of child and adolescent development is peer-group relations. Although controversy exists whether negative peer relations (e.g., rejection) are related to subsequent psychopathology (Parker & Asher, 1987), recent studies by Rubin et al. (1990) and Olweus (1993) provide evidence that negative peer relations are associated with greater risk for depression and suicide attempts. As a group, shy children and adolescents appear to be more likely to experience negative peer relations. A chief reason for this difficulty is that the shy child's inhibition and withdrawal is perceived as deviant from age-appropriate social behavior by the peer group and reacted to by responses of neglect, rejection, or victimization (e.g., bullying). For instance, Olweus (1993) found that a disproportionally large number of children who are classified as "victims" by teachers are described as socially isolated, withdrawn, anxious, and inhibited. Gilmartin's (1987a) interview study of extremely shy adult men also provides support for an association between shyness and negative peer relations. His results showed that approximately 88% of the shy men compared to none of the nonshy men, recalled being bullied and harassed during both childhood and adolescence. Likewise, Ishiyama (1984) found that shy adults reported that childhood incidents of being teased, picked on, and ridiculed contributed greatly to maintaining their shyness problems into adulthood.

Although informative, data from the previous studies are cross-sectional and cannot address the reciprocal properties of shyness and peer relations. A recent prospective study by Vernberg, Abwender, Ewell, and Beery (1992), however, provides some insight about the possible transactional nature of shyness and peer relations. These investigators examined, at three intervals over a 9-month period, relationships between social anxiety, friendship qualities, and rejection experiences for 68 early adolescents who had recently relocated. Adolescents in the midst of an intercommunity relocation were selected to provide a more powerful test of the possible impact of peer relations on social anxiety and vice versa. The measure of social anxiety used assessed the components of fear of negative evaluation, social avoidance–distress in new situations, and general social avoidance–distress.

Results from analyses of social anxiety components as predictors of friendship qualities (e.g., degree of intimacy) showed that general social avoidance–distress was associated with subsequently less intimacy and companionship. However, none of the social anxiety components predicted subsequent experiences of rejection (i.e., direct aggression and exclusion from desired activities) as expected by the researchers. Analyses of the reciprocal association between friendship qualities plus rejection experiences and subsequent change in social anxiety were equally interesting. Vernberg et al. (1992) report that lower levels of intimacy and companionship were related to increased fear of negative evaluation but not to increases in general or new situation social avoidance–distress for the first half of the school year. Likewise, rejection experiences were associated with increases in fear of negative evaluation early in the school year. However, rejection experiences during the second half of the school year were associated with higher scores on the general social avoidance–distress scale but not the other two social anxiety components. These findings are consistent with the notion that shyness and negative peer-group relations involve reciprocal processes but fail to support the hypothesized antecedent role of shyness in evoking peer rejection. Although preliminary, the pattern of associations between peer relations and specific social anxiety components is intriguing and suggests, for instance, that degree of dispositional shyness may have a greater impact on friendship formation, while rejection experiences may trigger an increase in cognitive aspects of shyness (i.e., fear of negative evaluation).

DISTURBANCE IN SELF-ESTEEM AND SHYNESS

Cheek and Melchior (1990) note that cross-sectional research consistently shows a substantial negative correlation between measures of shyness and global self-esteem in samples ranging from children to the elderly. However, the consistent finding of an inverse relation does not clarify whether shyness is an antecedent or consequence of low self-esteem. Such ambiguity naturally leads to the question "Which comes first, shyness or low self-esteem?" From the perspective of personality development, the answer may depend on what type of shyness is manifested by the individual and which model of self-esteem is employed. Relative to shyness, Buss's (1980, 1986) subtype of early-developing shyness is influenced by temperaments that result in fearfulness and behavioral inhibition. Because the consequences of these temperaments precede the development of the child's self-concept, Buss (1980) excludes low self-esteem as a likely antecedent of early-developing shyness. In contrast, later-developing shyness first appears around age 4 or 5, when the cognitive self has begun to develop, and peaks between 14 and 17, as adolescents transition from cognitive egocentrism to relativistic thinking (i.e., other-perspective thinking). Therefore, unlike early-developing shyness and its associated symptoms of behavioral and physiological anxiety, later-developing shyness involves primarily cognitive disturbances such as negative self-referent thinking. In turn, Buss (1980) theorizes that factors contributing to low self-esteem in middle childhood could contribute to the person's susceptibility to later-developing shyness in late childhood and adolescence; hence, with this type of shyness, low self-esteem may precede problems of shyness.

Relative to self-esteem, recent tests (Fleming & Courtney, 1984) of multidimensional models of self-esteem provide support for the notion that particular facets of self-esteem (e.g., academic) are better predictors of functioning in relevant domains than is a global self-esteem score. In this research, self-esteem pertains to an internal self-appraisal process that reflects an individual's resultant confidence with respect to such dimensions as one's academic, physical, and social self (Fleming & Courtney, 1984; Shavelson, Hubner, & Stanton, 1976). Given this conceptualization, the question can be raised of whether shy persons are low in self-esteem for most self-dimensions or only for those related to the social self. Using Fleming and Courtney's (1984) Self-Rating Scale to measure facets of self-esteem, Mamries, O'Connor, and Cheek (1983) found that shyness scores were more highly correlated with esteem for one's physical appearance ($-.44$ and $-.55$, men and women respectively) than with academic self-esteem ($-.16$ and $-.39$, men and women respectively). This pattern of relations was recently replicated by Bruch (1993), who found in a male sample that shyness correlated $-.52$ with esteem for physical appearance and $-.50$ with esteem for social acceptability, but only $-.18$ with academic self-esteem. Thus, the relation between shyness and low self-esteem probably resides primarily in low self-confidence with regard to the domain of social behavior.

Presumably, another antecedent of shyness is the personality dimension of public self-consciousness (Buss, 1980). Public self-consciousness is the tendency to focus one's attention on the self as a social object, but not to necessarily become anxious as a result of this focus. However, for some individuals high in public self-consciousness, evaluative concerns may elicit feelings of threat leading to shyness. Thus, Buss (1980) argues that all shy people should be high in public self-consciousness, but only some people high in public self-consciousness will be shy. For the later-developing type of shyness, Buss (1980) suggests that heightened public self-consciousness may develop prior to shyness because the individual becomes more sensitized to the public self through parental admonitions about physical appearance, dress, and manners.

What determines whether someone high in public self-consciousness will also become shy? In other words, what mechanism(s) determine when a person's attention to the public self will also lead to concern about negative evaluation (i.e., shyness)? In answering this question, we may arrive at a more explicit conceptualization of how low self-esteem operates as an antecedent of shyness. Bruch (1993) has proposed that one mediator may be the person's self-esteem. Because self-esteem involves an internal evaluative process, this appraisal process is likely to be activated when the individual's attention is focused on the public self, which is open to the scrutiny of others. However, as previously shown, shy and nonshy persons differ only on self-esteem dimensions open to the scrutiny of others. Therefore, Bruch (1993) predicted that self-esteem for dimensions only in the social domain (e.g., physical appearance) should mediate the relation between public self-consciousness and shyness. To test this prediction, Bruch (1993) administered Fleming and Courtney's (1984) Self-Rating Scale, which measures global, social, physical, and academic components of self-esteem, along with measures of shyness and public self-consciousness, to 115 male undergraduates. According to Baron and Kenny (1986) a mediating variable substantially reduces the effect of an independent variable on a dependent variable, in this case the bivariate correlation between public self-consciousness and shyness. Consequently when the dependent variable (i.e., shyness) is regressed on both the independent (public self-consciousness) and mediating (i.e., facets of self-esteem) variables, the size of the partial coefficient between public self-consciousness and shyness should be nonsignificant and approach zero. Five aspects of self-esteem were assessed: physical appearance, physical ability (e.g., "think of self as more athletic than most people"), academic ability (e.g., "think of self as a good student"), global (e.g., "think of self as generally worthwhile"), and social acceptance (e.g., "think of self as getting along well with others"). It was expected that physical appearance, physical ability, and social acceptance would be mediators but that the other two facets would not.

Analyses yielded the following results. The simple correlation between public self-consciousness and shyness was $r(115) = .27, p < .01$. The partial correlations between public self-consciousness and shyness with the self-esteem variables of physical appearance, physical ability, social acceptance, academic ability, and global esteem as mediators were, respectively, .09, .28, .03, .25, and .16, indicating that two of the predicted reductions occurred. As evident from these results, self-esteem about one's physical attractiveness and social acceptability to others acted as mediators of the public self-consciousness and shyness relation. In other words, for persons high in public self-consciousness, if they also possess high regard for their own physical and social attractiveness to others, it is unlikely that they will concurrently experience feelings of shyness. While needing replication, these results are consistent with the notion that enhancing a child's esteem toward his or her physical and social attributes will likely reduce the occurrence of shyness in later stages of development.

CONCLUSIONS

Although the relation between shyness and social phobia is unclear, as Turner, Beidel, and Townsley (1990) suggest, there may be one or more common vulnerabilities underlying both conditions. In this chapter a number of candidates emerge as possible factors contributing to such vulnerability. Certainly one factor is an inherited temperament involving wariness, emotionality, and behavioral inhibition. As described, the negative consequences of this temperament (e.g., bullying) might be diminished by a family context that does not overcompensate for the child's shyness by use of ineffective parenting approaches (e.g., overprotection, withholding affection) and that permits expression of emotion among family members. However, regardless of the role of temperament, by middle and late childhood three other factors become possible sources of vulnerability for shyness and/or social phobia. These factors alone or in combination include inappropriate parental child-rearing attitudes, negative peer relations, and disturbance in social facets of self-esteem. Evidence reviewed suggests that parental and societal emphasis on traditional sex-role behaviors (particularly with boys) may produce additional sources of conflict for shy children and adolescents, which in turn leads to maladaptive coping responses (e.g., avoidance of self-disclosure). Likewise, rejection and victimization by one's peers, especially for those high in affiliation motivation, appears to foster increased preoccupation with possible negative evaluation by others. Furthermore, if life experiences (e.g., peer rejection) lead to misinterpretation of one's physical and social acceptability, the individual may be more prone to developing symptoms of shyness and social phobia. Clearly, each of these vulnerability factors needs further conceptualization and empirical study regarding their possible contribution to shyness and social phobia. Particularly needed are longitudinal studies that directly compare shy children who eventually develop symptoms of social phobia versus those who remain shy or whose shyness abates. Given a more sophisticated understanding of these two conditions, it now appears possible to conduct such research.

REFERENCES

Adams, G. R., Abraham, K. G., & Markstrom, C. A. (1987). The relations among identity development, self-consciousness, and self-focusing during middle and late adolescence. *Developmental Psychology, 23,* 292–297.

Arcus, D. M. (1991). *The experiential modification of temperamental bias in inhibited and uninhibited children.* Unpublished doctoral dissertation, Harvard University, Cambridge, MA.

Arrindell, W. A., Emmelkamp, P. M. G., Monsma, A., & Brilman, E. (1983). The role of perceived parental rearing practices in the etiology of phobic disorders: A controlled study. *British Journal of Psychiatry, 143,* 183–187.

Arrindell, W. A., Kwee, M. G. T., Methorst, G. J., Van Der Ende, J., Pol, E., & Moritz, B. J. M. (1989). Perceived parental rearing styles of agoraphobic and socially phobic inpatients. *British Journal of Psychiatry, 155,* 526–535.

Bacon, M. K., & Ashmore, R. D. (1985). How mothers and fathers categorize descriptions of social behavior attributed to daughters and sons. *Social Cognition, 3*, 193–217.

Baldwin, J. M. (1984). Bashfulness in children. *Educational Review, 8*, 434–441.

Baron, R. M., & Kenny, D. A. (1986). The moderator–mediator variable distinction in social psychological research: Conceptual, strategic, and statistical considerations. *Journal of Personality and Social Psychology, 51*, 1173–1182.

Bem, S. L. (1981). *Bem Sex-Role Inventory professional manual*. Palo Alto, CA: Consulting Psychologists Press.

Berko, E. H. (1993). *Gender role conflict as a mediator of the impact of shyness, physical self-esteem, and sex-role attitudes on men's intimate self-disclosure*. Unpublished doctoral dissertation, State University of New York, Albany.

Bronson, W. C. (1966). Control orientations: A study of behavior organization from childhood to adolescence. *Child Development, 37*, 125–155.

Bruch, M. A. (1989). Familial and developmental antecedents of social phobia: Issues and findings. *Clinical Psychology Review, 9*, 37–47.

Bruch, M. (1993). [Facets of self-esteem that mediate the relation of public self-consciousness and shyness]. Unpublished data, State University of New York, Albany.

Bruch, M. A., Giordano, S., & Pearl, L. (1986). Differences between fearful and self-conscious shy subtypes in background and adjustment. *Journal of Research in Personality, 20*, 172–186.

Bruch, M. A., & Heimberg, R. G. (1994). Differences in perceptions of parental and personal characteristics between generalized and nongeneralized social phobics. *Journal of Anxiety Disorders, 8*, 155–168.

Bruch, M. A., Heimberg, R. G., Berger, P., & Collins, T. M. (1989). Social phobia and perceptions of early parental and personal characteristics. *Anxiety Research, 2*, 57–63.

Buss, A. H. (1980). *Self-consciousness and social anxiety*. San Francisco, CA: Freeman.

Buss, A. H. (1984). A conception of shyness. In J. A. Daly & J. C. McGroskey (Eds.), *Avoiding communication: Shyness, reticence, and communication apprehension* (pp. 39–50). Beverly Hills, CA: Sage.

Buss, A. H. (1986). A theory of shyness. In W. H. Jones, J. M. Cheek, & S. R. Briggs (Eds.), *Shyness: Perspectives on research and treatment* (pp. 39–46). New York: Plenum Press.

Buss, A. H., & Plomin, R. (1984). *Temperament: Early developing personality traits*. Hillsdale, NJ: Erlbaum.

Campbell, H. (1896). Morbid shyness. *British Medical Journal, 2*, 805–807.

Caspi, A., Elder, G. H., & Bem, D. J. (1988). Moving away from the world: Life-course patterns of shy children. *Developmental Psychology, 24*, 824–831.

Cheek, J. M., Carpentieri, A. M., Smith, T. G., Rierdan, J., & Koff, E. (1986). Adolescent shyness. In W. H. Jones, J. M. Cheek, & S. R. Briggs (Eds.), *Shyness: Perspectives on research and treatment* (pp. 105–115). New York: Plenum Press.

Cheek, J. M., & Melchior, L. A. (1990). Shyness, self-esteem, and self-consciousness. In H. Leitenberg (Ed.), *Handbook of social and evaluative anxiety* (pp. 47–82). New York: Plenum Press.

Cheek, J. M., & Zonderman, A. B. (1983, August). Shyness as a personality temperament. In J. M. Cheek (Chair), *Progress in research on shyness*. Symposium conducted at the meeting of the American Psychological Association, Anaheim, CA.

Engfer, A. (1993). Antecedents and consequences of shyness in boys and girls: A 6-year longitudinal study. In K. H. Rubin & J. B. Asendorpf (Eds.), *Social withdrawal, inhibition, and shyness in childhood* (pp. 49–79). Hillsdale, NJ: Erlbaum.

Fleming, J. S., & Courtney, B. E. (1984). The dimensionality of self-esteem: II. Hierarchical facet model for revised measurement scales. *Journal of Personality and Social Psychology, 46,* 404–421.

Fyer, A. J., Mannuzza, S., Chapman, T. F., Liebowitz, M. R., & Klein, D. F. (1993). A direct interview family study of social phobia. *Archives of General Psychiatry, 50,* 286–293.

Gilmartin, B. G. (1987a). Peer group antecedents of severe love-shyness in males. *Journal of Personality, 55,* 467–489.

Gilmartin, B. G. (1987b). *Shyness and love: Causes, consequences, and treatment.* Lanham, MD: University Press of America.

Heimberg, R. G., Holt, C. S., Schneier, F. R., Spitzer, R. L., & Liebowitz, M. R. (1993). The issue of subtypes in the diagnosis of social phobia. *Journal of Anxiety Disorders, 7,* 249–269.

Ishiyama, F. J. (1984). Shyness, anxious social sensitivity, and self-isolating tendency. *Adolescence, 19,* 903–911.

James, W. (1890). *The principles of psychology* (Vol. 2). New York: Holt.

Jones, W. H., Briggs, S. R., & Smith, T. G. (1986). Shyness: Conceptualization and measurement. *Journal of Personality and Social Psychology, 51,* 629–639.

Kagan, J., & Reznick, S. J. (1986). Shyness and temperament. In W. H. Jones, J. M. Cheek, & S. R. Briggs (Eds.), *Shyness: Perspectives on research and treatment* (pp. 81–90). New York: Plenum Press.

Kagan, J., Reznick, J. S., Snidman, N., Gibbons, J., & Johnson, M.O. (1988). Childhood derivatives of inhibition and lack of inhibition to the unfamiliar. *Child Development, 59,* 1580–1589.

Kagan, J., Snidman, N., & Arcus, D. (1993). On the temperamental categories of inhibited and uninhibited children. In K. H. Rubin & J. B. Asendorpf (Eds.), *Social withdrawal, inhibition, and shyness in childhood* (pp. 19–28). Hillsdale, NJ: Erlbaum.

Kendler, K. S., Heath, A. C., Martin, N. G., & Eaves, L. J. (1987). Symptoms of anxiety and symptoms of depression: Same genes, different environments? *Archives of General Psychiatry, 44,* 451–457.

Kendler, K. S., Neale, M. C., Kessler, R. C., Heath, A. C., & Eaves, L. J. (1992). The genetic epidemiology of phobias in women: The interrelationship of agoraphobia, social phobia, situational phobia, and simple phobia. *Archives of General Psychiatry, 49,* 273–281.

Mamries, L. M., O'Connor, C., & Cheek, J. M. (1983, April). *Vocational certainty as a dimension of self-esteem in college women.* Paper presented at the meeting of the Eastern Psychological Association, Philadelphia.

McCroskey, J. C., Daly, J. A., & Sorenson, G. A. (1976). Personality correlates of communication apprehension. *Human Communication Research, 2,* 376–380.

Mills, R. S. L., & Rubin, K. H. (1993). Socialization factors in the development of social withdrawal. In K. H. Rubin & J. B. Asendorpf (Eds.), *Social withdrawal, inhibition, and shyness in childhood* (pp. 117−148). Hillsdale, NJ: Erlbaum.

Moos, R. H. (1986). *Family Environment Scale.* Palo Alto, CA: Consulting Psychologists Press.

Morris, D. P., Soroker, M. A., & Burruss, G. (1954). Follow-up studies of shy, withdrawn children: I. Evaluation of later adjustment. *American Journal of Orthopsychiatry, 24,* 743−754.

Moskowitz, D. S., Ledingham, J. E., & Schwartzman, A. E. (1985). Stability and change in aggression and withdrawal in middle childhood and adolescence. *Journal of Abnormal Psychology, 94,* 30−41.

Olweus, D. (1993). Victimization by peers: Antecedents and long-term outcomes. In K. H. Rubin & J. B. Asendorpf (Eds.), *Social withdrawal, inhibition, and shyness in childhood* (pp. 315−341). Hillsdale, NJ: Erlbaum.

O'Neil, J. M. (1981). Patterns of gender role conflict and strain: Sexism and fear of femininity in men's loves. *Personnel and Guidance Journal, 59,* 203−210.

Parker, G. (1979). Reported parental characteristics of agoraphobics and social phobics. *British Journal of Psychiatry, 135,* 555−560.

Parker, J. G., & Asher, S. R. (1987). Peer relations and later personal adjustment: Are low-accepted children at risk? *Psychological Bulletin, 102,* 289−357.

Plomin, R., & Daniels, D. (1986). Genetics and shyness. In W. H. Jones, J. M. Cheek, & S. R. Briggs (Eds.), *Shyness: Perspectives on research and treatment* (pp. 63−80). New York: Plenum Press.

Plomin, T., & Rowe, D. C. (1979). Genetic and environmental etiology of social behavior in infancy. *Developmental Psychology, 15,* 62−72.

Reznick, J. S. (Ed.). (1989). *Perspectives on behavioral inhibition.* Chicago: University of Chicago Press.

Rothbart, M. K., & Mauro, J. A. (1990). Temperament, behavioral inhibition, and shyness in childhood. In H. Leitenberg (Ed.), *Handbook of social and evaluation anxiety* (pp. 139−160). New York: Plenum Press.

Rubin, K. H., LeMare, L., & Lollis, S. (1990). Social withdrawal in childhood: Developmental pathways to rejection. In S. R. Asher & J. D. Coie (Eds.), *Peer rejection in childhood* (pp. 217−249). New York: Cambridge University Press.

Scarr, S. (1987). Personality and experience: Individual encounters with the world. In J. Aronoff, A. I. Rabin, & R. A. Zucker (Eds.), *The emergence of personality* (pp. 49−78). New York: Springer.

Schneier, F. R., Johnson, J., Hornig, C. D., Liebowitz, M. R., & Weissman, M. M. (1992). Social phobia: Comorbidity and morbidity in an epidemiologic sample. *Archives of General Psychiatry, 49,* 282−288.

Shavelson, R. J., Hubner, J. J., & Stanton, G. C. (1976). Self-concept: Validation of construct interpretation. *Review of Educational Research, 46,* 407−441.

Shedlack, S. M. (1987). *The definition and development of shyness.* Unpublished bachelor's honors thesis, Wellesley College, Wellesley, MA.

Stevenson-Hinde, J., & Hinde, R. A. (1986). Changes in associations between characteristics and interactions. In R. Plomin & J. Dunn (Eds.), *The study of temperament: Changes, continuities, and challenges* (pp. 115−129). Hillsdale, NJ: Erlbaum.

Turner, S. M., Beidel, D. C., & Townsley, R. M. (1990). Social phobia: Relationship to shyness. *Behaviour Research and Therapy, 28,* 297–305.

Vernberg, E. M., Abwender, D. A., Ewell, K. K., & Beery, S. H. (1992). Social anxiety and peer relationships in early adolescence: A prospective analysis. *Journal of Clinical Child Psychology, 21,* 189–196.

PART III

Assessment

CHAPTER NINE

The Clinical Interview

JOHN H. GREIST
KENNETH A. KOBAK
JAMES W. JEFFERSON
DAVID J. KATZELNICK
ROBIN L. CHENE

"Clinical" pertains to "a sick bed or death bed" or clinic (*Webster's New Collegiate Dictionary*, 1956, p. 155). It also differentiates "investigation of disease in the living subject by observation" from controlled experiment (*Webster's New Collegiate Dictionary*, 1956, p. 155).

There are as many interviewing styles as there are interviewers. From casual to compulsive, from nondirective to controlling, from relaxed to pressured, from pole to pole on these and many other dimensions, clinicians interview patients to learn what they can of patients' problems. These clinician characteristics interact with patient characteristics that facilitate or frustrate the interviewing process. This amalgam of fluctuating variables, clinician curiosity, persistence, and good manners yield diagnoses that guide treatment. The clinical interview itself is the cornerstone of effective treatment. Despite rapid advances in understanding psychopathology and pathophysiology and the development of effective treatments, it is still the relationship with a caring clinician that is most precious to the patient.

The sequence of elements in the clinical interview and technical issues such as note taking or its absence are less important than is thoroughness, which permits a comprehensive understanding of the patient. Remembering that the map is not the territory and that our understandings are always incomplete and should be improved by new information, we seek to obtain enough information to permit reasonable predictions regarding prognosis and recommendations about treatment.

Diagnosis of a prominent disorder is often easy. Obtaining information needed for comprehensive management of the patient's problems is often difficult. Few patients approach the ideal of three hours with Osler and three hours with Freud. Many clinical interviews are constrained by "the therapeutic hour," however defined. Seeing patients over time permits more complete history taking. Certain information may be obtained through questionnaires or computer interviews that patients complete before or after the clinical interview, but good clinical interviewing takes time.

INTERVIEW TECHNIQUE

Clinicians must be aware of the distress that many social phobic individuals experience in coming to their first interview with a new clinician. For a sizable proportion, their discomfort is so great that they cancel or simply fail to attend that first appointment although they want help desperately. Others may prime themselves with alcohol or tranquilizers.

By contrast, the setting in which the clinical interview is conducted is not of critical importance. Outpatient office, clinic consultation room, or hospital ward are all satisfactory. It may be better to have more space rather than less between patient and interviewer because the social comfort distance may be greater for those with social phobia. In a similar vein, muted lighting may help individuals with social phobia feel less "in the spotlight." More important than the physical setting is assurance that there will be no disturbances (e.g., telephone calls, knocks on the door) during the interview and that ample time is allotted. Time is a nonrenewable resource, and "talk time" is expensive. Ideally, we would gather necessary data in a minimum of time. But arbitrary time limits in interviewing are an illusory advantage. Missing critical data and failing to establish rapport and gain the patient's trust lead to less complete understanding of the patient's problems and the best approaches to alleviating them. Although all clinicians are pressed for time, the best clinicians leave patients feeling that the interview has been unhurried and that the patient has been the center of the clinician's undivided attention.

Being nonjudgmental is never more important than when interviewing social phobic individuals because they are exquisitely sensitive and fear they are always being judged. Time and experience have shown the merit of emphasizing open-ended questions at the beginning of the clinical interview: "What is the nature of your difficulty?"; "What problem are you having?"; or, more simply, "How can I help?" Such nondirective inquiry leaves patients free to lead in whatever directions they wish and conveys respect for the patients' ability to communicate as a partner in the process of defining their disorder. Patients are, after all, experts on their distress, and without their collaboration, clinicians cannot come to a proper appreciation of the patient's disorder in all its contexts. Questions beginning with the words "what," "when," "where," "who," and "how" yield large returns. Those beginning with "why" have an immediate pejorative connotation that impedes disclosure.

Sometimes, however, open-ended questions are difficult for the social phobic individual because such questions keep them "on stage" longer. Balancing the open-ended ideal is the need to gather information for decision making. Changing interviewing technique to maximize data acquisition is the practical ideal in all clinical interviewing. A tactical retreat to closed questions can be reversed as patient comfort increases, and advances can then be made into more open-ended discussion, which is itself therapeutic.

The *chief complaint* should be recorded in the patient's own words and used as a referent in other questions. Social phobic individuals' chief complaints range widely but usually identify essential elements of their disorder: "I've been shy as long as I can remember." "I'm always nervous around people." "I blush all the time and it's embarrassing." "I avoid things I'd like to do in order to be comfortable." "Speaking in front of others is a terrible ordeal for me."

The *history of present illness* follows naturally and logically from the chief complaint. It is usually a mistake to bypass present illness and move directly from the chief complaint to other elements of the interview that, while important to the clinician's overall understanding, are less obviously so to the patient. The history of present illness should also proceed from open questions to more closed ones. When did the disorder begin? What has been its course (continuous, waxing and waning without remission, remissions and relapses, etc.)? What subjective symptoms and objective signs of distress does the patient notice and in what temporal sequence? How frequently do these symptoms and signs occur? What is their severity? What are the circumstances with which symptoms are associated? Usual situations are *social* interactions or encounters involving *public* speaking, performance (e.g., reading, playing a musical instrument, singing, acting), eating, writing or voiding. What has the patient found that aggravates and alleviates his or her symptoms and signs?

One chart entry summary of present illness recorded:

> Social anxiety first noticed in grade school worsened in high school and has persisted to the present, interfering with functioning and causing distress in work and nonfamily social interactions. The course has been continuous, with a constant low-grade anticipatory anxiety leading to avoidance of most social encounters where avoidance is possible. "Public speaking" involving demonstrations to groups of more than five of tasks

George performs alone every day is always avoided, if necessary by feigning illness. Even "teaching" an apprentice how to set up his machine induces distressing anticipatory anxiety if announced before the event. Symptoms and signs predictably emerge in these occupational situations and include increased heart rate, flushing with sweating, quavering voice, trembling of hands, blocking of thoughts, and, in anticipation of such encounters, nausea, sometimes progressing to vomiting, urinary frequency, and sometimes diarrhea. Symptoms and signs accumulate in proportion to the duration of interpersonal interactions up to an hour, but in an interaction that continued for lengthy periods (as when he trained an apprentice), they diminished but never abated over the weeks he worked with the apprentice. George has refused to serve in church or "stand up" in his brother's wedding but has usually attended close family functions unless "outsiders" are invited. He does not join colleagues for meals at work or after work but does exchange dinners with a couple he and his wife have known since high school. George is particularly perturbed because he missed the recognition ceremony when their son was the distinguished student in his sophomore class in high school. George has difficulty dealing with clerks in stores and would find it virtually impossible to return a purchase he found unsatisfactory. He prefers not to write in public for fear his hand will shake but was able to sign their mortgage 20 years ago. His wife does all of their banking while George reconciles their checking account in the privacy of their home. George's anxiety is increased by social exposures and diminished by avoiding them. He did find that prolonged contact with an apprentice led to reduction of discomfort but feels the length of time required and his distress during that time are too great to use this approach unless his work requires it. He thought about quitting his job at the time he was assigned the apprentice but would have had to seek another job which seemed even more frightening. George has found that alcohol diminished but did not relieve his anxiety and because it impaired his coordination, was a danger in his work and was also unacceptable to his wife.

Ideally, data collection would include all of the elements described by McNeil, Ries, and Turk and by Elting and Hope (Chapters 10 and 11, this volume), but, at a minimum, the clinician should understand the patient's salient thoughts, feelings, and behaviors in social settings. Across the domains of the history of present illness, past medical and psychiatric history, family history, social and marital history, educational history, occupational history, medical review of systems, and mental status examination, the focus should be on gathering data to permit a comprehensive psychiatric diagnosis according to Axes I–V of the fourth edition of the *Diagnostic and Statistical Manual of Mental Disorders* (DSM-IV; American Psychiatric Association, 1994) and to permit a thoughtful differential diagnosis between social phobia, simple phobia, and panic disorder alone and with agoraphobia. Common comorbid conditions, including depression and substance abuse, should also be carefully examined. Each of these domains contributes important elements to the comprehensive picture of a patient suffering from social phobia.

Working along a continuum from open-ended to closed questions, some interviewers proceed with tight rein through each topic while others maintain a looser rein but guide the patient along important interview pathways. Family, social, marital, educational, and occupational histories should yield relevant information about family patterns of social anxiety and specific information about the patient's social functioning in important areas where social anxiety often emerges. A review of the patient's early developmental history regarding shyness, indicators of behavioral inhibition, and possible events preceding the onset of social phobia is also appropriate in developing a comprehensive understanding of the patient's problems.

The patient's family history chart entry noted:

> Family history is positive for excessive social anxiety in his father, a paternal uncle, and in his younger sister, Henrietta, three years his junior. George met his wife-to-be in kindergarten and except for his family, has a very small group of acquaintances in addition to one couple whom he met through his wife's close friendship with the wife of that pair. George never dated anyone but his wife and their marriage has been satisfactory, although his wife would like a larger social network but "accepts" George as he is. None of their three children, ages 23, 21, and 15, has excessive social anxiety, and each has been academically and socially successful. George made As and Bs throughout high school, where he carefully maneuvered to avoid classes in which oral presentations were required. Although several teachers encouraged him to consider college, he felt the demands for social interactions would be more than he could tolerate and chose, instead, to work in a machine shop. He apprenticed in one shop and worked there until it closed, transferring to his present employment 15 years ago. He has been an "excellent" employee with attendance marred only by absences associated with group situations he could anticipate and avoid through feigned illness.[1]

STRUCTURED DATA GATHERING

Information should be gathered both about the specific *target problems* the patient experiences and through a *standardized assessment* to permit

---

[1] Because four of this chapter's five authors are physicians, we describe clinical interviewing from a medical tradition and perspective but recognize that clinicians from different training backgrounds may use different interview formats.

comparisons of the patient's distress and dysfunction with that of other social phobic individuals.

The target problem approach is straightforward and should identify issues that are of greatest importance to the patient and that may become targets of treatment.

> "What is the major problem or difficulty for which you are seeking help?"
> "How does _____ show up?"
> "How do you act or behave differently when _____ occurs?"
> "How often does _____ occur?"
> "On a scale of 0–10, where 0 is no distress and 10 the worst imaginable distress, what is the worst distress you have experienced because of _____ ?"
> "What is the average level of distress you experienced because of _____ during the last week?"
> "How would you be or act differently if _____ were not a problem for you?"

The target symptom approach defines issues of greatest importance to the patient and helps the clinician focus on problems for which the patient most wants help.

PATIENT SELF-REPORT QUESTIONNAIRES

The first and simplest standardized assessment of social phobia was the Fear Questionnaire developed by Marks and Matthews (1979). This 15-item questionnaire has five items for agoraphobia, five for blood–injury phobia, and five for social phobia. The Fear Questionnaire has been evaluated in several anxiety disorder populations and recently was again found to be an accurate indicator of severity of social phobia symptoms (Cottraux, Bouvard, & Messy, 1987; Cox, Swinson, & Shaw, 1991). A full review of self-report assessment of social phobia is provided by McNeil and colleagues (Chapter 10, this volume).

SEMISTRUCTURED CLINICAL INTERVIEWS

Semistructured interviews provide a framework for conducting the interview while allowing the clinician the flexibility of going beyond the structure in order to obtain more complete information. This flexibility permits the clinician to draw upon his or her clinical experience in order to adapt the questions to fit the patient's language, expand the questions to obtain further information, challenge the patient's inconsistencies, make inferences as to whether the patient's account of symptoms matches the intent of specified diagnostic criteria, and use clinical judgment in evaluating symptom severity (Spitzer, Williams, Gibbon, & First, 1992).

Semistructured clinical interviews can be conceptualized as falling under one of two broad categories: those used for diagnostic purposes and those used to quantify symptom severity. Semistructured diagnostic instruments include the Schedule for Affective Disorders and Schizophrenia (SADS; Endicott & Spitzer, 1978), the SADS—Lifetime Anxiety version (SADS-LA; Mannuzza, Fyer, Klein, & Endicott, 1986), the Structured Clinical Interview for DSM-III-R (SCID; Spitzer et al., 1992; Williams et al., 1992), and the Anxiety Disorders Interview Schedule—Revised (ADIS-R; Di Nardo & Barlow, 1988; Di Nardo, Moras, Barlow, Rapee, & Brown, 1993). Symptom rating scales include the Brief Social Phobia Scale (BSPS; Davidson et al., 1991) and the Liebowitz Social Anxiety Scale (LSAS; Liebowitz, 1987). What follows is a overview of the diagnostic interviews, followed by a review of the symptom rating scales for social phobia.

Diagnostic Interviews

The SADS (Endicott & Spitzer, 1978) was developed prior to the third edition of the *Diagnostic and Statistical Manual of Mental Disorders* (DSM-III; American Psychiatric Association, 1980) in order to increase the reliability of diagnostic evaluations. It was developed in conjunction with the Research Diagnostic Criteria (RDC; Spitzer, Endicott, & Robins, 1978) in an attempt to standardize both the information obtained in determining a diagnosis (information variance) and the inclusion and exclusion criteria used in determining diagnoses (criterion variance) (Endicott & Spitzer, 1978). While it has been criticized as not providing sufficient detail for the differential diagnosis of anxiety disorders (Di Nardo, O'Brien, Barlow, Woddell, & Blanchard, 1983), the authors report correlation coefficients of $r = .67$ for test–retest and $r = .94$ for interrater reliability for the Anxiety Summary scale scores (Endicott & Spitzer, 1978). Because the SADS provides diagnoses for a wide range of disorders, the administration time is rather lengthy (1½ to 2 hours). As with all diagnostic interviews, limiting features include the need for training in its administration and requiring administration by clinicians experienced in evaluating psychopathology and in clinical interviewing (Endicott & Spitzer, 1978).

With the development of DSM-III and of its revised version, DSM-III-R (American Psychiatric Association, 1987), came well-defined inclusion and exclusion criteria, greatly improving diagnostic reliability. The

SCID (Spitzer et al., 1992; Williams et al., 1992) was developed to provide a standardized procedure for determining diagnoses according to DSM-III-R criteria. Unlike the SADS, diagnostic algorithms are built into the structure of the interview, with branching logic to pass over items of no diagnostic significance (Spitzer et al., 1992). In addition, the interview consists of separate modules for different classes of disorders—such as anxiety disorders, mood disorders, and so on—thus allowing for the administration of only those modules of interest. Agreement between raters for the combined sample for social phobia, expressed in terms of kappa, were .47 for current diagnosis and .57 for lifetime diagnosis. Generally, kappas of .7 or above indicate good agreement, kappas ranging from .5 to .7 indicate fair agreement, and kappas below .5 are poor (Williams et al., 1992). As discussed by Di Nardo et al. (1993), the relatively low kappas might be attributed to the use of a heterogeneous sample. A sample consisting solely of patients with anxiety disorders would provide the potential for a larger kappa value (Di Nardo et al., 1993). As with the SADS, the SCID requires extensive training on both its administration and on the intent of the various diagnostic criteria (Williams et al., 1992).

The SADS-LA (Mannuzza et al., 1986) is a modification of the Lifetime version of the SADS, designed specifically for the lifetime diagnosis of anxiety disorders. It allows for diagnoses to be made according to RDC, DSM-III, and DSM-III-R criteria. Its emphasis is on the lifetime sequence and interrelationship between various symptoms and disorders (Mannuzza et al., 1986). It also provides a severity rating for 10 social phobia situations, based on both fear and avoidance. Other improvements include items helping with the conceptual differentiation between the anxiety disorders, provisions for identifying subthreshold symptoms and syndromes, codes for identifying episodes limited to concurrent affective disorder, and items aimed at clarifying the nature and course of generalized anxiety disorder. Kappas for diagnostic agreement are .68 for current and .71 for lifetime social phobia (Mannuzza et al., 1986); kappas for agreement on level of individual symptom severity range from .36 to .61 (Fyer et al., 1989). A concurrent diagnosis of major depression was found to slightly reduce reliability for lifetime diagnosis of social phobia (kappa = .82 without, .63 with comorbid major depression), although this difference was not significant.

The ADIS-R (Di Nardo et al., 1993) is a revision of the Anxiety Disorders Interview Schedule (Di Nardo et al., 1983), adapted for DSM-III-R criteria. In addition to providing diagnoses of current DSM-III-R anxiety and selected affective disorders, it provides detailed information on clinically relevant aspects of the disorder, such as situational and cognitive cues for anxiety, intensity of anxiety, extent of avoidance, precipitating events, and history of the problem (Di Nardo et al., 1983). Hamilton Anxiety

(Hamilton, 1959) and Depression (Hamilton, 1960) items are embedded within the interview, yielding scores on both of these scales. Each diagnosis is also given a severity rating, based on level of distress and functional impairment. Kappas for social phobia as a principal and additional diagnosis were .79 and .66, respectively (Di Nardo et al., 1993). As with the SADS and SCID, clinical judgment is required in determining ratings. As a result, the authors suggest the scale only be administered by experienced clinicians familiar with DSM-III-R criteria (Di Nardo et al., 1983, 1993). Administration time is approximately 90 minutes.

All of these interviews are being (or will be) updated to shift from DSM-III-R to DSM-IV and will need further study of reliability and validity at that time (even if the small extent of the changes in criteria should make this a relatively straightforward issue).

Symptom Rating Scales

The LSAS (Liebowitz, 1987) was the first clinician-administered scale to evaluate the wide range of social situations that social phobics have difficulty with. The scale contains 24 items, 13 for performance situations and 11 for social interaction situations (see Figure 9.1). Each item is rated separately for fear (0 = none, 1 = mild, 2 = moderate, 3 = severe) and for avoidance behavior (0 = never [0%], 1 = occasionally [10%], 2 = often [33–67%], 3 = usually [67–100%]). Thus, in addition to an overall severity rating, the scale yields scores on four subscales: performance fear, performance avoidance, social fear, and social avoidance. The scale has demonstrated good clinical utility (Holt, Heimberg, & Hope, 1992) and criterion validity (Brown, Heimberg, & Juster, 1995; Holt, Heimberg, Hope, & Liebowitz, 1992). As an outcome measure, it has been used successfully in several pharmacological trials for social phobia (Davidson et al., 1993; Liebowitz et al., 1992; Munjack et al., 1991; Reich & Yates, 1988), as well as in studies of cognitive-behavioral treatment (Brown et al., 1995). As designed by its author, the LSAS requires clinician judgment for completing ratings, and it is therefore not intended for use as a self-report measure. However, its wording is similar to that of a self-rated instrument, and it has in fact been used in this manner in pharmacological research (R. Katz, personal communication, November 16, 1992). A study on the construct validity of the scale found that the two-factor solution (performance/social) was not the best fit for the data; rather, items tended to group into four categories: interaction with strangers, formal performance/center of attention, eating and drinking while being observed, and behavior in parties and other informal situations (Slavkin, Holt, Heimberg, Jaccard, & Liebowitz, 1990). Other research with the scale found performance fear more highly

	Fear or anxiety	Avoidance
	0 = none	0 = never (0%)
	1 = mild	1 = occasionally (10%)
	2 = moderate	2 = often (33–67%)
	3 = severe	3 = usually (67–100%)

1 Telephone in public (P) _____

2 Participating in small groups (P) _____

3 Eating in public places (P) _____

4 Drinking with others in public places (P) _____

5 Talking to people in authority (S) _____

6 Acting, performing, or giving a talk in front
   of an audience (P) _____

7 Going to a party (S) _____

8 Working while being observed (P) _____

9 Writing while being observed (P) _____

10 Calling someone you don't know very
   well (S) _____

11 Talking with people you don't know very
   well (S) _____

12 Meeting strangers (S) _____

13 Urinating in a public bathroom (P) _____

14 Entering a room when others are already
   seated (P) _____

15 Being the center of attention (S) _____

16 Speaking up at a meeting (P) _____

17 Taking a test (P) _____

18 Expressing a disagreement or disapproval
   to people you don't know very well (S) _____

19 Looking at people you don't know very well
   in the eyes (S) _____

20 Giving a report to a group (P) _____

21 Trying to pick up someone (P) _____

22 Returning goods to a store (S) _____

23 Giving a party (S) _____

24 Resisting a high-pressure salesperson (S) _____

Total score _____

Performance (P) anxiety subscore _____

Social (S) anxiety subscore _____

FIGURE 9.1. The Liebowitz Social Anxiety Scale. From Liebowitz (1987, p. 152). Copyright 1987 by S. Karger. Reprinted by permission.

correlated with self-reported fear of being scrutinized than with interactional fear, while the reverse was true for the social fear score (Heimberg, Mueller, Holt, Hope, & Liebowitz, 1992).

The BSPS (Davidson et al., 1991) was developed to provide a brief (11-item) observer-rated assessment of symptom severity, to measure changes due to treatment over time, and to detect differences between active and inactive treatments (Davidson et al., 1991). The scale consists of 7 items measuring specific phobia situations from the perspective of both fear and avoidance and 4 additional items evaluating physiological symptoms experienced while in contact with or thinking about the phobia situation (see Figure 9.2). Thus, the scale yields three subscales (fear, avoidance, and physiologic), as well as a total score.

Instructions: It is recommended that the interviewer give a copy of this scale to the client for the interview. The time period will cover the previous week, unless otherwise specified (e.g., at the initial evaluation interview, when it could be the previous month).

Part I. (Fear/Avoidance)
How much do you fear and avoid the following situations? Please give separate ratings for fear and avoidance.

	Fear rating	Avoidance rating
	0 = None	0 = Never
	1 = Mild	1 = Rare
	2 = Moderate	2 = Sometimes
	3 = Severe	3 = Frequent
	4 = Extreme	4 = Always
	Fear (F)	Avoidance (A)
1. Speaking in public or in front of others	_____	_____
2. Talking to people in authority	_____	_____
3. Talking to strangers	_____	_____
4. Being embarrassed or humiliated	_____	_____
5. Being criticized	_____	_____
6. Social gatherings	_____	_____
7. Doing something while being watched (this does not include speaking)	_____	_____

Part II. Physiologic (P)
When you are in a situation that involves contact with other people, or when you are thinking about such a situation, do you experience the following symptoms?

	0 = None
	1 = Mild
	2 = Moderate
	3 = Severe
	4 = Extreme
8. Blushing	_____
9. Palpitations	_____
10. Trembling	_____
11. Sweating	_____

_____ Total scores   F =   A =   P =   Total =

FIGURE 9.2. The Brief Social Phobia Scale. From Davidson et al. (1991, *Journal of Clinical Psychiatry, 52*, p. 49). Copyright 1991 by Physicians Postgraduate Press. Reprinted by permission.

The authors recommend the scale be used after a clinical or semistructured interview, after which the scale is administered in a checklist fashion, with the patient looking at a copy of the scale. As with the LSAS, the wording is similar to that of a self-report instrument, although no published reports of its use in this manner have been found. The first seven items cover much of the same territory as the Fear Questionnaire (Marks & Mathews, 1979), with two items worded identically.

In a small ($N = 17$) validation study of the scale, the authors report good test–retest ($r = .986$) (time interval not reported) and interrater ($r = .998$) reliability (Davidson et al., 1991). Internal consistency (Cronbach's alpha) of the overall scale was .86, with internal consistencies of .78, .86, and .34 for the fear, avoidance, and physiologic subscales, respectively. The scale possesses good concurrent validity, demonstrating high correlations with both the clinician-administered LSAS ($r = .761$) and with several self-report measures of social phobia, such as the Fear Questionnaire (Marks & Mathews, 1979) ($r = .624$), the Fear of Negative Evaluation Scale (Watson & Friend, 1969) ($r = .766$), and the Social Phobia and Anxiety Inventory (Turner, Beidel, Dancu, & Stanley, 1989) ($r = .863$). Finally, the scale was able to detect both within- and between-treatment changes in a double-blind study of clonazepam and placebo (Davidson et al., 1993).

Reliable standardized symptom severity scales are of critical importance in the conduct of controlled research trials. They are also of great benefit to clinicians and patients as they work together to assess the initial intensity and subsequent change in severity and frequency of distress and dysfunction in response to treatment. However, there is a substantial time cost for clinicians to administer these standardized measures, and because most clinicians are not compensated for this time, these measures are little used despite their great merit.

Each of these measures has been programmed for direct patient-computer administration. Careful evaluations of these and other severity and change measures usually administered by clinicians have found that patients gave ratings to the computer that correlate highly with ratings obtained by skilled human interviewers. For example, in a recent crossover study of sertraline in social phobia (Katzelnick, Greist, Jefferson, & Kobak, 1994), computer- and clinician-administered versions of the LSAS were found to be highly correlated, $r = .89$, with no significant difference found between the forms. For the Hamilton Depression Rating Scale (Kobak, Reynolds, Rosenfeld, & Greist, 1990), correlations with the clinician-administered version of the scale were .96, and the mean score difference between the two forms for the total sample was nonsignificant. The scale also demonstrated high internal consistency (.91) and test–retest reliability (.94). Computer-administered versions of the Yale–Brown Obsessive Compulsive Scale (Rosenfeld, Dar, Anderson, Kobak, & Greist, 1992) and the Hamilton Anxiety Scale (Kobak, Reynolds, & Greist, 1993) have also yielded high correlations (.88 and .92, respectively) when compared with clinician ratings.

It is probably a poor use of clinicians to have them do repetitive tasks that computers do as well and at a much lower cost. The computer also ensures perfect "interrater" reliability and is available at all hours and in any setting where a microcomputer is installed. There is evidence that, as patients are asked to disclose sensitive information, they often find it easier to do so in the computer interview (Greist et al., 1974; Greist & Klein, 1980; Kobak, Reynolds, & Greist, 1994; Lucas, Mullins, Luna, & McInroy, 1977). Patients want their clinician to have sensitive information but sometimes have difficulty disclosing it directly to another person. Social phobic persons may have even more reticence in face-to-face interviews than do non–social phobics. For example, in a recent study utilizing both clinician- and computer-administered versions of several social phobia rating scales, the percentage of patients with social phobia who preferred being interviewed by the computer (64%) was significantly greater than either the percentage of those who preferred being interviewed by the clinician (9%) or the percentage of those who expressed no preference (28%). This is in contrast to our previous findings in patients with affective and other anxiety disorders, where a significantly greater percentage of patients (52%) preferred the clinician to the computer (6%).

The computer interview moves at the patient's pace and does not boss the patient or appear impatient. Clinicians are provided with symptom scores and histograms showing change over time, which they may chose to share with the patient. These change measures permit clinician and patient to review progress and to emphasize effective measures while eliminating or minimizing less-beneficial approaches. While some may object to the intrusion of the computer into clinical interviewing, the use of inhuman devices is not inhumane. Two "heads" are better than one, and the computer's utterly reliable systematic coverage of important dimensions frees clinicians from an onerous task, permitting them to emphasize things that they do uniquely well.[2]

Other Sources of Information

The *medical review of systems* will probably identify physiological manifestations of anxiety occurring in social situations or in anticipation of them as

---

[2] Computerized evaluations are a particular interest of our group and, although of potentially great value to the field, have not been widely used at this time.

well as any other organ system symptoms and signs. One needs to rule out competing explanations, such as comorbid Axis III disorders (e.g., Parkinson's) or the use of caffeine, stimulants, cocaine, or alcohol.

Observations of behavior often provide a wealth of specific information relevant to the patient's social phobia. Is the patient's gaze averted when meeting the clinician? Are the patient's eyes hidden behind hair or hand ("peek-a-boo" visage)? Are eyelids fluttering not to enrapture the clinician but to permit the patient a partial barrier behind which to hide? Does the patient blush or flush? Is the hand the clinician shakes moist? Is perspiration visible? Is tremor apparent in the outstretched hand? Is the patient's voice high pitched, quavering, or breaking? Does the patient appear tense and frightened? Is anxiety so severe that thoughts are blocked? It is always appropriate to ask how the patient is feeling during the interview and to inquire about specific symptoms that are perceived only by the patient. Thus, a positive response to a question about rapid or irregular heart beat might lead to palpation of the pulse both to measure rate and to search for irregularities of rhythm.

Specific questions should cover common social phobia problems involving public speaking, performing in public, eating with others, writing in front of others, and using public bathrooms—if they have not been covered already. The LSAS provides a good guide to specific social phobia problem areas. Asking whether patients have only one or a few areas of social discomfort or feel uncomfortable most or all of the time helps distinguish between discrete and generalized forms of social phobia. The overarching themes of embarrassment and/or humiliation, or synonyms such as feeling "dumb" or "stupid," pervade all kinds of social phobia. DSM-IV criteria for social phobia are found in Table 1.1 in Heckelman and Schneier (Chapter 1, p. 9, this volume).

It is also useful, from both a diagnostic and treatment perspective, to assess the extent of avoidance behavior associated with the illness, as well as the degree of impairment the illness causes in the person's life.

One clue to social phobia in its various forms is a common social awkwardness in conversation that makes the clinician uncomfortable. This communication dissonance is socially discomfiting for the interviewer rather than saddening as would be the case in the presence of a depressed patient, or bizarre and eerie, as would be the case with a psychotic patient.

The clinical interview should yield a clear understanding of the patient's problems, which are encapsulated in a formal diagnosis. The clinical interview should also determine targets for treatment and include a standardized measure of severity to permit examination of change in response to treatment. These goals are seldom reached in a single session, but the careful acquisition of information about the patient through a series of clinical interviews forms the foundation for treatment and the relationship through which effective treatment is provided.

REFERENCES

American Psychiatric Association. (1980). *Diagnostic and statistical manual of mental disorders* (3rd ed.). Washington, DC: Author.

American Psychiatric Association. (1987). *Diagnostic and statistical manual of mental disorders* (3rd ed., rev.). Washington, DC: Author.

American Psychiatric Association. (1994). *Diagnostic and statistical manual of mental disorders* (4th ed.). Washington, DC: Author.

Brown, E. J., Heimberg, R. G., & Juster, H. R. (1995). Social phobia subtype and avoidant personality disorder: Effect on severity of social phobia, impairment, and outcome of cognitive-behavioral treatment. *Behavior Therapy, 26,* 467–486.

Cottraux, J., Bouvard, M., & Messy, P. (1987). Validation and factor analysis of a phobia scale: The French version of the Marks–Mathews Fear Questionnaire [in French; English abstract]. *Encephale, 13,* 23–29.

Cox, B. J., Swinson, R. P., & Shaw, B. F. (1991). Value of the Fear Questionnaire in differentiating agoraphobia and social phobia. *British Journal of Psychiatry, 159,* 842–845.

Davidson, J. R. T., Potts, N. L. S., Richichi, E. A., Krishnan, R., Ford, S. M., Smith, R. D., & Wilson, W. (1991). The Brief Social Phobia Scale. *Journal of Clinical Psychiatry, 52,* 48–51.

Davidson, J. R. T., Potts, N. L. S., Richichi, E. A., Krishnan, R. R., Ford, S. M., Smith, R. D., & Wilson, W. (1993). The treatment of social phobia with clonazepam and placebo. *Journal of Clinical Psychopharmacology, 13,* 423–428.

Di Nardo, P. A., & Barlow, D. H. (1988). *The Anxiety Disorders Interview Schedule—Revised (ADIS-R).* Albany, NY: Graywind.

Di Nardo, P. A., Moras, K., Barlow, D. H., Rapee, R. M., & Brown, T. A. (1993). Reliability of DSM-III-R anxiety disorder categories: Using the Anxiety Disorders Interview Schedule-Revised (ADIS-R). *Archives of General Psychiatry, 50,* 251–256.

Di Nardo, P. A., O'Brien, G. T., Barlow, D. H., Waddell, M. T., & Blanchard, E. B. (1983). Reliability of DSM-III anxiety disorder categories using a new structured interview. *Archives of General Psychiatry, 40,* 1070–1074.

Endicott, J., & Spitzer, R. L. (1978). A diagnostic interview: The Schedule for Affective Disorders and Schizophrenia. *Archives of General Psychiatry, 35,* 837–844.

Fyer, A. J., Mannuzza, S., Martin, L., Gallops, M. S., Endicott, J., Schleyer, B., Gorman, J. M., Liebowitz, M. R., & Klein, D. F. (1989). Reliability of anxiety assessment: II. Symptom agreement. *Archives of General Psychiatry, 46,* 1102–1110.

Greist, J. H., Gustafson, D. H., Stauss, F. F., Rowse, G. L., Laughren, T. P., & Chiles, J. A. (1974). Suicide risk prediction: A new approach. *Life Threatening Behavior, 4,* 212–223.

Greist, J. H., & Klein, M. H. (1980). Computer programs for patients, clinicians, and researchers in psychiatry. In J. B. Sidowski, J. H. Johnson, & T. A. Williams (Eds.), *Technology in mental health care delivery systems* (pp. 161–182). Norwood, NJ: Ablex.

Hamilton, M. (1959). The assessment of anxiety states by rating. *British Journal of Medical Psychology, 32,* 50–55.

Hamilton, M. (1960). A rating scale for depression. *Journal of Neurology, Neurosurgery, and Psychiatry, 23,* 56–62.

Heimberg, R. G., Mueller, G. P., Holt, C. S., Hope, D. A., & Liebowitz, M.R. (1992). Assessment of anxiety in social interaction and being observed by others: The Social Interaction Anxiety Scale and the Social Phobia Scale. *Behavior Therapy, 23,* 57–73.

Holt, C. S., Heimberg, R. G., & Hope, D. A., (1992). Avoidant personality disorder and the generalized subtype of social phobia. *Journal of Abnormal Psychology, 101,* 318–325.

Holt, C. S., Heimberg, R. G., Hope, D. A., & Liebowitz, M. R. (1992). Situational domains of social phobia. *Journal of Anxiety Disorders, 6,* 63–77.

Katzelnick, D. J., Greist, J. H., Jefferson, J. W., & Kobak, K. A. (1994, May). *Sertraline in social phobia: A double-blind placebo-controlled crossover pilot study.* Paper presented at the annual meeting of the American Psychiatric Association, Philadelphia.

Kobak, K. A., Reynolds, W. R., & Greist, J. H. (1993). Development and validation of a computer administered Hamilton Anxiety Scale. *Psychological Assessment: A Journal of Consulting and Clinical Psychology, 5,* 487–492.

Kobak, K. A., Reynolds, W. R., & Greist, J. H. (1994). Computerized assessment of depression and anxiety: Respondent evaluation and satisfaction. *Journal of Personality Assessment, 63,* 173–180.

Kobak, K. A., Reynolds, W. M., Rosenfeld, R., & Greist, J. H. (1990). Development and validation of a computer-administered version of the Hamilton Depression Rating Scale. *Psychological Assessment: A Journal of Consulting and Clinical Psychology, 2,* 56–63.

Liebowitz, M. R. (1987). Social phobia. *Modern Problems of Pharmacopsychiatry, 22,* 141–173.

Liebowitz, M. R., Schneier, F., Campeas, R., Hollander, E., Hatterer, J., Fyer, A., Gorman, J. M., Papp, L., Davies, S., Gully, R., & Klein, D. F. (1992). Phenelzine vs atenolol in social phobia: A placebo-controlled comparison. *Archives of General Psychiatry, 49,* 290–300.

Lucas, R. W., Mullins, P. J., Luna, C. B., & McInroy, D. C. (1977). Psychiatrists and a computer as interrogators of patients with alcohol-related illnesses: A comparison. *British Journal of Psychiatry, 131,* 160–167.

Mannuzza, S., Fyer, A. J., Klein, D. F., & Endicott, J. (1986). Schedule for Affective Disorders and Schizophrenia—Lifetime version (modified for the study of anxiety disorders): Rationale and conceptual development. *Journal of Psychiatric Research, 20,* 317–325.

Marks, I. M., & Mathews, A. M. (1979). Brief standard self-rating for phobic patients. *Behaviour Research and Therapy, 17,* 263–267.

Munjack, D. J., Bruns, J., Baltazar, P. L., Brown, R., Leonard, M., Nagy, R., Koek, R., Crocker, B., & Schafer, S. (1991). A pilot study of buspirone in the treatment of social phobia. *Journal of Anxiety Disorders, 5,* 87–98.

Reich, J., & Yates, W. (1988). A pilot study of the treatment of social phobia with alprazolam. *American Journal of Psychiatry, 145,* 590–594.

Rosenfeld, R., Dar, R., Anderson, D., Kobak, K. A., & Greist, J. H. (1992). A computer administered version of the Yale–Brown Obsessive Compulsive Scale. *Psychological Assessment: A Journal of Consulting and Clinical Psychology, 4,* 329–332.

Slavkin, S. L., Holt, C. S., Heimberg, R. G., Jaccard, J. J., & Liebowitz, M. R. (1990, November). *The Liebowitz Social Phobia Scale: An exploratory analysis of construct validity.* Paper presented at the annual meeting of the Association for Advancement of Behavior Therapy, Washington, DC.

Spitzer, R. L., Endicott, J., & Robins, E. (1978). Research diagnostic criteria: Rationale and reliability. *Archives of General Psychiatry, 35,* 773–782.

Spitzer, R. L., Williams, J. B., Gibbon, M., & First, M. B. (1992). Structured Clinical Interview for DSM-III-R (SCID): History, rationale, and description. *Archives of General Psychiatry, 49,* 624–629.

Turner, S. M., Beidel, D. C., Dancu, C. V., & Stanley, M. A. (1989). An empirically derived inventory to measure social fears and anxiety: The Social Phobia and Anxiety Inventory. *Psychological Assessment: A Journal of Consulting and Clinical Psychology, 1,* 35–40.

Watson, D., & Friend, R. (1969). Measurement of social-evaluative anxiety. *Journal of Consulting and Clinical Psychology, 33,* 448–457.

Webster's new collegiate dictionary (2nd ed.). (1956). Springfield, MA: G. & C. Merriam.

Williams, J. B. W., Gibbon, M., First, M. B., Spitzer, R. L., Davies, M., Borus, J., Howes, M. H., Kane, J., Pope, H. G., Rounsaville, B., & Wittchen, H. (1992). Structured Clinical Interview for DSM-III-R (SCID): Multisite test–retest reliability. *Archives of General Psychiatry, 49,* 630–636.

CHAPTER TEN

Behavioral Assessment: Self-Report, Physiology, and Overt Behavior

DANIEL W. McNEIL

BARRY J. RIES

CYNTHIA L. TURK

Contemporary behavioral assessment of social phobia, in its ideal form, is multimodal and multimethod (Lang, 1968; 1993). In devising assessment strategies and evaluating the need for new and improved evaluation instruments, it is important to work from a theoretical perspective. Both historically (Lang, 1968) and currently (Lang, 1993; Miller & Kozak, 1993), the three-response-systems approach (i.e., overt behavior, physiology, and self-report) has been embraced. The three-response-systems approach has had a tremendous impact on assessment, not only with social phobia and other anxiety disorders but also with other emotional problems as well. Although this approach has been criticized, both methodologically and conceptually (e.g., Eifert & Wilson, 1991), it is a useful framework around which to organize this chapter. Comprehensive behavioral assessment of social phobia should therefore include attention to each of the three response modes: self-reports (and reports of others), overt behavior, and physiology. This chapter will not include references to self-reports of thinking or self-statements, or measures reflecting processing of information, as these areas are covered by Elting and Hope (Chapter 11, this volume). Additionally, since Albano, DiBartolo, Heimberg, and Barlow (Chapter 16, this volume) address social phobia among children, this chapter will focus on adult assessment.

It must be recognized that there is relative independence among the three response systems. Typically, low correlations have been found among overt behavior, physiology, and self-reports in three-systems research (e.g., Rachman & Hodgson, 1974). The lack of concordance, however, may often be due to methodological inadequacies (Cone, 1979). Rather than being a problem, the independence of these systems may reflect important individual differences in response manifestation.

This chapter is also written from the theoretical position that social anxieties (and other anxieties and fears as well) exist along a continuum, ranging from no anxiety, or fearlessness (cf. Rachman, 1990), to social phobia (cf. McNeil, Turk, & Ries, 1994). One implication is that any distinctions between social anxiety and social phobia are quantitative rather than qualitative. It is important for assessment strategies to be able to detect whether individuals meet standard criteria for diagnosis of social phobia. Nevertheless, in assessing social anxiety and phobia, one is still measuring the same sorts of self- and other-report, motoric, and physiological responses. Measures of social phobia can be used to assess social anxiety and vice versa (but not to indicate whether diagnostic criteria have been met). This chapter also considers social anxiety and phobia from a broad perspective, rejecting arbitrary distinctions within psychology and related fields concerning nomenclature and definitional issues. Consequently, we extend Cheek and Melchior's (1990) argument that the intercorrelations among measures of shyness and social anxiety suggest that the "same global psychological construct" (p. 56) is being measured. We agree, and we contend that researchers in clinical and counseling psychology and psychiatry measuring social phobia, in social and personality psychology assessing shyness and social anxiety, and in speech communication departments evaluating communication apprehension are all measuring parts of the same global construct. Consequently, we will endeavor to include various behavioral assessment measures from all these areas of research.

This chapter follows previous integrative writings on behavioral assessment of social phobia, including reviews (Donohue, Van Hasselt, & Hersen, 1994; Glass & Arnkoff, 1989) and chapters (Barlow, 1988, Chap. 14; Scholing & Emmelkamp, 1990). Works on social skills assessment are referenced as well (e.g., Becker & Heimberg, 1988).

GENERAL STRATEGIES FOR SOCIAL PHOBIA ASSESSMENT

A structured clinical interview, such as the Anxiety Disorders Interview Schedule–IV (ADIS-IV; Brown, Di Nardo, & Barlow, 1994), is quite important early in the initial assessment process. This formal interview may follow a more general screening interview or an unstructured clinical interview. Structured interviews are preferred, even in purely clinical service settings, given their breadth of assessment and known psychometric properties. Since social phobia exists comorbidly with a variety of Axis I and Axis II disorders (Turner, Beidel, Borden, Stanley, & Jacob, 1991), it is important that a comprehensive psychosocial evaluation be conducted. It should be noted that these interviews involve both social contact and evaluation and so may produce significant anxiety for social phobia patients. As interview strategies and clinician-administered scales are specifically covered in Greist, Kobak, Jefferson, Katzelnick, and Chene (Chapter 9, this volume), they will not be further considered here. A medical examination may be appropriate for some patients to rule out medical conditions that mimic anxiety (see Hollandsworth, 1986).

Various general fear/anxiety and depression instruments, along with one or more questionnaires that specifically target social anxiety and phobia, may also be administered following the structured interview. Given the numerous social anxiety and phobia verbal report instruments currently available, it is important to choose among them wisely. The issue of incremental validity is raised with the abundance of these instruments (i.e., whether adding one more questionnaire to a battery will indeed contribute much new information).

Overt behaviors are often evaluated informally (e.g., by observing patient interactions with support staff) and formally (e.g., by simulating social situations in the laboratory or clinic). These latter behavioral assessment tests typically include measures of social skill and self-reports of distress, although it is recommended that avoidance/escape behavior and psychophysiological response be evaluated as well. Even in purely clinical service settings, role-play scenarios can be utilized in behavioral assessment.

SELF-REPORTS

Since there are numerous social anxiety and phobia instruments currently available, only the ones believed to be most important in terms of their impact on the field, both currently and historically, will be highlighted in this chapter. As noted by Scholing and Emmelkamp (1990), social phobia self-report instruments can be divided into those that are targeted directly toward the signs and symptoms that are a part of social phobia and those that are more general measures of anxiety and fear.

Self-Report Questionnaires Specific to Social Anxiety and Phobia

Table 10.1 contains various descriptive and psychometric data about selected scales discussed in this section.

Social Phobia Scale and Social Interaction Anxiety Scale

Mattick and Clarke (1989) developed the Social Phobia Scale (SPS) and the Social Interaction Anxiety Scale (SIAS) as companion measures to assess two separate domains of social anxiety. The initial data on the SPS and the SIAS (Mattick & Clarke, 1989) are currently unpublished. Heimberg, Mueller, Holt, Hope, and Liebowitz (1992), however, offer a summary of these scales' psychometric development. SPS items pertain to situations that involve being observed by others (e.g., eating in a restaurant). SIAS statements describe the individual's affective, behavioral, or cognitive responses to a variety of situations that require social interaction (e.g., speaking with someone in authority).

Both the SPS and SIAS have demonstrated reliability. Mattick and Clarke (1989) reported that internal consistency for each scale exceeded alpha = .88 across five patient and control groups. Test–retest reliability for social phobia patients was $r = .91–.93$ for both scales after intervals of 1 month and 3 months.

In terms of validity, Mattick and Clarke (1989) found that SPS and SIAS scores from a social phobia sample had significant positive correlations ($rs = .54–.69$) with other standard measures of social anxiety and with each other ($r = .72$). Heimberg et al. (1992) investigated the divergent and convergent validity of these companion scales. In a social phobia sample, the SPS only correlated significantly with a measure of fear/anxiety about and avoidance of performance situations. The SIAS was more highly correlated with a similar measure associated with social interaction, relative to the performance measure.

Ries et al. (1995) found that the SPS and the SIAS correlated positively and significantly with another standard measure of social anxiety and phobia, as well as with each other. Also, scores on the SIAS were related to measures of negative thoughts and inversely related to measures of positive self-statements following speech and conversation behavioral assessment tests. SPS scores had a significant, although slight, negative relationship with time spent in a speech task.

The SPS and SIAS have shown good discriminative validity, being used to differentiate social phobia patients from community volunteers and patients with other anxiety disorders; subtypes of social phobia have been uniquely identified as well. Mattick and Clarke (1989) reported that social phobia patients scored higher than did undergraduates, community samples, patients with simple phobia, and agoraphobic samples on both instruments. In a study of a variety of anxiety disorder patients, the SIAS differentiated social phobia patients from others (Rapee, Brown, Antony, & Barlow, 1992). Comparing social phobia patients to a matched healthy community sample (Heimberg et al., 1992) or to other anxiety patients and normal

TABLE 10.1. Psychometric Information on Selected Social Anxiety and Phobia Self-Report Instruments

Instrument[a]	Number of items	Format[b]	Scoring[c]	Range[d]	Social phobia patients[e]		Community controls[f]	Undergraduate controls[g]
SPS	20	L-T (0–4)	Unidirectional	0–80	M	31.1 (16.8)	9.0 (6.5)	12.1 (8.9)
					F	35.4 (10.9)	16.1 (14.2)	15.6 (10.7)
					B	32.8 (14.8)	12.5 (11.5)	13.4 (9.6)
SIAS	20	L-T (0–4)	Bidirectional	0–80	M	46.1 (16.0)	16.8 (9.5)	20.2 (12.2)
					F	53.4 (14.2)	22.9 (17.4)	18.1 (8.1)
					B	49.0 (15.6)	19.9 (14.2)	19.5 (10.9)
SPAI Social	45 13	L-T (1–7)	Unidirectional	0–192	M	101.2 (—)	—	56.3 (—)
					F	111.4 (—)	—	42.3 (—)
					B	109 (38.3)	31 (17.7)	—
Agoraphobia	32			0–78	M	10.4 (—)	—	16.6 (—)
					F	14.9 (—)	—	18.5 (—)
					B	14 (11.4)	4 (3.0)	—
Difference				−78–192	M	90.8 (—)	—	39.6 (—)
					F	96.5 (—)	—	23.8 (—)
					B	95 (32.8)	27 (16.4)	—
SAD	28	T-F	Bidirectional	0–28	M	—	—	11.2 (—)
					F	—	—	8.2 (—)
					B	18.7 (7.8)	—	9.1 (8.0)
FNE	30	T-F	Bidirectional	0–30	M	—	—	14.0 (—)
					F	—	—	16.1 (—)
					B	25.7 (5.3)	—	15.5 (8.0)
IAS	15	L-T (0–4)	Bidirectional	15–75	M	—	—	—
					F	—	—	—
					B	—	—	—

AAS	12	L-T (0-4)	Bidirectional	12-60	M	—	—	14.4 (7.1)
					F	—	—	15.0 (7.3)
					B	—	—	—
PRCS	30	T-F	Bidirectional	0-30	M	—	—	—
					F	—	—	—
					B	23.4 (4.7)	—	—
FQ (Social)	5	L-T (0-8)	Unidirectional	0-40	M	21.4 (5.4)	—	—
					F	15.9 (8.7)	—	—
					B	18.0 (8.5)	—	—

Note. M, male scores; F, female scores; B, both male and female scores. Values for patients and both controls are means, with standard deviations in parentheses. Dashes indicate that data were not available from the articles referenced in this chapter. For all instruments, higher scores are indicative of greater anxiety. The referenced articles from which the means and standard deviations are drawn should be consulted for specific demographic and other characteristics of the samples.

[a] SPS, Social Phobia Scale (Mattick & Clarke, 1989); data are from Heimberg, Mueller, Holt, Hope, and Liebowitz (1992). SIAS, Social Interaction Anxiety Scale (Mattick & Clarke, 1989); data are from Heimberg et al. (1992). SPAI, Social Phobia and Anxiety Inventory, its two subscale scores, and one derived score (Turner, Beidel, Dancu, & Stanley, 1989); patient data are from Turner and Beidel (in press); undergraduate data are from Beidel, Turner, Stanley, and Dancu (1989); for the patients, the male/female and both data represent differing samples. SAD, Social Avoidance and Distress Scale (Watson & Friend, 1969); patient data are from Holt, Heimberg, and Hope (1992); undergraduate data are from Watson and Friend (1969). FNE, Fear of Negative Evaluation Scale (Watson & Friend, 1969); patient data are from Holt et al. (1992); undergraduate data are from Watson and Friend (1969). IAS, Interaction Anxiety Scale (Leary, 1983b). AAS, Audience Anxiety Scale (Leary, 1983b). PRCS, Personal Report of Confidence as a Speaker (Paul, 1966); patient data are from Cook, Melamed, Cuthbert, McNeil, and Lang (1988); undergraduate data are from Klorman, Weerts, Hastings, Melamed, and Lang (1974). FQ (Social), Social Phobia subscale of the Marks and Mathews Fear Questionnaire (Marks & Mathews, 1979); patient data for males and females separately are from Oei, Moylan, and Evans (1991); patient data for both males and females are from Cook et al. (1988).

[b] L-T is a Likert-type scale; numerals in parentheses refer to the range of choices on the scale. T-F indicates a true-false scale.

[c] In unidirectional scoring, all items are worded in such a way that endorsing them indicates anxiety. With bidirectional scoring, some items suggest little or no anxiety, while others indicate the presence of anxiety.

[d] Range indicates the theoretically possible lowest to highest scores.

[e] Social phobia patients are individuals diagnosed with social phobia. The means in this table reflect a sample that either combines subtypes of social phobia or includes individuals with generalized social phobia without avoidant personality disorder. Referenced articles should be consulted for further information about each sample.

[f] Community controls are individuals from the general community who do not have identified psychological disorders. For the SPAI sample, however, these individuals were identified only as "normal controls."

[g] Undergraduate controls are students who participated in a general screening with questionnaires. For all instruments except the SPAI, these students were unselected, being included without regard to anxiety level or psychological disorder. For the SPAI sample, these students were selected as being low in social anxiety.

controls (Brown, Turovsky, Heimberg, Brown, & Barlow, 1994), the SIAS correctly categorized 82% or more of the social phobia patients. Similarly, the SPS properly categorized 73% or more of the social phobia patients. A clear minority of other anxiety disorder patients or normal controls were incorrectly classified.

Patients with both generalized social phobia and avoidant personality disorder, with generalized social phobia but no avoidant personality disorder, and with circumscribed speech phobia have been assessed with the SPS and SIAS (Ries et al., 1995). Utilizing the SPS, the group with both generalized social phobia and avoidant personality disorder reported greater anxiety than did the circumscribed speech phobia group, but neither group was different from the generalized social phobia group. On the SIAS, both generalized social phobia groups reported more anxiety than did the circumscribed speech phobia group. Heimberg et al. (1992) found that the SIAS, but not the SPS, differentiated generalized versus nongeneralized subtypes of social phobia. The SPS and the SIAS have also been shown to be sensitive to the effects of cognitive and behavioral treatments in clinical outcome studies (Mattick & Peters, 1988; Mattick, Peters, & Clarke, 1989).

In summary, the SPS and the SIAS have strong psychometric properties and are promising new instruments. They appear to measure different, yet related, aspects of social anxiety and phobia.

Social Phobia and Anxiety Inventory

The Social Phobia and Anxiety Inventory (SPAI; Turner, Beidel, Dancu, & Stanley, 1989; Turner & Beidel, in press) was specifically designed to assess cognitions, somatic symptoms, and avoidance and escape behaviors in various situations that people with social phobia typically find anxiety evoking. The SPAI includes two subscales: Social Phobia and Agoraphobia. The Agoraphobia subscale assesses anxiety associated with classic agoraphobia situations (e.g., waiting in lines). A score is produced for each subscale, and a Difference (or Total) score is derived by subtracting the Agoraphobia score from the Social Phobia score. Various factor scores (Turner, Stanley, Beidel, & Bond, 1989), as well as cognitive and behavioral dimensions (Beidel, Turner, Stanley, & Dancu, 1989), have also been identified.

Details of the construction and scoring of the SPAI are outlined by Turner, Beidel, et al. (1989). The SPAI is innovative in that separate ratings of response are given for four different aspects (i.e., with strangers, authority figures, opposite sex, and people in general) of many of the listed situations. The SPAI is longer than other social anxiety and phobia instruments and so requires more administration time. Its scoring is also complex and time-consuming. However, programs for computer administration and scoring are available, which may help to resolve these concerns. Although Turner, Beidel, et al. (1989) suggest that diagnosis should be based on clinical decisions rather than on test results alone, they indicate that a SPAI Difference score above 60 should occasion evaluation for social phobia. A cutoff score of 80 maximizes the identification rate, although it may lead to some false negatives.

Turner, Beidel, et al. (1989) tested 51 college students with social phobia and demonstrated test–retest reliability ($r = .86$) for the Difference score over a 2-week period. Internal consistency was alpha $= .96$ for the Social Phobia subscale and .85 for the Agoraphobia subscale. Various types of validity have also been tested for the SPAI. Specifically, Turner, Stanley, et al. (1989) reported on the SPAI's construct validity, suggesting that the subscales are unique and useful in differentiating various anxious and normative groups. The concurrent validity of the SPAI has been demonstrated in an undergraduate sample (Beidel, Turner, Stanley, & Dancu, 1989). In a social phobia patient sample, Beidel, Borden, Turner, and Jacob (1989) found that the SPAI Difference score was significantly correlated ($r = .43$) with ratings of daily social distress from self-monitoring forms.

The SPAI has also been shown to distinguish social phobia patients from those with other anxiety disorders. Turner, Beidel, et al. (1989) found that social phobia patients had significantly higher SPAI Difference scores than did patients with panic disorder with or without agoraphobia or obsessive–compulsive disorder. In another study that explored the discriminative ability of the SPAI, both the Social Phobia subscale and the Difference score differentiated three subtypes of social phobia in a clinical sample (Ries et al., 1995).

Investigators have also explored the SPAI as a measure of treatment outcome with social phobia patients. Beidel, Turner, and Cooley (1993) reported that the SPAI reliably measured clinically significant changes following treatment. The SPAI has also been incorporated into a composite measure to determine the functional status of social phobia patients after treatment (Turner, Beidel, Long, Turner, & Townsley, 1993).

There is a current debate as to which of the SPAI scores is the best measure of social phobia. Turner, Beidel, et al. (1989) suggest that the Difference score is the best measure of social phobia since it controls for the anxiety associated with agoraphobia situations. Herbert, Bellack, and Hope (1991) found that both the Social Phobia score and the Difference score had similar correlations with other measures of social anxiety, while the Agoraphobia score was not related to any of them. They concluded that independent use of the SPAI Social Phobia and Agoraphobia subscale scores may be preferred over use of the Difference score, as this latter index is based on theoretical assumptions about the relationship of social phobia and agoraphobia. In response, Beidel and Turner (1992) criticized Herbert et al.'s (1991) lack of empirical support for their position and offered further theoretical reasons to support the use of the Difference score. Herbert, Bellack, Hope, and Mueser (1992) suggested that the choice of which SPAI score(s) to use may best be based on the investigator's purpose, either for information about diagnosis or pure measurement of social phobia symptoms. Ries et al. (1995) further examined these issues and found that the SPAI Social Phobia and Difference scores performed very similarly in assessing social phobia patients.

The SPAI has been tested across a wide age range. In addition to data on adult clinic patients and college students, there is information for adolescents, ages 12 to 18 (Clark et al., 1994). Moreover, the Social Phobia and Anxiety Inventory for Children is a similar version of the instrument, designed for children ages 8 through 17 (Beidel, Turner, & Morris, 1995).

In conclusion, there is a great deal of psychometric data on the SPAI. The research with this instrument from Turner and Beidel and their colleagues is broad and of high quality, spanning a breadth of ages and populations. A need exists for additional research on the SPAI, by investigators other than its authors, to confirm its generalizability. Further research should examine which of the SPAI scores is the best measure, and in what instances.

Social Avoidance and Distress Scale and Fear of Negative Evaluation Scale

The Social Avoidance and Distress (SAD) and Fear of Negative Evaluation (FNE) scales, developed together by Watson and Friend in 1969, are among the most widely used measures of social anxiety. The SAD scale includes items about anxiety and avoidance associated with social interactions (e.g., "I often find social situations upsetting," "I try to avoid situations which force me to be very sociable"). Items pertaining to psychophysiological response and impaired performance were excluded. The SAD scale has avoidance and distress subscales that are rarely considered.

The FNE assesses one's expectation of being evaluated negatively by others (e.g., "If someone is evaluating me I tend to expect the worst"). A shorter, 12-item version is available, using a five-point Likert-type scale (Leary, 1983a). It correlates highly with the original scale ($r = .96$); its brevity makes it amenable for use in repeated administrations.

Watson and Friend (1969) provide details about the development of the SAD and FNE scales and report on their psychometric properties. In terms of reliability, a *KR-20* reliability coefficient of .94 was found for both instruments. Test–retest reliability coefficients after a 1-month interval were $r = .68$ for the SAD and $r = .78$ for the FNE in a college student sample.

A variety of studies provide support for the validity of the SAD and FNE scales. SAD scores have been found to be significantly related to global ratings of social skills obtained from familiar peers ($r = -.70$) and to specific behavioral measures of social skills, including gaze time ($r = -.34$), speech latency ($r = .48$), and number of words spoken ($r = -.31$) during social interaction tests (Arkowitz, Lichtenstein, McGovern, & Hines, 1975). Significant positive correlations have been observed between the SAD and other social anxiety questionnaires, including one that assesses perceived ability to initiate interactions with the opposite gender ($r = .54$; Wallander, Conger, Mariotto, Curran, & Farrell, 1980). Smith and Sarason (1975) found that individuals with high FNE scores felt worse about receiving negative feedback and rated themselves as more likely to receive negative evaluations than did those with low FNE scores. Individuals with high FNE scores have also been shown to avoid threatening social comparison information (Friend & Gilbert, 1973).

The appropriateness of the SAD and FNE scales for social phobia patients has been debated in the literature. Turner, McCanna, and Beidel (1987) criticized these instruments as lacking in discriminative validity. Specifically, they found that these instruments failed to differentiate patients with a principal diagnosis of social phobia from groups of patients with other anxiety disorders. Additionally, they reported that the SAD and FNE correlate significantly with general measures of emotional distress and proposed that these instruments do not have particular relevance for social phobia.

Heimberg, Hope, Rapee, and Bruch (1988) offered alternative explanations for the results obtained by Turner et al. (1987) and concluded that the SAD and FNE are useful in the assessment of social phobia. Moreover, Heimberg et al. (1988) suggested that these scales would not necessarily discriminate social phobia patients from those with other anxiety disorders because clinically significant social anxiety may be manifested in all anxiety disorders and because social phobia patients can be very heterogeneous in terms of level of anxiety. Additionally, they suggested that social anxiety may be an important component of trait anxiety, depression, and general emotional distress, and that the significant correlations obtained by Turner et al. (1987) should not necessarily be interpreted as evidence that the SAD and FNE measure emotional distress in general rather than social anxiety in particular.

In response, Turner and Beidel (1988) reaffirmed their position that the SAD and FNE have questionable utility as assessment and treatment outcome measures in social phobia research. While acknowledging that the SAD and FNE may measure social anxiety, which is present in many clinical syndromes, they stated that these instruments do not appear to be adequate in identifying social phobia. Furthermore, they proposed that, if the SAD and FNE are measuring unique constructs other than trait anxiety, depression, and general distress, these scales should be able to differentiate among patient groups despite high correlations with these other measures.

Overall, the SAD and FNE scales are valuable in the assessment of social anxiety because of their long history of use in research. While much of the research with these instruments in the past has been conducted with college populations, they are increasingly being used with patient populations. While both of these instruments are limited by their true–false format, their continued use with social phobia populations is advocated. The brief FNE should be considered for use, given its shorter, Likert-type format. Reviews are available for the FNE (Ammerman, 1988; Fisher & Corcoran, 1994) and for both the SAD and FNE (Heimberg, 1988). There is a need for additional psychometric and validational information on these instruments with clinically anxious individuals, particularly including reliability data. These scales have tremendous historical value, which will allow comparison of new results with older studies.

Interaction Anxiousness Scale and Audience Anxiousness Scale

The Interaction Anxiousness Scale (IAS) and the Audience Anxiousness Scale (AAS) were developed by Leary (1983b). The IAS measures anxiety concerning social behavior that is contingent upon the ongoing responses of another in a situation (e.g., conversations). The AAS, on the other hand, assesses anxiety in noncontingent situations, in which there is little or no immediate feedback from the social responses of others (e.g., delivering a prepared speech). The scales include items that refer to affective, cognitive, and physiological content; Leary (1983b) specifically excluded overt behavior items. Leary (1983b) reports reliability and validity data; a brief review is also available (Fisher & Corcoran, 1994).

Personal Report of Confidence as a Speaker

Paul (1966) modified Gilkinson's (1942) Personal Report of Confidence as a Speaker (PRCS) into the current inventory. Gilkinson (1942) originally intended this scale to assess both fear and confidence about speaking, including before, during, and after a speech. The current version of the test contains a mixture of both fear and confidence items across the three temporal dimensions. Psychometric data from a college sample are available and indicate high internal consistency (Klorman, Weerts, Hastings,

Melamed, & Lang, 1974). The test–retest reliability of the 30-item version, however, is unknown. Validity data are available (cf. Lombardo, 1988). Lombardo's (1988) review suggested that the PRCS, while developed as a research instrument, is suitable for clinical use. The PRCS is important because of its status as the major, and perhaps only, instrument from the field of psychology that specifically measures anxiety in public speaking situations. The PRCS remains a valuable instrument, although it is limited by its true–false format.

Other Instruments

There are a variety of other self-report instruments in the area of social anxiety and phobia, as broadly defined in this chapter, and they cannot all be identified here. Nevertheless, some additional ones are worth mentioning. The Situation Questionnaire (Rehm & Marston, 1968) was developed to assess heterosexual social anxiety; its reliability and validity were examined by Heimberg, Harrison, Montgomery, Madsen, and Sherfey (1980). There are a number of instruments that assess shyness and social anxiety from the perspective of social and personality psychology (Briggs & Smith, 1986), including the Stanford Shyness Survey (Zimbardo, 1977) and the Social Reticence Scale (Jones, Briggs, & Smith, 1986). Also from social and personality psychology is the Self-Consciousness Scale, developed by Fenigstein, Scheier, and Buss (1975), including subscales for both private and public self-consciousness, as well as for social anxiety. Finally, there is a variety of tools available from the field of communication apprehension, including McCroskey's Shyness Scale and the Personal Report of Communication Apprehension (Richmond & McCroskey, 1992). In fact, there are 11 of these instruments found in Richmond and McCroskey's (1992) book. This area is very closely related to that of social anxiety and social phobia. Hope, Gansler, and Heimberg (1989) encouraged the "cross-fertilization" of social anxiety research from social psychology with other specialty areas. Likewise, this crossover should include communication apprehension research.

Self-Report General Fear and Anxiety Instruments with Social Anxiety and Phobia Components

A Social Phobia subscale is included in the 24-item Marks and Mathews (1979) Fear Questionnaire (FQ), which is a very commonly used general inventory in social phobia research. Among other FQ subscales, that for social phobia is comprised of five social anxiety/phobia situations (e.g., "being watched or stared at") that are rated for degree of *avoidance*. Psychometric data specifically for social phobia are available (e.g., Oei, Moylan, & Evans, 1991), as are reliability and validity data, along with information on sensitivity to clinical change (see Fisher & Corcoran, 1994; Lelliott, 1988).

There are a number of other general instruments containing subscales relating to social anxiety and phobia that can be used in clinical screening applications. A Social Fears factor, comprised of 13 items, has been identified (e.g., Arrindell, Kolk, Pickersgill, & Hageman, 1993) in the Fear Survey Schedule (FSS; Wolpe & Lang, 1977). The Minnesota Multiphasic Personality Inventory–2 (MMPI-2; Butcher, Dahlstrom, Graham, Tellegen, & Kaemmer, 1989) contains the 69-item Scale 0 (Social Introversion). There are three MMPI-2 Scale 0 subscales developed by Ben-Porath, Hostetler, Butcher, and Graham (1989): Shyness/Self-Conciousness (14 items), Social Avoidance (8 items), and Self/Other Alienation (17 items). There is also a 24-item MMPI-2 content scale, Social Discomfort (Butcher, Graham, Williams, & Ben-Porath, 1990). The Symptom Checklist-90-R (Derogatis, 1983) contains a 9-item Interpersonal Sensitivity subscale. A 9-item Behavioral Social Avoidance subscale is contained in the Lehrer–Woolfolk Anxiety Symptom Questionnaire (Lehrer & Woolfolk, 1982). Finally, the 25-item Willoughby Personality Schedule (see Steketee & Freund, 1988) primarily assesses interpersonal anxiety but also includes dysphoric mood and various questions about nonsocial concerns, yielding a single total score.

MOTORIC ASSESSMENT

Observation and systematic measurement of overt motoric behavior is the sine qua non of behavioral assessment. Examples of social behaviors to be evaluated include entering a frightening social situation, degree of eye contact with an audience in a speech, and number of pauses in a conversation. Glass and Arnkoff (1989) regard such evaluation as "almost a requirement for a comprehensive assessment" (pp. 80–81). Scholing and Emmelkamp (1990) regard these methods as "useful" but are more cautious about them because of methodological questions. Behaviors related to social anxiety and social phobia are most commonly evaluated in the clinic or laboratory by arranging simulated social situations that involve role-plays. Kern (1994) provides a helpful review of role-play assessment.

Glass and Arnkoff (1989) carefully reviewed behavioral observation of social anxiety and social phobia. They identified five important issues in this area, including (1) nature of situation or interaction, (2) type of role-play assessment, (3) identity of partner or audience, (4) raters for observation and coding, and (5) choice of behavior being evaluated. This last point is extremely important to investigations of social anxiety and social phobia. A considerable literature exists on the conceptualization, assessment, and treatment of social skills deficits that is somewhat separate from that of social anxiety and social phobia. Becker and Heimberg (1988) provide an excellent review of social skills assessment. The relationship between social anxiety/social phobia and social skills is complex. While there is some overlap between these constructs, it is clear that there is some independence too, as many individuals with high social anxiety and social phobia have excellent social skills, and some people with deficient skills experience little or no social anxiety (cf. Lewin, McNeil, & Lipson, 1995).

In clinical practice, evaluation of overt motoric behaviors is often based on the patient's retrospective oral accounts, given practical considerations hindering use of other methods. Self-monitoring forms, however, provide greater standardization and are readily employed. Observation by others, particularly independent raters, is also frequently used, often involving the coding or rating of role-played behaviors. Increasingly, comprehensive Behavioral Assessment Test (BAT) strategies are being used, including evaluation of motoric behaviors, as well as assessment of psychophysiological response and self- and other-reports.

Self-Monitoring Forms

Self-monitoring is an efficient, highly practical method for assessing social behavior in an individual's natural environment, outside of the clinic or laboratory. It is an integral component of contemporary cognitive-behavioral treatments (Heimberg, 1991) and behavioral treatments (Turner, Beidel, Cooley, Woody, & Messer, 1994) for social phobia. Daily logs, recording forms, and diaries are among the formats that can be used in self-monitoring. Various parameters of interactions can be coded, such as number and duration, but feelings, thoughts, and perceived physiological arousal can be detailed as well.

Little research in the social anxiety or social phobia literature addresses the psychometric properties of self-monitoring or the correspondence of these data with those from other assessment methods. Nevertheless, self-monitoring diary forms have been successfully included in assessment research. Dodge, Heimberg, Nyman, and O'Brien (1987) studied opposite-sex interactions of undergraduates high or low in social anxiety. The duration of each interaction was recorded, along with details about the event, the relationship, and the topic of conversation. Anxiety, performance, and satisfaction were rated for each event as well. Subjects were reminded about the self-recording several times over the 2-week study period. Low anxiety subjects participated in more interactions and gave more positive ratings. Self-monitoring has a valuable assessment function, including its utility in treatment planning.

Mattick et al. (1989) collected some similar measures in a treatment outcome study over 6 weeks of therapy. At each treatment session, patients were interviewed about their activities, independent from data in their diary, as an accuracy check. In their diaries, patients also recorded the number of cognitive restructuring exercises completed, demonstrating the utility of self-monitoring in assessing treatment adherence.

As in other assessment modalities, self-monitoring can be individually tailored, which can be helpful in assessing idiosyncratic social anxieties (e.g., of same-sex authority figures) because broadly assessing all social interactions may be cumbersome. For general details about the clinical implementation of self-monitoring, such as frequency and timing of recording, the reader is referred to Cormier and Cormier (1991), and specifically for social behavior recording, to Becker and Heimberg (1988).

The reactivity of behavior to self-monitoring (i.e., changes in the behavior as a result of self-observation and recording) is an important consideration (Becker & Heimberg, 1988). In treatment applications, however, reactivity that prompts positive behavior change is a lesser concern. Nevertheless, reactivity raises questions about reliability and validity. For self-recordings of social behavior, the psychometric data are scant (e.g., Twentyman & McFall, 1975). With the advent of standardized treatment packages for social phobia that provide self-monitoring forms (Heimberg, 1991; Turner et al., 1994), research to further develop these forms and to assess their psychometric properties will be more feasible.

Role-Play Tests Assessing Skill and Anxiety

Formal tests are available for standardized observation of social skills and anxiety, although none has a sufficient body of research. In these tests, individuals role-play with one or more confederates or respond to standard stimuli presented on audiotape. Glass and Arnkoff (1989) classified role-play tests as either brief or extended in nature. Some assess general social skills, but a number specifically focus on heterosocial and dating situations.

The Simulated Social Interaction Test (SSIT; e.g., Monti, Wallander, Ahern, Abrams, & Munroe, 1984) examines behavior in eight brief social interactions (e.g., involving interpersonal warmth). A narrator first describes a social situation. A male and a female confederate, who are actually present, then each deliver brief (one to three sentences) prompts in four of the situations. Subjects respond orally, and then rate themselves on two global scales (i.e., skill and anxiety); their responses are videotaped and later evaluated by trained, independent judges on the same scales. The SSIT has a considerable amount of psychometric data suggesting its generalizability, discriminative validity, and interrater reliability (Curran, 1982). The SSIT is limited, however, in its focus on males as subjects. Other brief tests are similar in nature but typically present social prompts in audiotape format, without the presence of live confederates. The 22-item Heterosocial Adequacy Test (Perri & Richards, 1979), 24-situation Dating Behavior Assessment Test (Glass, Gottman, & Shmurak, 1976), and 10-item Taped Situation Test (Rehm & Marston, 1968) all focus on dating or other heterosocial interactions, such as dealing with the opportunity to propose going out on a date. Responses are audiotaped in each of these tests, with later evaluation by independent judges for anxiety and "adequacy." Other variables, including self-ratings, are part of certain tests.

In extended role-play tests, interactions typically are longer but less structured. Among these is the Social Interaction Test (SIT; Trower, Bryant, & Argyle, 1978), which involves an assessment of conversation skills with a male and a female confederate who are unfamiliar to the subject (see Gershenson & Morrison, 1988). The conversation takes place in groups of three and consists of three, 4-minute phases. Unknown to the subject, the confederates have prescribed roles. Retrospective evaluations are made by the confederates and other judges of videotapes of the sessions using three methods. In one, there are 29 ratings of verbal (e.g., clarity), nonverbal (e.g., gesture), and other categories (e.g., turn-taking) of social behavior. Second, global ratings on 13 bipolar adjective scales (e.g., like–dislike) are completed. Finally, there are descriptions of two areas that were most problematic. There are data on the SIT's discriminative validity, interrater agreement, and sensitivity to treatment outcome (see Gershenson & Morrison, 1988). There are other extended role-play tests that involve heterosocial and dating interactions. Twentyman and McFall (1975), for example, utilized six Social Behavior Situations in which male subjects interacted with female confederates over an intercom, role-playing situations that involved meeting and proposing dates.

Aside from the format of role-play tests, various strategies have been used to rate specific behaviors and patterns of behavior, including social skill. These coding systems are reviewed by Scholing and Emmelkamp (1990). There are three levels of measurement that have been employed, differing in terms of their degree of specificity (Becker & Heimberg, 1988). Molecular approaches assess highly specific behaviors (e.g., pauses, dysfluencies). Macro, or molar, systems evaluate complex groups of actions in terms of global ratings (e.g., overall social skills; Herbert, Hope, & Bellack, 1992). Intermediate or "midi-level" measurement systems (Monti et al., 1984) have been developed that collapse some molecular categories (e.g., rate and pressure of speech). Coding systems are available at all these levels and for different formats, including Paul's (1966) Timed Behavioral Checklist for public speaking and Kolko and Milan's (1985) Heterosocial Skill Observational Rating System for heterosocial skills in females. There presently are no widely accepted coding systems, however, which leads to problems in cross-study comparisons.

There is now less emphasis on role-play tests that rely solely upon verbal reports (from the participant[s] and/or independent raters) about skill and anxiety (cf. Kern, 1994). Currently, interest focuses on the use of more comprehensive BAT strategies that include evaluation of all modes of response using multiple methods. Some earlier investigations, however, also included avoidance and physiological measures in comprehensive assessments (e.g., Twentyman & McFall, 1975). The newer BATs are similar to the older tests in that they, too, involve role-play of different social situations, as well as ratings of skill and anxiety.

Behavioral Assessment Tests

BATs are best regarded as an assessment strategy rather than as a particular type of test (McGlynn, 1988). Indeed, the BATs used in social anxiety and social phobia research have a great number of variations. Primary among these is the choice of using standardized (e.g., Turner, Beidel, & Larkin, 1986) or individually tailored (e.g., Heimberg, Hope, Dodge, & Becker, 1990) BATs. There have been three primary types of standardized BATs: conversation with a same-gender stranger, conversation with an opposite-gender stranger, and an impromptu speech to a small audience (e.g., Beidel, Turner, & Dancu, 1985). The idiographic BATs have included such situations as interacting in a group conversation or starting a conversation with someone who is attractive and romantically interesting (Brown, Heimberg, & Juster, 1995). The number of items in a BAT has also differed, along with whether the ordering was stepwise (e.g., Mattick et al., 1989). Other variations involve the degree that the BAT situation(s) are role-played and the degree of instructional control of interactions (e.g., whether participants are provided with choices of speech topics or not). Some studies instruct subjects to converse with a stranger in the laboratory and to try to get to know that person (e.g., McNeil & Lewin, 1995). Although the situation is contrived, there are no artificial roles for the participants to play. Other investigations instruct subjects to play a specific role, such as acting as if one is interacting with a new neighbor (Hope, Herbert, & White, 1995). Additional variations include the amount of preparation allowed for speeches and other interactions, whether there are interruptions for anxiety ratings, the number and familiarity of interaction partners or audiences, and whether these confederates are socially interactive or not.

Yet another important BAT variation is the measurement of avoidance (i.e., never entering a situation) and escape (i.e., entering the situation but leaving it prematurely). Earlier investigations did not allow avoidance or escape, but more recent ones have used them successfully as a measure to differentiate groups (e.g., Hofmann, Newman, Ehlers, & Roth, 1995). Many studies have provided a motoric response (e.g., grasping a "stop sign") to allow subjects to terminate a BAT step, since they may not have the social skill to so indicate orally (e.g., Carter, McNeil, Turk, Ries, & Boone, 1995). It should be noted that avoidance and escape are not the only overt anxiety behaviors. Others identified by Marks (1987) include immobility (e.g., "freezing" during delivery of a speech), camouflage (e.g., hiding by being a "wallflower" in a social gathering), and submission (e.g., social appeasement).

Relatedly, the instructional set for allowing or encouraging avoidance and escape is another important BAT variable, for it has been shown that experimental instructions in part determine the length of time a subject will endure (Miller & Bernstein, 1972). The maximum duration for each part or step of a BAT has varied as well, typically ranging from 2 minutes (e.g., McNeil & Lewin, 1995) to 10 minutes (e.g., Beidel, Turner, Jacob, & Cooley, 1989).

One of the strengths of the BAT strategy is that not only can overt behaviors be directly assessed, but psychophysiological and self-report measures can be included as well. In fact, BATs now often include measurement of avoidance or escape, self- and other-ratings of skill and anxiety, cardiovascular reactivity, and reports about self-statements (e.g., Turner, Beidel, & Townsley, 1992). The reliability of these various measures (i.e., self-reports of affect and cognition, physiology, or overt behavior) in a 10-minute impromptu-speech BAT has been found to be acceptable (Beidel, Turner, Jacob, & Cooley, 1989). Issues surrounding the validity of BAT measures have been examined directly (Monti et al., 1984) and indirectly through an evaluation of their concordance and discordance (Matias & Turner, 1986).

BATs represent an extremely useful research assessment strategy for social anxiety and social phobia. They allow direct evaluation of motoric behavior in a multimodal fashion. Self-monitoring forms and role-play tests are helpful, too, and are particularly amenable for use in clinical practice settings. Developments in motoric assessment call for its increased use in clinical and research settings.

PHYSIOLOGICAL ASSESSMENT

Measurement of physiological processes is an extremely important part of the behavioral assessment of social anxiety and social phobia. Possible psychophysiological (e.g., Hofmann et al., 1995) and psychobiological differences (Tancer, 1994) between individuals with social phobia and those with other psychological disorders, between social phobia patients and normal controls, and among patients with subtypes of social phobia have been the matter of some interest. Certain physiological responses have been found to differentiate related disorders from social phobia (e.g., Rapee et al., 1992), but there are few data to suggest that there are biological markers unique to social phobia (Tancer, 1994).

There has been relatively little examination of resting, baseline levels of psychophysiology in social phobia. Possible modest differences between individuals with social phobia and comparison groups may be masked by the typically small number of subjects in clinical investigations. Most research has focused on response to some sort of stimulation, whether that be imagery (e.g., McNeil, Vrana, Melamed, Cuthbert, & Lang, 1993), biological challenge (e.g., Rapee et al., 1992), or social challenge in the laboratory (e.g., Heimberg et al., 1990). It is in this latter example that psychophysiological evaluation interacts with the motoric assessment mentioned earlier, particularly in BATs. There has been very little attention paid to psychophysiological assessment in the natural environment. Advances in ambulatory monitoring technology, however, should allow future research to include unobtrusive physiological assessment in social situations in patients' everyday lives.

In planning psychophysiological investigations, there are a number of principles, both conceptual and technical, to be considered that are beyond the scope of this chapter (cf. Hollandsworth, 1986). For example, the placement and length of baselines, the use of raw versus change scores, and sampling rates are all important considerations. Psychophysiology texts (e.g., Coles, Donchin, & Porges, 1986) are recommended for further reading.

The selection of physiological and/or biological measures is another important consideration. Most psychophysiological social anxiety and social phobia research has focused on autonomic nervous system (ANS) measures, particularly the change in cardiovascular indices such as heart rate and blood pressure to social anxiety situations (e.g., Turner et al., 1986). Heart rate response fairly reliably distinguishes among subtypes of social phobia (e.g., Heimberg et al., 1990), as well as between certain social phobia subtypes and normal controls (Hofmann et al., 1995). Blushing is a common response among individuals with social phobia (Amies, Gelder, & Shaw, 1983), can be measured with a photoplethysomograph, and has been shown to be sensitive to an embarrassing (as opposed to another arousing) situation and to audience size (Shearn, Bergman, Hill, Abel, & Hinds, 1992).

In general, measures of psychophysiological activity increase when social stimuli are present for socially anxious individuals, suggesting activation of the ANS and other systems (e.g., Dimberg, Fredrikson, & Lundquist, 1986). Notably, embarrassment may be an example of competing sympathetic and parasympathetic ANS influences, as it has been associated with heart rate decrease (e.g., Buck, Parke, & Buck, 1970).

Electrodermal activity, including skin conductance responses and level, has also been shown to be relevant to social phobia. Skin conductance responses of individuals with social phobia, like those of some other patient groups, have been shown to habituate more slowly and to have more spontaneous fluctuations than those of a normative control group, even in response to mild, nonsocial stimuli such as tone presentations (Lader, 1967). Slower habituation and greater magnitude of response are also related to degree of social anxiety in the presence of social stimuli (Dimberg et al., 1986).

There are some possible respiratory activity differences in social phobia that merit further investigation (cf. Rapee et al., 1992). Neuroendocrine indices (e.g., epinephrine, norepinephrine, and cortisol collected from urine or plasma) have shown sensitivity to situational effects such as private versus public performance (Fredrikson & Gunnarsson, 1992) and stages of a speech task (Levin et al., 1993) but have not demonstrated differences among subject groups. Finally, preliminary investigation of brain imaging in individuals with social phobia versus normal controls suggests its promise as an investigatory method (Davidson et al., 1993).

Psychophysiological assessment in general applications has been shown to be reliable and stable (Waters, Williamson, Bernard, Blouin, & Faulstich, 1987). Specifically, too, there are data suggesting adequate test–retest reliability of pulse rate and blood pressure during an impromptu speech task, which is regarded as a useful all-purpose behavioral task for individuals with various kinds of social anxiety (Beidel, Turner, Jacob, & Cooley, 1989). The validity of psychophysiological measures raises important questions about the choice of a "gold standard" as the criterion against which psychophysiological responses are measured. From a three-systems perspective, comparing physiology to self-report or overt behavior may be problematic, given the relative independence of response systems. Turpin (1991) provides a valuable discourse on the conceptual validity of psychophysiological responses and their relationship to treatment outcome.

One of the difficulties in psychophysiological assessment of social anxiety is that many social situations inherently include task demands, occasioning the mobilization of cardiovascular and other systems (McNeil et al., 1993). There may be no differences between social phobia and other subjects on certain measures (e.g., cardiovascular) *during* social situations such as speeches because of the similar physical requirements (e.g., the cardiovascular demands of voice projection and gesturing) for both groups (cf. Knight & Borden, 1979). Nevertheless, with some methodological savvy, differences can be detected with certain physiological measures at other temporal points, such as during anticipation of delivering a speech (Knight & Borden, 1979).

Physiological measures have been instrumental in advancing the conceptual understanding of anxiety disorders (Turpin, 1991), including social phobia. Using physiological and self-report measures, Cook, Melamed, Cuthbert, McNeil, and Lang (1988) found social phobia to be distinct from simple phobia and agoraphobia, suggesting important differences among diagnostic groups in response organization and phobic memories. Social phobia appears to fall in between simple phobia (which is highly organized in memory and has a robust physiological response to cue stimuli) and agoraphobia (which is less coherently structured in memory and is inconsistently reactive in a physiological sense). Physiological measures (i.e., heart rate and skin conductance level) were also found to differentiate individuals with simple and/or social phobia in McNeil et al. (1993): Social phobia subjects were less consistently physiologically responsive in imagery. Moreover, subjects were divided into fearful and anxious subgroups based on questionnaire measures. It was suggested that *fear* responding is physiologically robust and closely tied to specific stimulus situations, while *anxiety* responses are more variable and inconsistent with measures of psychopathology and cognition. One implication from this research is that certain kinds of social distress may be related to *fear* (e.g., specific phobia of public speaking) and others may be related to *anxiety* (e.g., generalized social phobia).

Relatedly, research using heart rate as a measure suggests an interesting difference in the cardiac response of individuals with specific public speaking phobia compared to that of those with generalized social phobia (Carter et al., 1995; Heimberg et al., 1990). Specifically, the public speaking phobia patients showed a greater cardiac response to behavioral challenge. These subjects may be manifesting a specific *fear* response, in comparison to the more general *anxiety* response in the generalized social phobia group. Both Levin et al. (1993) and Hofmann et al. (1995) found a similarly greater heart rate elevation across a speech task for individuals with discrete social phobia than for those who had generalized social phobia or for controls. Turner and Beidel (1985) divided socially anxious individuals based on their physiological reactivity and self-statements. While virtually all reported negative thinking patterns, systolic blood pressure was found to differentiate these individuals into more and less reactive groups. Finally, physiological variables such as pulse rate have been shown to be important dependent measures in treatment outcome research (e.g., Turner, Beidel, Long, & Greenhouse, 1992).

Our view is that psychophysiological measurement is an integral component of the behavioral assessment of social anxiety and phobia, consistent with the views of Lang (1968, 1993) and of Eifert and Wilson (1991). Contrary to Scholing and Emmelkamp (1990), we are optimistic about the use of physiological measures in social phobia assessment. As with any assessment measures, they must be used cautiously and appropriately, with both conceptual and methodological sophistication.

CONCLUSIONS AND RECOMMENDATIONS

Behavioral assessment of social anxiety and social phobia is currently alive with methodological advances. It is, however, beset with some conceptual murkiness, like that in other areas of behavioral assessment, in which content and method of assessment are confused (cf. Eifert & Wilson, 1991). Moreover, difficulties also persist in the lack of integration among overlapping areas of research (e.g., shyness) and in barriers between areas within psychology and related disciplines (e.g., communication apprehension). Another area in need of conceptual development is the relationship between social-related anxiety and fear. Distinctions between these states are of tremendous potential importance in terms of the understanding of the nature of social phobia. The relationships between social anxiety and social skills remain unclear and in need of conceptual and empirical work (cf. Lewin et al., 1995). Finally, new ways of viewing and assessing social anxiety and phobia should be considered, such as impact on quality of life (e.g., Schneier et al., 1994).

In spite of the present methodological focus, most instruments need readily available (i.e., published) psychometric data, including means and standard deviations, for both normative and patient populations. The paucity of data in Table 10.1 demonstrates this need. This information is required both for instruments specifically targeted toward social anxiety and social phobia, and for instruments that are more broadly focused. Moreover, assessment research is needed with diverse populations, including ethnic minority groups and older persons. Thereby, the scope of available normative data will be extended, and knowledge about possibly unique manifestations of social phobia will be enhanced.

Kendall (1990) has noted that scale development is currently the primary focus of behavioral assessment. Given the available data, this view would certainly seem to hold true for social anxiety and social phobia. While there are certainly benefits to the present emphasis, scale development seems to be advancing at the expense of other approaches. Much work remains to be accomplished in the areas of motoric and physiological assessment of social anxiety and phobia, particularly in terms of bringing these methods into the mainstream of clinical research and practice.

Finally, more advances in behavioral assessment of social anxiety and phobia will provide information on current topics of interest, including research on subtypes of social phobia (see Heimberg, Holt, Schneier, Spitzer, & Liebowitz, 1993). Improved assessment methodologies will also assist both researchers and clinicians to scientifically inquire about social phobia and anxiety in order to select the best treatments for these prevalent and debilitating problems.

REFERENCES

Amies, P. L., Gelder, M. G., & Shaw, P. M. (1983). Social phobia: A comparative clinical study. *British Journal of Psychiatry, 142,* 174–179.

Ammerman, R. T. (1988). Fear of Negative Evaluation. In M. Hersen & A. S. Bellack (Eds.), *Dictionary of behavioral assessment techniques* (pp. 214–215). New York: Pergamon Press.

Arkowitz, H., Lichtenstein, E., McGovern, K., & Hines, P. (1975). The behavioral assessment of social competence in males. *Behavior Therapy, 6,* 3–13.

Arrindell, W. A., Kolk, A. M., Pickersgill, M. J., & Hageman, W. J. J. M. (1993). Biological sex, sex-role orientation, masculine sex-role stress, dissumulation and self-reported fears. *Advances in Behaviour Research and Therapy, 15,* 103–146.

Barlow, D. H. (1988). *Anxiety and its disorders: The nature and treatment of anxiety and panic.* New York: Guilford Press.

Becker, R. E., & Heimberg, R. G. (1988). Assessment of social skills. In A. S. Bellack & M. Hersen (Eds.), *Behavioral assessment: A practical handbook* (3rd ed., pp. 365–395). New York: Pergamon Press.

Beidel, D. C., Borden, J. W., Turner, S. M., & Jacob, R. G. (1989). The Social Phobia and Anxiety Inventory: Concurrent validity with a clinic sample. *Behaviour Research and Therapy, 27,* 573–576.

Beidel, D. C., & Turner, S. M. (1992). Scoring the Social Phobia and Anxiety Inventory: Comments on Herbert et al. (1991). *Journal of Psychopathology and Behavioral Assessment, 14,* 377–379.

Beidel, D. C., Turner, S. M., & Cooley, M. R. (1993). Assessing reliable and clinically significant change in social phobia: Validity of the Social Phobia and Anxiety Inventory. *Behaviour Research and Therapy, 31,* 331–337.

Beidel, D. C., Turner, S. M., & Dancu, C. V. (1985). Physiological, cognitive and behavioral aspects of social anxiety. *Behaviour Research and Therapy, 23,* 109–117.

Beidel, D. C., Turner, S. M., Jacob, R. G., & Cooley, M. R. (1989). Assessment of social phobia: Reliability of an impromptu speech task. *Journal of Anxiety Disorders, 3,* 149–158.

Beidel, D. C., Turner, S. M., & Morris, T. L. (1995). A new inventory to assess childhood social anxiety and phobia: The Social Phobia and Anxiety Inventory for Children. *Psychological Assessment, 7,* 73–79.

Beidel, D. C., Turner, S. M., Stanley, M. A., & Dancu, C. V. (1989). The Social Phobia and Anxiety Inventory: Concurrent and external validity. *Behavior Therapy, 20,* 417–427.

Ben-Porath, Y. S., Hostetler, K., Butcher, J. N., & Graham, J. R. (1989). New subscales for the MMPI-2 Social Introversion (Si) scale. *Psychological Assessment, 1*, 169–174.

Briggs, S. R., & Smith, T. G. (1988). The measurement of shyness. In W. H. Jones, J. M. Cheek, & S. R. Briggs (Eds.), *Shyness: Perspectives on research and treatment* (pp. 47–62). New York: Plenum Press.

Brown, E. J., Heimberg, R. G., & Juster, H. R. (1995). Social phobia subtype and avoidant personality disorder: Effect on severity of social phobia, impairment, and outcome of cognitive-behavioral treatment. *Behavior Therapy, 26*, 467–486.

Brown, E. J., Turovsky, J., Heimberg, R. G., Brown, T. A., & Barlow, D. H. (1994). *Validation of the Social Interaction Anxiety Scale and the Social Phobia Scale across the anxiety disorders.* Manuscript submitted for publication.

Brown, T. A., Di Nardo, P. A., & Barlow, D. H. (1994). *Anxiety Disorders Interview Schedule for DSM-IV (ADIS-IV).* Albany, NY: Graywind.

Buck, R. W., Parke, R. D., & Buck, M. (1970). Skin conductance, heart rate, and attention to the environment in two types of stressful situations. *Psychonomic Science, 18*, 95–96.

Butcher, J. N., Dahlstrom, W. G., Graham, J. R., Tellegen, A., & Kaemmer, B. (1989). *Minnesota Multiphasic Personality Inventory–2 (MMPI-2): Manual for administration and scoring.* Minneapolis: University of Minnesota Press.

Butcher, J. N., Graham, J. R., Williams, C. L., & Ben-Porath, Y. S. (1990). *Development and use of the MMPI-2 content scales.* Minneapolis: University of Minnesota Press.

Carter, L. E., McNeil, D. W., Turk, C. L., Ries, B. J., & Boone, M. L. (1995). *Differential treatment response among social phobia subtypes.* Manuscript submitted for publication.

Cheek, J. M., & Melchior, L. A. (1990). Shyness, self-esteem, and self-consciousness. In H. Leitenberg (Ed.), *Handbook of social and evaluation anxiety* (pp. 47–82). New York: Plenum Press.

Clark, D. B., Turner, S. M., Beidel, D. C., Donovan, J. E., Kirisci, L., & Jacob, R. G. (1994). Reliability and validity of the Social Phobia and Anxiety Inventory for adolescents. *Psychological Assessment, 6*, 135–140.

Coles, M. G. H., Donchin, E., & Porges, S. W. (Eds.). (1986). *Psychophysiology: Systems, processes, and applications.* New York: Guilford Press.

Cone, J. D. (1979). Confounded comparisons in triple response mode assessment research. *Behavioral Assessment, 1*, 85–95.

Cook, E. W., III, Melamed, B. G., Cuthbert, B. N., McNeil, D. W., & Lang, P. J. (1988). Emotional imagery and the differential diagnosis of anxiety. *Journal of Consulting and Clinical Psychology, 56*, 734–740.

Cormier, W. H., & Cormier, L. S. (1991). *Interviewing strategies for helpers: Fundamental skills and cognitive behavioral interventions* (3rd ed.). Pacific Grove, CA: Brooks/Cole.

Curran, J. P. (1982). A procedure for the assessment of social skills: The Simulated Social Interaction Test. In J. P. Curran & P. M. Monti (Eds.), *Social skills training: A practical handbook for assessment and treatment* (pp. 348–373). New York: Guilford Press.

Davidson, J. R. T., Krishnan, K. R. R., Charles, H. C., Boyko, O., Potts, N. L. S., Ford, S. M., & Patterson, L. (1993). Magnetic resonance spectroscopy in social phobia: Preliminary findings. *Journal of Clinical Psychiatry, 54*, 19–25.

Derogatis, L. R. (1983). *SCL-90-R administration, scoring, and procedures manual.* Towson, MD: Clinical Psychometric Press.

Dimberg, U., Fredrikson, M., & Lundquist, O. (1986). Autonomic reactions to social and neutral stimuli in subjects high and low in public speaking fear. *Biological Psychology, 23,* 223–233.

Dodge, C. S., Heimberg, R. G., Nyman, D., & O'Brien, G. T. (1987). Daily heterosocial interactions of high and low socially anxious college students: A diary study. *Behavior Therapy, 18,* 90–96.

Donohue, B. C., Van Hasselt, V. B., & Hersen, M. (1994). Behavioral assessment and treatment of social phobia: An evaluative review. *Behavior Modification, 18,* 262–288.

Eifert, G. H., & Wilson, P. H. (1991) The triple response approach to assessment: A conceptual and methodological reappraisal. *Behaviour Research and Therapy, 29,* 283–292.

Fenigstein, A., Scheier, M. F., & Buss, A. H. (1975). Public and private self-consciousness: Assessment and theory. *Journal of Consulting and Clinical Psychology, 43,* 522–527.

Fisher, J., & Corcoran, K. (Eds.). (1994). *Measures for clinical practice: A sourcebook: Vol. 2. Adults.* New York: Free Press.

Fredrikson, M., & Gunnarsson, R. (1992). Psychobiology of stage fright: The effect of public performance on neuroendocrine, cardiovascular and subjective reactions. *Biological Psychology, 33,* 51–61.

Friend, R., & Gilbert, J. (1973). Threat and fear of negative evaluation as determinants of locus of social comparison. *Journal of Personality, 41,* 328–340.

Gershenson, B., & Morrison, R. L. (1988). Social Interaction Test. In M. Hersen & A. S. Bellack (Eds.), *Dictionary of behavioral assessment techniques* (pp. 427–429). New York: Pergamon Press.

Gilkinson, H. (1942). Social fears as reported by students in college speech classes. *Speech Monographs, 9,* 141–160.

Glass, C. R., & Arnkoff, D. B. (1989). Behavioral assessment of social anxiety and social phobia. *Clinical Psychology Review, 9,* 75–90.

Glass, C. R., Gottman, J. M., & Shmurak, S. H. (1976). Response-acquisition and cognitive self-statement modification approaches to dating-skills training. *Journal of Counseling Psychology, 23,* 520–526.

Heimberg, R. G. (1988). Social Avoidance and Distress Scale and Fear of Negative Evaluation Scale. In M. Hersen & A. S. Bellack (Eds.), *Dictionary of behavioral assessment techniques* (pp. 425–427). New York: Pergamon Press.

Heimberg, R. G. (1991). *Cognitive behavioral treatment of social phobia in a group setting: A treatment manual* (2nd ed.). (Available from Social Phobia Program, Center for Stress and Anxiety Disorders, Pine West Plaza, Bldg. 4, Washington Avenue Extension, Albany, NY 12205.)

Heimberg, R. G., Harrison, D. F., Montgomery, D., Madsen, C. H., Jr., & Sherfey, J. A. (1980). Psychometric and behavioral analysis of a social anxiety inventory: The Situation Questionnaire. *Behavioral Assessment, 2,* 403–415.

Heimberg, R. G., Holt, C. S., Schneier, F. R., Spitzer, R. L., & Liebowitz, M. R. (1993). The issue of subtypes in the diagnosis of social phobia. *Journal of Anxiety Disorders, 7,* 249–269.

Heimberg, R. G., Hope, D. A., Dodge, C. S., & Becker, R. E. (1990). DSM-III-R subtypes of social phobia: Comparison of generalized social phobics and public speaking phobics. *Journal of Nervous and Mental Disease, 178*, 172–179.

Heimberg, R. G., Hope, D. A., Rapee, R. M., & Bruch, M. A. (1988). The validity of the Social Avoidance and Distress Scale and the Fear of Negative Evaluation Scale with social phobic patients. *Behaviour Research and Therapy, 26*, 407–410.

Heimberg, R. G., Mueller, G., Holt, C. S., Hope, D. A., & Liebowitz, M. R. (1992). Assessment of anxiety in social interaction and being observed by others: The Social Interaction Anxiety Scale and the Social Phobia Scale. *Behavior Therapy, 23*, 53–73.

Herbert, J. D., Bellack, A. S., & Hope, D. A. (1991). Concurrent validity of the Social Phobia and Anxiety Inventory. *Journal of Psychopathology and Behavioral Assessment, 13*, 357–368.

Herbert, J. D., Bellack, A. S., Hope, D. A., & Mueser, K. T. (1992). Scoring the Social Phobia and Anxiety Inventory: Reply to Beidel and Turner. *Journal of Psychopathology and Behavioral Assessment, 14*, 381–383.

Herbert, J. D., Hope, D. A., & Bellack, A. S. (1992). Validity of the distinction between generalized social phobia and avoidant personality disorder. *Journal of Abnormal Psychology, 101*, 332–339.

Hofmann, S. G., Newman, M. G., Ehlers, A., & Roth, W. T. (1995). Psychophysiological differences between subgroups of social phobia. *Journal of Abnormal Psychology, 104*, 224–231.

Hollandsworth, J. G., Jr. (1986). *Physiology and behavior therapy: Conceptual guidelines for the clinician.* New York: Plenum Press.

Holt, C. S., Heimberg, R. G., & Hope, D. A. (1992). Avoidant personality disorder and the generalized subtype of social phobia. *Journal of Abnormal Psychology, 101*, 177–189.

Hope, D. A., Gansler, D. A., & Heimberg, R. G. (1989). Attentional focus and causal attributions in social phobia: Implications from social psychology. *Clinical Psychology Review, 9*, 49–60.

Hope, D. A., Herbert, J. D., & White, C. (1995). Diagnostic subtype, avoidant personality disorder, and efficacy of cognitive behavioral group therapy for social phobia. *Cognitive Therapy and Research, 19*, 285–303.

Jones, W. H., Briggs, S. R., & Smith, T. G. (1986). Shyness: Conceptualization and measurement. *Journal of Personality and Social Psychology, 51*, 629–639.

Kendall, P. C. (1990). Behavioral assessment and methodology. In C. M. Franks, G. T. Wilson, P. C. Kendall, & J. P. Foreyt, *Review of behavior therapy: Theory and practice* (Vol. 12, pp. 44–71). New York: Guilford Press.

Kern, J. M. (1994). The use of role-plays in behavioral assessment. In M. Hersen, R. Eisler, & P. Miller (Eds.), *Progress in behavior modification* (Vol. 29, pp. 73–97). Pacific Grove, CA: Brooks/Cole.

Klorman, R., Weerts, T. C., Hastings, J. E., Melamed, B. G., & Lang, P. J. (1974). Psychometric description of some specific-fear questionnaires. *Behavior Therapy, 5*, 401–409.

Knight, M. L., & Borden, R. J. (1979). Autonomic and affective reactions of high and low socially-anxious individuals awaiting public performance. *Psychophysiology, 16*, 209–213.

Kolko, D. J., & Milan, M. A. (1985). A women's heterosocial skills observational rating system: Behavior-analytic development and validation. *Behavior Modification, 9,* 165–192.

Lader, M. H. (1967). Palmar skin conductance measures in anxiety and phobic states. *Journal of Psychosomatic Research, 11,* 271–281.

Lang, P. J. (1968) Fear reduction and fear behavior: Problems in treating a construct. In J. M. Shlien (Ed.), *Research in psychotherapy* (Vol. 3, pp. 90–102). Washington, DC: American Psychological Association.

Lang, P. J. (1993). The three-system approach to emotion. In N. Birbaumer & A. Ohman (Eds.), *The structure of emotion* (pp. 18–30). Seattle, WA: Hogrefe & Huber.

Leary, M. R. (1983a). A brief version of the Fear of Negative Evaluation Scale. *Personality and Social Psychology Bulletin, 9,* 371–375.

Leary, M. R. (1983b). Social anxiousness: The construct and its measurement. *Journal of Personality Assessment, 47,* 66–75.

Lehrer, P. M., & Woolfolk, R. L. (1982). Self-report assessment of anxiety: Somatic, cognitive, and behavioral modalities. *Behavioral Assessment, 4,* 167–177.

Lelliott, P. (1988). Marks and Mathews Fear Questionnaire. In M. Hersen & A. S. Bellack (Eds.), *Dictionary of behavioral assessment techniques* (pp. 293–294). New York: Pergamon Press.

Levin, A. P., Saoud, J. B., Strauman, T., Gorman, J. M., Fyer, A. J., Crawford, R., & Liebowitz, M. R. (1993). Responses of "generalized" and "discrete" social phobics during public speaking. *Journal of Anxiety Disorders, 7,* 207–221.

Lewin, M. R., McNeil, D. W., & Lipson, J. M. (1995). *Enduring without avoiding: Verbal dysfluencies and pauses in public speaking anxiety.* Manuscript submitted for publication.

Lombardo, T. W. (1988). Personal Report of Confidence as a Speaker. In M. Hersen & A. S. Bellack (Eds.), *Dictionary of behavioral assessment techniques* (pp. 347–348). New York: Pergamon Press.

Marks, I. M. (1987). *Fears, phobias, and rituals: Panic, anxiety, and their disorders.* New York: Oxford University Press.

Marks, I. M., & Mathews, A. M. (1979). Brief standard rating for phobic patients. *Behaviour Research and Therapy, 17,* 263–267.

Matias, R., Jr., & Turner, S. M. (1986). Concordance and discordance in speech anxiety assessment: The effects of demand characteristics on the tripartite assessment method. *Behaviour Research and Therapy, 24,* 537–545.

Mattick, R. P., & Clarke, J. C. (1989). *Development and validation of measures of social phobia scrutiny fear and social interaction anxiety.* Unpublished manuscript.

Mattick, R. P., & Peters, L. (1988). Treatment of severe social phobia: Effects of guided exposure with and without cognitive restructuring. *Journal of Consulting and Clinical Psychology, 56,* 251–260.

Mattick, R. P., Peters, L., & Clarke, J. C. (1989). Exposure and cognitive restructuring for social phobia: A controlled study. *Behavior Therapy, 20,* 3–23.

McGlynn, F. D. (1988). Behavioral Avoidance Test. In M. Hersen & A. S. Bellack (Eds.), *Dictionary of behavioral assessment techniques* (pp. 59–60). New York: Pergamon Press.

McNeil, D. W., & Lewin, M. R. (1995). *Behavioral avoidance and escape in circumscribed speech and generalized social anxiety.* Manuscript in preparation.

McNeil, D. W., Turk, C. L., & Ries, B. J. (1994). Anxiety and fear. In V. S. Ramachandran (Ed.), *Encyclopedia of human behavior* (Vol. 1, pp. 151–163). San Diego, CA: Academic Press.

McNeil, D. W., Vrana, S. R., Melamed, B. G., Cuthbert, B. N., & Lang, P. J. (1993). Emotional imagery in simple and social phobia: Fear vs. anxiety. *Journal of Abnormal Psychology, 102*, 212–225.

Miller, B. V., & Bernstein, D. A. (1972). Instructional demand in a behavioral avoidance test for claustrophobic fears. *Journal of Abnormal Psychology, 80*, 206–210.

Miller, G. A., & Kozak, M. J. (1993). Three-systems assessment and the construct of emotion. In N. Birbaumer & A. Ohman (Eds.), *The structure of emotion* (pp. 31–47). Seattle, WA: Hogrefe & Huber.

Monti, P. M., Boice, R., Fingeret, A. L., Zwick, W. R., Kolko, D., Munroe, S., & Grunberger, A. (1984). Midi-level measurement of social anxiety in psychiatric and non-psychiatric samples. *Behaviour Research and Therapy, 22*, 651–660.

Monti, P. M., Wallander, J. L., Ahern, D. K., Abrams, D. B., & Munroe, S. M. (1984). Multimodal measurement of anxiety and social skills in a behavioral role-play test: Generalizability and discriminant validity. *Behavioral Assessment, 6*, 15–25.

Oei, T. P. S., Moylan, A., & Evans, L. (1991). Validity and clinical utility of the Fear Questionnaire for anxiety-disorder patients. *Psychological Assessment, 3*, 391–397.

Paul, G. (1966). *Insight vs. desensitization in psychotherapy*. Stanford, CA: Stanford University Press.

Perri, M. G., & Richards, C. S. (1979). Assessment of heterosocial skills in male college students: Empirical development of a behavioral role-playing test. *Behavior Modification, 3*, 337–354.

Rachman, S. J. (1990). *Fear and courage* (2nd ed.). New York: Freeman.

Rachman, S., & Hodgson, R. (1974). I. Synchrony and desynchrony in fear and avoidance. *Behaviour Research and Therapy, 12*, 311–318.

Rapee, R. M., Brown, T. A., Antony, M. A., & Barlow, D. H. (1992). Response to hyperventilation and inhalation of 5.5% carbon dioxide-enriched air across the DSM-III-R anxiety disorders. *Journal of Abnormal Psychology, 101*, 538–552.

Rehm, L. P., & Marston, A. R. (1968). Reduction of social anxiety through modification of self-reinforcement: An instigation therapy technique. *Journal of Consulting and Clinical Psychology, 32*, 565–574.

Richmond, V. P., & McCroskey, J. C. (1992). *Communication: Apprehension, avoidance, and effectiveness* (3rd ed.). Scottsdale, AZ: Gorsuch Scarisbrick.

Ries, B. J., McNeil, D. W., Boone, M. L., Turk, C. L., Carter, L. E., & Heimberg, R. G. (1995). *Assessment of contemporary social phobia verbal report instruments*. Manuscript in preparation.

Schneier, F. R., Heckelman, L. R., Garfinkel, R., Campeas, R., Fallon, B. A., Gitow, A., Street, L., Del Bene, D., & Liebowitz, M. R. (1994). Functional impairment in social phobia. *Journal of Clinical Psychiatry, 55*, 322–331.

Scholing, A., & Emmelkamp, P. M. G. (1990). Social phobia: Nature and treatment. In H. Leitenberg (Ed.), *Handbook of social and evaluation anxiety* (pp. 269–324). New York: Plenum Press.

Shearn, D., Bergman, E., Hill, K., Abel, A., & Hinds, L. (1992) Blushing as a function of audience size. *Psychophysiology, 29,* 431–436.

Smith, R. E., & Sarason, I. G. (1975). Social anxiety and the evaluation of negative interpersonal feedback. *Journal of Consulting and Clinical Psychology, 43,* 429.

Steketee, G., & Freund, B. (1988). Willoughby Personality Schedule. In M. Hersen & A. S. Bellack (Eds.), *Dictionary of behavioral assessment techniques* (pp. 492–494). New York: Pergamon Press.

Tancer, M. E. (1994). Neurobiology of social phobia. *Journal of Clinical Psychiatry, 54,* 26–30.

Trower, P., Bryant, B., & Argyle, M. (1978). *Social skills and mental health.* Pittsburgh: University of Pittsburgh Press.

Turner, S. M., & Beidel, D. C. (1985). Empirically derived subtypes of social anxiety. *Behavior Therapy, 16,* 384–392.

Turner, S. M., & Beidel, D. C. (1988). Some further comments on the measurement of social phobia. *Behaviour Research and Therapy, 26,* 411–413.

Turner, S. M., & Beidel, D. C. (in press). *Social Phobia and Anxiety Inventory Manual.* Toronto: Multi-Health Systems.

Turner, S. M., Beidel, D. C., Borden, J. W., Stanley, M. A., & Jacob, R. G. (1991). Social phobia: Axis I and II correlates. *Journal of Abnormal Psychology, 100,* 102–106.

Turner, S. M., Beidel, D. C., Cooley, M. R., Woody, S. R., & Messer, S. C. (1994). A multicomponent behavioral treatment for social phobia: Social effectiveness therapy. *Behaviour Research and Therapy, 32,* 381–390.

Turner, S. M., Beidel, D. C., Dancu, C. V., & Stanley, M. A. (1989). An empirically derived inventory to measure social fears and anxiety: The Social Phobia and Anxiety Inventory. *Psychological Assessment, 1,* 35–40.

Turner, S. M., Beidel, D. C., & Larkin K. T. (1986). Situational determinants of social anxiety in clinic and nonclinic samples: Physiological and cognitive correlates. *Journal of Consulting and Clinical Psychology, 54,* 523–527.

Turner, S. M., Beidel, D. C., Long, P. J., & Greenhouse, J. (1992). Reduction of fear in social phobics: An examination of extinction patterns. *Behavior Therapy, 23,* 389–403.

Turner, S. M., Beidel, D. C., Long, P. J., Turner, M. W., & Townsley, R. M. (1993). A composite measure to determine the functional status of treated social phobics: The Social Phobia Endstate Functioning Index. *Behavior Therapy, 24,* 265–275.

Turner, S. M., Beidel, D. C., & Townsley, R. M. (1992). Social phobia: A comparison of specific and generalized subtypes and avoidant personality disorder. *Journal of Abnormal Psychology, 101,* 326–331.

Turner, S. M., McCanna, M., & Beidel, D. C. (1987). Discriminative validity of the Social Avoidance and Distress and Fear of Negative Evaluation Scales. *Behaviour Research and Therapy, 25,* 113–115.

Turner, S. M., Stanley, M. A., Beidel, D. C., & Bond, L. (1989). The Social Phobia and Anxiety Inventory: Construct validity. *Journal of Psychopathology and Behavioral Assessment, 11,* 221–234.

Turpin, G. (1991). The psychophysiological assessment of anxiety disorders: Three-systems measurement and beyond. *Psychological Assessment, 3,* 366–375.

Twentyman, C. T., & McFall, R. M. (1975). Behavioral training of social skills in shy males. *Journal of Consulting and Clinical Psychology, 43*, 384–395.

Wallander, J. L., Conger, A. J., Mariotto, M. J., Curran, J. P., & Farrell, A. D. (1980). Comparability of selection instruments in studies of heterosexual–social problem behaviors. *Behavior Therapy, 11*, 548–560.

Waters, W. F., Williamson, D. A., Bernard, B. A., Blouin, D. C., & Faulstich, M. E. (1987). Test–retest reliability of psychophysiological assessment. *Behaviour Research and Therapy, 25*, 213–221.

Watson, D., & Friend, R. (1969). Measurement of social-evaluative anxiety. Journal of Consulting and Clinical Psychology, 33, 448–457.

Wolpe, J., & Lang, P. J. (1977). *Manual for the Fear Survey Schedule*. San Diego, CA: Educational and Industrial Testing Service.

Zimbardo, P. G. (1977). *Shyness: What it is and what to do about it*. Reading, MA: Addison-Wesley.

CHAPTER ELEVEN

Cognitive Assessment

DIRK TAYLOR ELTING
DEBRA A. HOPE

The cardinal feature of social phobia—fear of negative evaluation—is essentially a cognitive construct. Social phobics fear scrutiny by others and worry that they will be humiliated or embarrassed by their own actions. Thus, when social phobics are in the presence of others, they *believe* their performance is inadequate and they *think* they are being judged or criticized. By definition, *thoughts* play a central role in their disorder. In addition to thoughts, other cognitive constructs also play an important role in the pathogenesis of social phobia. For instance, cross-situational expectations of threat in social settings may contribute to the avoidance exhibited by many social phobics. Atypical allocation of attention and biased memory processes may interfere with the execution of complex social exchanges or result in the misinterpretation of social cues. Thus, any comprehensive conceptualization of social phobia must incorporate an understanding of the disorder's relevant cognitive features.

However, it is difficult to discuss these features without first attempting to define what exactly is meant by the term "cognitive." Depending on one's orientation, the term "cognitive" can be used to describe anything from a treatment modality focused on changing dysfunctional thoughts and schemata (e.g., Beck & Emery, 1985) to the experimental paradigms associated with cognitive science (e.g., Posner, 1989) and cognitive neuroscience (e.g., Näätänen, 1992). Given this conceptual diversity, Ingram and Kendall and their colleagues (e.g., Ingram & Kendall, 1987; Ingram & Wisnicki, 1991; Kendall & Ingram, 1987) have developed a "meta-construct model of psychopathology" that can be usefully adapted to define the aspects of cognition relevant to this chapter.

Within the meta-construct model, two broad dimensions are conceptualized. The first of these is a "cognitive taxonomy" that delineates four levels intended to encompass the important components of a cognitive system. The most elemental of these is the *cognitive structural* level, which refers to the "architecture," or structural mechanisms, of the system. By definition cognitive structures are "contentless." Ingram and Wisnicki (1991) offer long- and short-term memory as examples of constructs represented at this level. However, from the perspective of cognitive neuroscience, one could logically also incorporate the actual physical structures of the central nervous system. *Cognitive propositions* are the bits of information stored and organized within the cognitive structures. Included at this level are both memory traces and the abstractions (e.g., beliefs, expectancies, schemata) used to organize memories into rules that guide the cognitive system. *Cognitive operations*, or the processes by which the system gathers and handles information, represent the third level in the taxonomy. Processes such as attention, encoding, and retrieval are examples of cognitive operations. Finally, *cognitive products* are the output of the system. Thoughts, self-statements, and specific attributions are all examples of cognitive products.

The second dimension in the Ingram–Kendall meta-construct framework is called the "component model of psychopathology." In this dimension, it is proposed that aspects of psychopathology can be partitioned into three basic components. The first of these encompasses *critical features*, or those aspects of psychopathology that are central to a specific disorder. The second component encompasses *common features*, or those aspects of psychopathology that are identifiable in a variety of different disorders. The final component involves features that vary unsystematically, such as individual differences. Ingram and Kendall group these features under the rubric of *error variance*. Since these features tend to be ideographic, the discussion of them vis-à-vis nomothetic assessment is inappropriate and will not be considered further.

By combining Ingram and Kendall's cognitive taxonomy and component models, it is possible to construct a matrix within which the different cognitive elements may be organized. As may be seen in Table 11.1, thoughts associated with a fear of negative evaluation (e.g., "They'll think I'm boring") would be placed at the intersection of cognitive products and critical features. More generic instances of dysfunctional thoughts (e.g., "I'm worthless") fall at the intersection of cognitive products and common features, since these thoughts may occur in both social phobia and other disorders such as depression. At a lower level, attentional processes favoring social threat cues fall at the intersection of cognitive operations and critical features, while less specific attentional process (e.g., excessive processing of task-irrelevant stimuli) would fall at the intersection of cognitive operations and common features.

This matrix will be utilized as a heuristic to organize the information presented in the remainder of this chapter and to facilitate a more coherent

TABLE 11.1. Elements of a Meta-Construct Model of Psychopathology Applied to Social Phobia

	Components of psychopathology	
Level of analysis	Critical features	Common features
Cognitive products	Thoughts associated with the fear of negative evaluation	Dysfunctional thoughts
Cognitive operations	Selective attention to cues of social threat	Allocation of attentional resources to task-irrelevant stimuli
Cognitive propositions	High expectancies of social threat, and low expectancies for the performance of socially relevant behaviors	Dysfunctional schemata and beliefs
Cognitive structures	Disregulation of monoamine pathways	Central nervous system disregulation

Note. Adapted from Ingram and Wisnicki (1991, p. 198). Copyright 1991 by Sage Publications. Adapted by permission.

and theoretically interesting discussion of the subject matter. This discussion will incorporate a review of assessment instruments and procedures that are useful at different levels of the cognitive taxonomy. Where it is logical to do so, the discussion will be further subdivided along the critical features versus common features distinction. As will become clear, these divisions are somewhat artificial, with some instruments and procedures falling into more than one category.

Unfortunately, the discussion will not include a review of assessment strategies useful at the cognitive structural level. No traditional psychometric or information-processing strategies currently exist for investigating constructs at this level, and the tools of cognitive neuroscience (e.g., animal modeling, neuroimaging) are well beyond the scope of this chapter. Interested readers are referred to Gray (1982) or Panksepp (1990) for excellent discussions of the role of structural elements in anxiety disorders.

COGNITIVE PROPOSITIONS

Cognitive propositions may be thought of as the informational content of the cognitive system. This logically includes representations of past and present events but, more important, involves abstractions pertaining to the meaning of such events. These abstractions allow the individual to organize sensory information drawn from the environment and to make predictions about both proximal and distal future events. If these abstractions are dysfunctional, it follows that the individual will be vulnerable to the development of a wide range of emotional problems. Such overlapping theoretical constructs as expectancies (Bandura, 1977), beliefs (Ellis, 1962), locus of control (Levenson, 1973), attributional style (Abramson, Seligman, & Teasdale, 1978), and schemata[1] (e.g., Beck & Emery, 1985) may be thought of as examples of cognitive propositions.

Expectancies

Expectancies play a central role in several theoretical formulations of social anxiety and social phobia (Leary & Kowalski, Chapter 5, this volume; Trower & Gilbert, 1989). However, a review of the literature reveals a paucity of empirical investigations addressing social phobics' expectancies and few options for expectancy assessment.

The Self-Efficacy Questionnaire for Social Skills (SEQSS; Moe & Zeiss, 1982) provides one option. With this instrument, subjects are presented with 12 social situations derived from combinations of three dimensions: (1) familiarity with others (close friend, acquaintance, stranger), (2) number of others (one, small group), and (3) interest of conversation (lively, dull). Subjects rate their expected social behavior in these situations across 12 positive attributes (e.g., assertiveness, humor, warmth). The authors present good reliability data (e.g., coefficient alphas > .80) for all but two situation subscales. All but one of the subscales yielded moderately high correlations ($r = .32 - .64$) with other measures of social anxiety, providing some evidence of construct validity. Unfortunately, these data were derived from analogue studies, and no psychometric data are available from clinical populations. Furthermore, a search of the literature found no empirical investigations of social phobia utilizing this instrument.

Another instrument, the Situational Expectancies Inventory (SEI; Gormally, Sipps, Raphael, Edwin, & Varvil-Weld, 1981) is a paper-and-pencil measure designed to assess risk expectancy in heterosocial situations. With this instrument, subjects are presented with four typical dating situations and required to rate each on two scales: (1) outcome (horrible to ecstatic), and (2) probability of rejection (not at all to highly likely). Risk scores for each situation are defined as the product of the two scales. The authors report good reliability for the instrument (Cronbach's alpha = .81), and

---

[1] Many theorists refer to schemata as cognitive structures, while Ingram and Wisnicki (1991) placed them in both the structural and propositional levels of the taxonomy. However, we prefer to view them simply as propositional constructs, since most definitions suggest schemata are abstractions that develop from experience.

evidence for validity comes from the moderately high negative correlation ($r = -.51$) with measures of dating confidence.

Both the SEQSS and the SEI appear to tap expectancies that are relevant to social phobia. However, the latter scale would be appropriate only for social phobics with dating fears. Because neither scale has been widely used, more research is needed to determine their utility in clinical samples.

In a report of preliminary data from an ongoing investigation, Franklin, Perry, Herbert, and Foa (1993) describe a questionnaire used to assess expectancies in treated and untreated generalized social phobics. The Probability–Cost Questionnaire (PCQ) requires subjects to rate the probability that 20 negative social events and 20 negative nonsocial events would happen to them. Subjects also rate the costs associated with these same events. An overall threat index is computed by multiplying the subjects' probability and cost judgments. Compared to normal control subjects and treated social phobics, untreated social phobics judged negative social events to be more likely *and* predicted that higher costs would be associated with these events. Consequently, the overall threat index for untreated social phobics was significantly greater than that for treated social phobics or normal controls, who did not differ on this measure. Unfortunately, psychometric data are not available for the PCQ at this time. Such data, which are currently being collected, will be necessary before a complete assessment of the utility of this measure can be made.

Beliefs

A more abundant literature exists regarding the assessment of irrational beliefs, though once again, few measures have been developed for this task. The Irrational Beliefs Test (IBT; Jones, 1969) has been used in at least five studies addressing social phobia treatment outcome, while the Rational Behavior Inventory (RBI; Shorkey, Reyes, & Whiteman, 1977) has been used in at least two (Heimberg, 1994). Both of these instruments are based on Ellis's (1962) rational–emotive theory and are designed for the assessment of irrational beliefs thought to be associated with psychopathology. Neither of these instruments was designed for the assessment of social phobia per se, but either may be a useful index of common features.

The IBT is a 100-item endorsement-type measure designed to tap 10 common irrational beliefs. Lohr and Bonge (1982) reported moderate evidence in support of the IBT's internal structure but found the reliability of the 10-subscale scoring system to be lacking. They propose an alternative 7-subscale system derived from principal components analysis. Similarly, the 70-item RBI was designed to assess 11 aspects of rational behavior, but a subsequent factor analysis by Himle, Thyer, and Papsdorf (1982) suggested that only 7 factors are represented by the measure. No one appears to have investigated whether the 7 factors of the two measures represent the same seven constructs.

While some empirical investigations indicate that different irrational beliefs are associated with different fears (Deffenbacher, Zwemer, Whisman, Hill, & Sloan, 1986) and that measures of irrational beliefs may be useful in research addressing social anxiety (e.g., Gormally et al., 1981), Heimberg (1994) noted that the IBT appears to lack discriminant validity (e.g., Smith, 1983; Smith & Zurawski, 1983) and may simply be a measure of negative affect. Smith (1989) argued that the apparent low validity of the IBT results from a failure to differentiate between irrational beliefs (i.e., cognitive propositions) and negative thinking (i.e., cognitive products). Since the RBI has very similar qualities, it may also have this particular shortcoming. Thus, a careful consideration of assessment goals should be made prior to selecting these particular measures of beliefs.

Locus of Control

Rotter (1966) postulated that people who believe that contingencies are related to their own behavior (internal locus of control) are less vulnerable to emotional distress than are people who believe contingencies are controlled by fate, chance, or powerful others (external locus of control). The Internal–External Locus of Control Scale (Rotter, 1966) was developed to test this hypothesis and has become one of the most widely used instruments in psychological assessment. Levenson (1973) modified the original scale in order to differentiate subsets of individuals with an external locus of control. Thus the Levenson Locus of Control Scale (LOCS) contains a subscale for Internality and two subscales for Externality: Powerful Others (contingencies are controlled by people who wield power) and Chance (contingencies are the result of random chance factors).

The LOCS contains 24 items (8 per subscale) and utilizes a six-point response format. Levenson (1973) reports acceptable internal consistency for the subscales, with Kuder–Richardson reliabilities of .67, .82, and .79 for the Internality, Powerful Others, and Chance subscales, respectively. Cloitre, Heimberg, Liebowitz, and Gitow (1992) found similar reliabilities, reporting Cronbach's alphas of .77, .72, and .69 for the same subscales, respectively. Factor analysis of the LOCS (Levenson, 1973) strongly supported the validity of the Chance and Powerful Others subscales, with seven out of eight items from each subscale loading solely on the appropriate factor. Moderate support for the validity of the Internality subscale was found, with four out of eight items loading solely on the appropriate factor.

Cloitre, Heimberg, Liebowitz, and Gitow (1992) used the LOCS to assess perceptions of control in individuals with social phobia and panic disorder. The LOCS was administered to 14 social phobics, 14 panic disordered subjects, and 14 normal controls. As expected, social phobics achieved significantly higher scores on the Powerful Others subscale than did either the normal control or panic disordered groups, which did not differ from each other. Likewise, the panic disordered group produced significantly higher scores on the Chance subscale than did the social phobics or normal controls, who did not differ from each other. All three groups were significantly different from each other on the Internality subscale, with normals achieving the highest scores, social phobics achieving the next highest scores, and panic disordered individuals achieving the lowest scores.

The findings reported by Cloitre, Heimberg, Liebowitz, and Gitow (1992) suggest the LOCS may be useful in assessing perceptions of control in social phobics. The Powerful Others subscale is conceptually related to social phobia, and it clearly is able to distinguish social phobia from panic disorder. However, since a large number of studies have shown locus of control to be related to many types of physical and emotional distress (e.g., Bates, Edwards, & Andersen, 1993; Nezu, 1986; Obitz & Oziel, 1978), it is difficult to determine if the LOCS assesses a truly critical feature of social phobia. It may, in fact, measure a construct that is in a somewhat gray area between common and critical features, an issue that arises again below.

Attributional Style

While the attributions an individual makes about specific events are clearly cognitive products, attributional style (i.e., the tendency to make certain types of attributions across situations) is a construct best represented at the propositional level of the cognitive taxonomy. Although attributional style is most often associated with research involving depression and the reformulated theory of learned helplessness (Abramson et al., 1978), some studies have demonstrated differences in attributional style between individuals who are low versus those who are high in social anxiety (e.g. Alden, 1987; Anderson & Arnoult, 1985; Girodo, Dotzenroth, & Stein, 1981). Irrespective of the disorder addressed by specific studies, most indicate that individuals whose attributional style favors internal, global, and/ or stable causal explanations for negative events are more vulnerable to emotional distress.

The Attributional Style Questionnaire (ASQ; Peterson et al., 1982) is easily the most widely used measure of attributional style. The ASQ utilizes 12 hypothetical events—6 with positive outcomes (e.g., "You do a project that is highly praised") and 6 with negative outcomes (e.g., "You go out on a date and it goes badly"). Half the events address interpersonal/ affiliative issues, and half address achievement-related issues, resulting in four types of events (i.e., good–achievement; good–affiliation; bad–achievement; bad–affiliation). For each event, subjects are asked to provide, through free response, one major cause for the event. They then rate that same cause on three seven-point scales addressing attributional style (internality–externality, globality–specificity, stability–instability), as well as a fourth seven-point scale addressing the importance of the event.

Peterson et al. (1982) reported acceptable psychometric properties for the ASQ. Cronbach's alpha coefficients of .75 and .72 were obtained for the composite scales addressing good and bad events, respectively. Interitem reliabilities for the three attributional dimensions range from .44 to .69 (mean = .54). Unfortunately, Peterson et al. (1982) report that the ASQ fails to discriminate between interpersonal/affiliative and achievement-related issues.

This failure is particularly disappointing for those interested in social phobia, as interpersonal/affiliative issues are central to the disorder. Nonetheless, Heimberg, Becker, Goldfinger, and Vermilyea (1985) reported that social phobics who received cognitive-behavioral therapy showed significant changes on the ASQ attributional dimensions of internality and stability. This finding, in concert with findings reporting the utility of the ASQ in depression research (e.g., Hamilton & Abramson, 1983; Persons & Rao, 1985), suggests the ASQ measures aspects of attributional style that are common to many disorders. This hypothesis was substantiated by Heimberg et al. (1989), who reported no systematic differences on the ASQ between social phobics, agoraphobics, and persons with dysthymic disorder.

It may be that attributional style dimensions other than those incorporated in the ASQ are necessary to address the critical features of social phobia. For instance, Anderson and Arnoult (1985) reported that attributions relating to controllability were the most robust predictor of shyness in college undergraduates. However, this same attribution was also an excellent predictor of loneliness and depression, suggesting that controllability is also an attributional dimension relevant to common rather than critical features. Clearly, further investigations will be necessary before the role of attributional styles specific to social phobia can be understood.

Self-Schemata

Higgins (1987) hypothesized that discrepancies between an individual's various representations of him- or herself are associated with specific types of emotional distress. In this formulation, known as "self-discrepancy theory," it is proposed that six self-state representations (i.e., self-schemata) are formed by a combination of two dimensions. The first dimension, *standpoints on the self*, consists of two positions—an individual's *own* standpoint and the standpoint of a significant *other*. Thus, it is argued that distinct representations of the self exist, based on internal and external perspectives. The second dimension, *domains of the self*, encompasses three basic positions. The *actual* self is the representation that an individual has of the attributes that someone (oneself or another) believes the individual actually possesses. The *ideal* self is the representation that an individual has of the attributes that someone (oneself or another) believes the individual should ideally possess, while the *ought* self is the representation that an individual has of the attributes that someone (oneself or another) believes the individual ought to possess. According to Higgins (1987), the distinction between the ideal and the ought representations is reflected in the distinction between an individual's "personal wishes" and his or her "sense of duty" (p. 320).

Six self-states (actual/own, actual/other, ideal/own, ideal/other, ought/own, ought/other) are formed by a combination of the two dimensions. It is thought that the intensity of emotional distress is related to the magnitude of discrepancy between self-states, whereas the quality of the distress (e.g., dissatisfaction, shame, guilt, apprehension) is a manifestation of discrepancies between two specific self-states.

The Selves Questionnaire (Higgins, Klein, & Strauman, 1985) quantifies the six self-states by asking subjects to list up to 10 attributes associated with each representation (e.g., "Please list the attributes of the type of person your parents or friends believe you ought to be"). Discrepancy scores are calculated by analyzing inconsistencies in the attributes listed across the different self-state categories. Higgins et al. (1985) report good interrater reliability for scoring of the questionnaire ($r = .81$). Moreover, as was hypothesized, specific patterns of discrepancy were associated with specific emotional states, supporting the measure's discriminant validity. For instance, discrepancies between actual/own and actual/other representations were associated with indecision and dependency, whereas an actual/own–ideal/other discrepancy was associated with dysphoria and loss of pride.

Consistent with the predictions of self-discrepancy theory, Strauman (1989) reported that social phobics have a discrepancy between their actual view of themselves and their beliefs of what significant others think they ought to be (actual/own versus ought/other; A-Own/Ogt-Oth). Such a discrepancy is congruent with the social phobics' fear of negative evaluation by others. In contrast, patients with major depression exhibited a discrepancy between their actual view of themselves and their view of how they would ideally like to be (actual/own versus ideal/own; A-Own/I-Own), suggesting emotional distress because of a failure to achieve personal goals. Thus, Strauman's findings further support the discriminant validity of the Selves Questionnaire by obtaining the hypothesized relationship between self-state, social phobia, and depression. Moreover, they indicate that the instrument should be useful in the assessment of cognitive propositions associated with social phobia.

However, Weilage and Hope (1993) failed to replicate Strauman's (1989) findings when comparing dysthymics, generalized social phobics, and nongeneralized social phobics. In this study, dysthymics' and nongeneralized social phobics' discrepancy scores did not differ, contrary to expectations. Moreover, generalized social phobics had larger discrepancies than did either group on *both* the A-Own/Ogt-Oth and A-Own/I-Own comparisons. The failure to replicate appears to have resulted from lower than expected A-Own/I-Own discrepancies in the dysthymic group, suggesting meaningful differences between dysthymia and major depression vis-à-vis the role of self-discrepancy.

The findings reported by Weilage and Hope (1993) suggest an actual/own–ought/other discrepancy is probably not a critical feature of social phobia. This is not surprising in light of Higgins's (1987) formulation, which predicts such discrepancies will be associated with "agitation from fear and threat" (p. 326), an emotional state clearly not unique to social phobia. Nonetheless, such discrepancies do seem to play an important role in social anxiety. Likewise, the larger discrepancies evidenced by generalized social phobics compared to nongeneralized social phobics are consistent with Higgins's (1987) formulation that the magnitude of discrepancy is associated with the intensity of distress. Thus, the Selves Questionnaire appears to be useful in assessing both self-schemata and the degree of pathology associated with social phobia.

In addition to the Selves Questionnaire, some researchers (e.g., Arnkoff & Glass, 1989; Parks & Hollon, 1988) have proposed that self-schemata may be assessed using information-processing paradigms such as depth-of-processing tasks and the modified Stroop procedure. Although these methods may reflect the impact of schemata and other types of cognitive propositions on the processing of information, they more clearly reflect the cognitive processes themselves. Thus, these techniques will be discussed in the following section on cognitive operations.

COGNITIVE OPERATIONS

Research on atypical information processing thought to be associated with psychopathology has blossomed in recent years (see Eysenck, 1992, or Magaro, 1991, for detailed discussions). Typically these investigations have adapted research paradigms from experimental cognitive psychology. Several of these methodologies have been used to explore the extent to which socially anxious individuals selectively attend to, encode, and recall threatening information.

Attentional Processes

Modified Stroop Tasks

One of the most widely used information-processing paradigms is a modification of the Stroop color-naming task (Stroop, 1935). In the original version of this task, subjects were asked to name the ink color in which either symbols or words were printed. Subjects were instructed to ignore semantic content and attend only to ink color. However, when the printed words were the names of incongruent colors (e.g., when the word "green" was printed in red ink), the time required to name ink color substantially increased. The exact mechanisms underlying this phenomenon are not clearly understood. The interested reader is referred to C. M. MacLeod (1992) for an excellent recent review.

When used to explore cognitive processes associated with social anxiety, the stimulus words in the Stroop task are selected to reflect social-evaluative concerns. These words may denote negative evaluation by others (e.g., "foolish" or "boring") or aspects of the feared social situations (e.g., "dating" or "speech"). Typically the words are matched with affectively neutral control words for frequency of usage and number of letters and syllables. However, because threat words are chosen to be central to subjects' fears, it seems possible that social threat words may be more familiar to subjects than to the general population. This makes the use of standard word frequency references (e.g., Carroll, Davies, & Richman, 1971) to control for frequency of usage somewhat questionable.

Usually the primary variable of interest is the "interference index," or the difference in color-naming latency between threat and control words. The interference index is intended to estimate the extra processing time associated with the emotional content of the words, after controlling for other factors such as word familiarity and overall intersubject differences in color-naming latencies. However, some researchers (e.g., Martin, Williams, & Clark, 1991) report only the actual color-naming latencies.

The use of raw latency scores may be problematic for two reasons. First, it fails to control for intersubject variability in overall color-naming latency within diagnostic groups, adding to the error variance. Second, Mattia, Heimberg, and Hope (1993) found that social phobics had longer latencies than did community controls, regardless of type of stimulus, suggesting a general performance deficit on the task. Use of the interference index separates this general deficit from specific effects associated with social threat stimuli. Clearly, further research on the validity of various scoring strategies is needed.

Several studies have supported the utility of the Stroop task with social phobics. Latency to color-name social threat stimuli versus panic-related and control stimuli distinguished social phobics from individuals with panic disorder (Hope, Rapee, Heimberg, & Dombeck, 1990) and from community controls (Mattia et al., 1993). Moreover, marked reductions in response latency to social threat stimulus sets were associated with a positive response to treatment for social phobia (Mattia et al., 1993). Excessive processing of social threat stimuli, as assessed by the Stroop task, appears to be associated with the critical features of social phobia.

McNeil et al. (1995) used three types of social threat stimuli—general social stimuli, speech stimuli, and negative social evaluative stimuli—to distinguish two groups of generalized social phobics (those with and without avoidant personality disorder [APD]) from a circumscribed speech phobia group. All groups showed interference from speech stimuli and negative social evaluative stimuli, but only generalized social phobics—with or without APD—evidenced interference from the general social stimuli. However, this study was unable to differentiate generalized social phobics with APD from those without APD. It is unknown whether this failure is attributable to the small number of APD subjects used in the study ($N = 9$), to lack of sensitivity of the Stroop task, or to poor validity of conceptualizations of APD (e.g., Widiger, 1992) according to the criteria of the third revised edition of the *Diagnostic and Statistical Manual of Mental Disorders* (DSM-III-R; American Psychiatric Association, 1987).

Although the modified Stroop task is hypothesized by many to demonstrate an attentional basis in favor of threat (e.g., Mathews & MacLeod, 1985; McNally, Reimann, & Kim, 1990), an alternative hypothesis that emotionality per se (positive or negative) produces the interference is also tenable. Recent studies (Martin et al., 1991; Mathews & Klug, 1993) provide empirical support for this position, though it appears that only words (positive or negative) associated with an anxious person's emotional concerns produce large amounts of interference. Along similar lines, Cloitre, Heimberg, Holt, and Liebowitz (1992) have suggested a more complex explanation for the interference reported in modified Stroop studies. They hypothesized that anxiety has differential effects on attentional and response mechanisms and suggest that although anxiety may facilitate the recognition of threatening stimuli, it may simultaneously inhibit responses to it. Thus, both attentional allocation and response inhibition may play a role in the observed interference with color-naming.

It is also unclear exactly what attentional processes the modified Stroop task assesses. Recent work by C. MacLeod and colleagues (C. MacLeod & Hagan, 1992; C. MacLeod & Rutherford, 1992) using the Stroop task in a backward masking paradigm indicated that preattentive processing plays a role in color-naming interference among individuals high in trait anxiety. Clearly, further research is necessary before a complete understanding of the cognitive processes assessed by the Stroop task is possible.

Visual Dot-Probe

Another paradigm that is potentially useful for the assessment of cognitive processes is the visual dot-probe task (C. MacLeod, Mathews, & Tata, 1986). This paradigm is particularly interesting because it may be useful in separating attentional allocation from response inhibition. Typically, this paradigm requires the subject to read aloud the top word of a pair of words presented briefly (500 msec) on a computer monitor. (However, a fixation cross may be used, thus allowing the investigator to counterbalance the word [top or bottom] that is read aloud.) The reading of the word focuses the subject's attention on that word, theoretically preventing the meaning of the second word from entering awareness. On critical trials, one word in the pair is neutral while the other has a high threat value. Immediately after such critical trials, a small dot appears in the location of one of the words. Subjects respond by pressing a button when they see the dot.

The primary variable of interest is latency of the button press in response to the dot-probe. Shorter response latencies to probes that replace threat cues are evidence of selective attention to threat stimuli. That is, if an individual attends more to a threatening stimulus than to a neutral stimulus, he or she will see the probe sooner and respond more quickly when the probe appears in the same location as did the threat stimulus (compared to the neutral word). Conversely, if there is no selective attention, response latencies to probes should not vary as a function of the stimuli preceding probe presentation.

The dot-probe paradigm has two important qualities. First, since the words that are not read aloud do not enter awareness, the task has the potential for separating preattentive from attentive processes. In other words, any facilitative effect of threatening words presented in the lower position would have to occur without the conscious processing of the words, providing persuasive evidence of a preattentive mechanism sensitive to threat cues. Second, this paradigm may separate attentional allocation from response inhibition because the subject makes a neutral response (button press) to a neutral stimulus (dot-probe). Thus, the paradigm overcomes the response inhibition confound associated with techniques, such as the modified Stroop task and dichotic listening, that require subjects to respond to a nonneutral stimulus (Williams, Watts, MacLeod, & Mathews, 1988).

In the only published study using the dot-probe paradigm with social phobics, Asmundson and Stein (1994) offer some evidence of its utility. As expected, social phobics' reaction time was enhanced when the probe followed words with high social threat value presented in the upper position. No reaction time enhancement was found for words associated with physical threat, and normal controls exhibited no differences in reaction time as a function of antecedent words. However, social phobics did not evidence an enhancement of reaction time to words and probes presented in the lower position. Whether this finding is attributable to the task or to the absence of preattentive processing of social threat stimuli is currently unknown. It should be noted that some evidence of a preattentive mechanism has been found in studies with other anxiety disorders (e.g., Asmundson, Sandler, Wilson, & Walker, 1992; C. MacLeod, & Hagan, 1992; C. MacLeod & Rutherford, 1992), but other investigators have found no evidence in support of this phenomenon (e.g., McNally et al., 1992).

Unfortunately, Asmundson and Stein (1994) did not include positive–neutral word pairs. Consequently, the possibility that emotionality per se, rather than threat value, guides the allocation of attentional resources cannot be ruled out. Also, only generalized social phobics were included in the sample. Thus, differential effects based on subtype were unassessed. Future research should address this issue and determine whether subtypes can be distinguished using this paradigm (as McNeil et al., 1995, reported for the Stroop task).

Lexical and Category Decision Tasks

Lexical decision tasks and category decision tasks are closely related paradigms that are useful for assessing the speed of cognitive processes under different circumstances. In lexical decision tasks, subjects view letter strings that form either words or nonsense syllables. The subject's task is to indicate whether or not the string is a word by pressing the appropriate button on a computer keyboard. Similarly, category decision tasks present subjects with a word and require them to determine if the word belongs to a certain semantic category (e.g., "Does this word refer to a feeling?"). As with the Stroop and dot-probe tasks, the variable of interest is response time. Faster response time is thought to be associated with facilitated processing of environmental stimuli as predicted by cognitive models of anxiety.

The one study using these two paradigms with social phobics (Cloitre, Heimberg, Holt, & Liebowitz, 1992) had unexpected results. It was hypothesized that, compared to normal controls, social phobics would recognize and categorize cues of social threat more quickly than they would positive or neutral cues. Surprisingly, social phobics made decisions significantly more *slowly* for words associated with social threat than for positive or neutral words, while controls showed no effect as a function of word type. Cloitre, Heimberg, Holt, and Liebowitz (1992) argued that these findings suggest that cognitive processes in social phobia may be more complex than previous studies had suggested, and that researchers must consider the role of both attentional and response processes in cognitive processing. More research is necessary to clarify this issue.

Memory Processes

Depth-of-Processing Tasks

Based on the work of Craik and Tulving (1975), depth-of-processing tasks are intended to assess cognitive processes that mediate the encoding and retrieval of information. A typical design (e.g., Smith, Ingram, & Brehm, 1983) requires subjects to listen to an audiotape recording of adjective lists and respond to a *single* question about each word as it is presented. For some adjectives the question will ask for superficial information (e.g., "Was the word read by a man or a woman?"), while on other trials the question requires semantic processing (e.g., "Does the word mean the same thing as _____ ?"). Other questions ask subjects to determine if the word is privately self-referent (e.g., "Does the word describe you?") or publicly self-referent (e.g. "Would your friends say the word describes you?"). Self-referent words are thought to be more deeply processed and are associated with superior performance on surprise tests of free recall (Craik & Tulving, 1975). Thus, the variable of interest in such tasks is number of words recalled across processing conditions and word type.

Smith et al. (1983) utilized the depth-of-processing paradigm with a sample of college undergraduates. Subjects were screened for level of social anxiety, and experimental conditions were manipulated to produce high or low levels of social stress. Subjects with high levels of social anxiety in the high stress condition recalled significantly more adjectives if they were processed with a *public* self-referent question. No other between group differences were found. Hope (1993) used a similar paradigm but subdivided the adjective list into social threat, depressive, and neutral control adjectives. Preliminary data from a group of social phobics indicated enhanced recall for adjectives associated with social threat when followed by a *private* self-referent question but not for other types of adjectives followed by such a question. Interestingly, no enhancement of recall was found for adjectives followed by public self-referent questions, thus failing to replicate the findings of Smith et al. (1983). Despite this divergence in results, both studies suggest that socially anxious individuals have enhanced encoding and recall of information relevant to social threat and self-reference, suggesting a possible role for memory processes in social phobia. However, other investigators (e.g., Rapee, McCallum, Melville, Ravenscroft, & Rodney, 1994) have failed to find memory biases in social phobics. Consequently, further research is necessary for an adequate understanding of the role of memory processes in social phobia.

COGNITIVE PRODUCTS

Cognitive products represent the portion of the cognitive taxonomy that has received the most investigation in studies of social phobia. Three main strategies have been utilized—questionnaires, thought production methods, and thought endorsement methods.

Questionnaires

The Fear of Negative Evaluation Scale (FNE; Watson & Friend, 1969) is the only widely used questionnaire suitable for the assessment of cognitive products thought to represent a critical feature of social phobia.[2] The original FNE is a 30-item true–false inventory. However, Leary (1983) developed a 12-item brief form using a five-point response format. Since scores on the brief form are highly correlated with the original scale (r = .96), it probably can be substituted for the original form. Moreover, the five-point response format may make it more sensitive to changes in clinical status. Both the original and brief forms have excellent interitem reliabilities (alpha coefficients = .94 and .92, respectively) and test–retest reliabilities (coefficients = .68 and .75, respectively).

Meaningful clinical change in social phobia treatment outcome studies has been associated with a reduction in FNE scores (e.g., Gelernter et al, 1991; Heimberg, Dodge et al., 1990). Likewise, Mattick and colleagues (Mattick & Peters, 1988; Mattick, Peters, & Clarke, 1989) found that FNE change scores were the best single predictor of end-state functioning in their assessment battery. Using a somewhat different methodology, Hope, Heimberg, and Bruch (1993) replicated this finding. Such data support the

---

[2] There are, of course, other paper-and-pencil questionnaires developed for the assessment of social anxiety and social phobia (e.g., the Social Phobia and Anxiety Inventory [Turner, Beidel, Dancu, & Stanley, 1989], the Social Interaction Anxiety Scale [Heimberg, Mueller, Holt, Hope, & Liebowtiz, 1992; Mattick & Clarke, 1989], the Social Phobia Scale [Heimberg et al., 1992; Mattick & Clarke, 1989], the Social Avoidance and Distress Scale [Watson & Friend, 1969]). However, only the FNE can be described realistically as a cognitive measure.

validity of the FNE and indicate that the instrument taps an important cognitive construct associated with social phobia. Despite this apparent utility, questions regarding the appropriateness of the instrument in social phobia research have been raised.

Originally developed with college populations, some researchers have suggested that the FNE is more appropriate for the measurement of common rather than critical features of social phobia. Turner, McCanna, and Beidel (1987) found that, when compared to groups with other anxiety disorders, social phobics differed only from simple phobics on FNE scores. Further, they reported that the FNE and measures of trait anxiety and depression were significantly correlated, suggesting that the instrument is simply a measure of emotional distress (i.e., common features). However, Heimberg, Hope, Rapee, and Bruch (1988) argued that the findings reported by Turner et al. (1987) can be interpreted as an indication that the FNE assesses critical features of social phobia but that these features are common in other anxiety disorders. In fact, social phobia is frequently seen as a secondary diagnosis among individuals with a primary diagnosis of another anxiety disorder (Sanderson, Di Nardo, Rapee, & Barlow, 1990). Moreover, Heimberg et al. (1988) pointed out that the mean FNE scores reported by Turner et al. (1987) were substantially lower than those typically found in samples of social phobics, suggesting potential sampling difficulties.

Finally, in factor analyses of a social phobia assessment battery (Elting, Hope, & Heimberg, 1994), the FNE loaded with broader measures of trait anxiety and depression on a General Pathology factor, but the FNE also loaded on a Social Anxiety factor that did not include these broader measures. Thus, it seems likely that the FNE may measure both critical and common features of social phobia.

Production Methods

Production methods typically require the subject to report thoughts that occurred to them prior to or during a social interaction. Several techniques exist to facilitate this process, but the goal of each is to produce a representative sampling of the subject's thoughts. Since each subject produces a unique record, the technique makes possible a richer, more ideographic understanding of the individual. A more typical approach, however, is to code the data and use it nomothetically.

Probably the most frequently used of the production methods is thought listing (Cacioppo, Glass, & Merluzzi, 1979). In this procedure, subjects are asked to write down all the thoughts they can recall having had during a particular time frame. In research settings, this period is usually associated with a simulated social interaction conducted in the laboratory. However, thought listing has also been used for naturally occurring social interactions (Dodge, Heimberg, Nyman, & O'Brien, 1987). Informal thought listing is commonly used by clinicians as part of cognitive-behavioral treatments (e.g., Heimberg, 1991).

A second production method is videotape-aided (e.g., Ickes, Robertson, Tooke, & Teng, 1986) or audiotape-aided (e.g., Johnson & Glass, 1989) thought recall. With these procedures, role-plays are recorded and then played back for subjects as an aid to their recall of thoughts. In a variation of this approach, Davison, Robins, and Johnson (1983) had subjects listen to an audiotape of a simulated social situation. The tape was interrupted at predetermined intervals to allow subjects to think aloud. No empirical investigations appear to have addressed which of these methods is superior.

Once the cued or uncued sampling of thoughts has been completed, the thoughts are typically coded for positive, negative, or neutral valence. One of the most robust findings of such analyses is that the number of negative thoughts is more highly correlated with psychopathology than is the number of positive thoughts, a phenomenon known as the "power of nonnegative thinking" (Kendall & Hollon, 1981). However, Schwartz and Garamoni (1986) argued that a state of mind (SOM) ratio—the ratio of positive (P) thoughts to the sum of positive and negative (N) thoughts $(P / [P + N])$—is a better predictor of psychological adjustment than the percentage of total thoughts that are negative $(N / [P + N + \text{Neutral}])$.

Schwartz and Garamoni (1986) have identified five different SOMs which coincide with different ratio ranges. SOM ratios that fall between .56 and .68, or approximately one negative for every two positive thoughts, are thought to reflect psychological adjustment. This range, labeled the *positive dialogue*, includes the "optimal" SOM ratio of .618. It is argued that ratios encompassed by the positive dialogue keep negative thoughts—which are important for the realistic assessment of a situation—salient, without disrupting appropriate coping. The *internal dialogue of conflict* is thought to reflect mild levels of psychopathology and encompasses SOM ratios between .45 and .55. Moderate degrees of psychopathology, such as those found with clinically anxious or depressed subjects, are associated with SOM ratios between .32 and .44, a range labeled the *negative dialogue*. Extreme SOM ratios that fall between .00 and .31, the *negative monologue*, or .69 and 1.00, the *positive monologue*, are thought to be associated with more severe forms of psychopathology.

Heimberg, Bruch, Hope, and Dombeck (1990) compared the SOM ratio with the simple percentage of negative thoughts among social phobics. The two ratios were highly correlated, but the SOM ratio proved to be somewhat more sensitive to differences on other measures of psychopathology. Bruch, Heimberg, and Hope's (1991) post hoc analysis of treatment outcome data for social phobics receiving either cognitive-behavioral group therapy (CBGT) or a credible attention-control treatment consisting of education and supportive group therapy (ES) supported the SOM ratio as an index of clinically significant change. Prior to treatment, subjects achieved an average SOM ratio of .287, falling in the negative monologue range. After treatment, both groups exhibited improvement and achieved SOM ratios in the internal dialogue of conflict range. However, at 6-month follow-up, subjects in the ES condition had fallen back to ratios in the negative dialogue range while subjects in the CBGT condition evidenced continued improvement, achieving ratios in the positive dialogue range.

One potential problem with the SOM model is that the ratio will always equal zero if subjects list no positive thoughts, or 1.0 if subjects list no negative thoughts. To overcome this problem, Amsel and Fichten (1990) recommend adding a constant of 1.0 to the frequency of positive or negative thoughts in the case that either, but not both, of these frequencies is zero. This correction has proven to be useful in samples using college undergraduates (Amsel & Fichten, 1990) and social phobics (Heimberg, Bruch et al., 1990). However, it is important to note that the use of such a correction will alter the shape of a sample distribution and should be carefully considered if a large proportion of subjects require the correction.

Although thoughts derived from production methods are typically coded only for valence, some studies (e.g., Burgio, Merluzzi, & Pryor, 1986; Johnson & Glass, 1989) have also coded for attentional focus (i.e., oneself, others). Stopa and Clark (1993) used a combination of valence and attentional focus in their coding of social phobics' thoughts. Social phobics' thoughts not only tended to be negative, but they also were predominantly self-focused. That is, social phobics tended to have more thoughts such as "I'm boring" (self-focused/negative) than thoughts such as "they think I'm boring" (other-focused/negative). This finding suggests the scoring of focus may add important information and should be considered as a potentially useful adjunct in future work.

Endorsement Methods

Endorsement methods are structured questionnaires that present subjects with a standardized set of potentially relevant thoughts. The subject's task is to rate either the impact, the degree of belief, or the frequency with which he or she had each thought during a specified time frame. Typically, thoughts were originally derived through production methods with an appropriate population and situation. The Social Interaction Self-Statement Test (SISST; Glass, Merluzzi, Biever, & Larsen, 1982) is clearly the most widely utilized endorsement instrument for social anxiety and social phobia.

The SISST contains 30 thoughts (15 positive, 15 negative) drawn from thought listings following a heterosocial interaction. Subjects use a 5-point scale to rate the relative frequency of each thought during the specified period. Glass et al. (1982) report item–total correlations from .58 to .77 for negative thoughts and from .45 to .75 for positive thoughts. Split-half reliability coefficients were .73 and .86 for the Negative and Positive subscales, respectively. Finally, Zweig and Brown (1985) found no correlation between the SISST and measures of social desirability, suggesting that this response bias is not a problem with the SISST.

Consistent with the pattern found for production methods, the Negative subscale of the SISST is a better predictor of social anxiety and emotional distress than the Positive subscale. Surprisingly, however, correlations between the positive and negative scores on the SISST and positive and negative thoughts on thought-listing tasks have not been high (e.g., Dodge, Hope, Heimberg, & Becker, 1988; Myszka, Galassi, & Ware, 1986), suggesting the two methods do not tap the same construct domains.

Most studies examining the relative merits of the SISST and production methods have found that the SISST is more highly correlated with other cognitive measures (e.g., Myszka et al., 1986). However, these correlations may be a measurement artifact resulting from similar task demands rather than evidence of greater convergent validity. One advantage of the SISST over production methods is that it may be particularly useful when individuals have difficulty spontaneously generating thoughts. On the other hand, the thoughts sampled are limited to heterosocial interactions and thus may not reflect the cognitive productions of individuals with fears in other social domains. Some researchers (e.g., Turner, Beidel, & Larkin, 1986) have changed "he/she" to "they" on several items of the SISST and used the instrument for same-sex interactions and speech situations. However, the psychometric consequences of this change have not been well investigated. In cases in which the SISST may not be appropriate, instruments designed to assess self-statements for nonassertiveness (Heimberg, Chiauzzi, Becker, & Madrazo-Peterson, 1983) and job interview anxiety (Heimberg, Keller, & Peca-Baker, 1986) may be relevant for some individuals.

Because negative thoughts are common across disorders (e.g., Beck & Emery, 1985), the SISST and coded data from production methods probably measure common features of psychopathology. However, examination of the social stimuli that trigger the thoughts and qualitative analysis of thought content may yield information about critical features of social phobia.

DISCUSSION

Cognitive assessment of social phobia has made considerable progress over the past 15 years. The assessment of cognitive products is particularly advanced. The FNE, the Brief FNE, the SISST, and thought-listing procedures all provide important and well-validated measures of cognitive products associated with social phobia. Nonetheless, a greater variety of measures would prove useful. For example, future research should focus on the development of instruments similar to the SISST for situations other than heterosocial interaction.

Assessment of cognitive processes has also developed significantly in recent years. Unfortunately, with a few exceptions, investigations of cognitive processes appear to have been driven more by the availability of research paradigms than by theory. This research has now reached the stage at which more sophisticated hypothesis testing can occur. Until then, research on the cognitive processes in social phobia will be difficult to integrate.

At this time, research on the assessment of cognitive propositions is particularly absent. Of the techniques reviewed, only the Selves Questionnaire and the Levenson LOCS have been shown to discriminate between social phobia and other forms of psychopathology. However, the ability of these measures to clearly distinguish critical features of social phobia is doubtful. Currently available measures of irrational beliefs have questionable psychometric properties and appear to lack discriminant validity. Likewise, measures of attributional style appear to assess features of psychopathology that are common to several disorders. Finally, the paucity of well-developed measures of expectancies is particularly disappointing, although the instruments currently being developed by Franklin et al. (1993) may help to fill this void. Given the central role that expectancies play in theoretical accounts of social phobia (e.g., Trower & Gilbert, 1989; Leary & Kowalski, Chapter 5, this volume), the current lack of suitable expectancy assessment techniques is an important impediment to the advancement of theory and treatment.

ACKNOWLEDGMENTS

Preparation of this chapter was supported in part by Grant No. MH48751 to Debra A. Hope from the National Institute of Mental Health.

REFERENCES

Abramson, L. Y., Seligman, M. E. P., & Teasdale, J. D. (1978). Learned helplessness in humans: Critique and reformulation. *Journal of Abnormal Psychology, 87,* 49–74.

Alden, L. (1987). Attributional responses of anxious individuals to different patterns of social feedback: Nothing succeeds like improvement. *Journal of Personality and Social Psychology, 52,* 100–106.

American Psychiatric Association. (1987). *Diagnostic and statistical manual of mental disorders* (3rd ed., rev.). Washington, DC: Author.

Amsel, R., & Fichten, C. S. (1990). Ratio versus frequency scores: Focus of attention and the balance between positive and negative thoughts. *Cognitive Therapy and Research, 14,* 257–277.

Anderson, C. A., & Arnoult, L. H. (1985). Attributional style and everyday problems in living: Depression, loneliness, and shyness. *Social Cognition, 3,* 16–35.

Arnkoff, D. B., & Glass, C. R. (1989). Cognitive assessment in social anxiety and social phobia. *Clinical Psychology Review, 9,* 61–74.

Asmundson, G. J. G., Sandler, L. S., Wilson, K. G., & Walker, J. R. (1992). Selective attention toward physical threat in patients with panic disorder. *Journal of Anxiety Disorders, 6,* 295–303.

Asmundson, G. J. G., & Stein, M. B. (1994). Selective attention for social threat in patients with generalized social phobia: Evaluation using a dot-probe paradigm. *Journal of Anxiety Disorders, 8,* 107–117.

Bandura, A. (1977). *Social learning theory.* Englewood Cliffs, NJ: Prentice-Hall.

Bates, M. S., Edwards, W. T., & Andersen, K. O. (1993). Ethnocultural influences on variation in chronic pain perception. *Pain, 52,* 101–112.

Beck, A. T., & Emery, G. (1985). *Anxiety disorders and phobias: A cognitive perspective.* New York: Basic Books.

Bruch, M. A., Heimberg, R. G., & Hope, D. A. (1991). States of Mind Model and cognitive change in social phobics. *Cognitive Therapy and Research, 15,* 429–441.

Burgio, K. L., Merluzzi, T. V., & Pryor, J. R. (1986). Effects of performance expectancy and self-focused attention on social interaction. *Journal of Personality and Social Psychology, 50,* 1216–1221.

Cacioppo, J. T., Glass, C. R., & Merluzzi T. V. (1979). Self-statements and self-evaluations: A cognitive-response analysis of heterosocial anxiety. *Cognitive Therapy and Research, 3,* 249–262.

Carroll, J. B., Davies, P., & Richman, B. (1971). *The American Heritage word frequency book.* Boston: Houghton Mifflin.

Cloitre, M., Heimberg, R. G., Holt, C. S., & Liebowitz, M. R. (1992). Reaction time to threat stimuli in panic disorder and social phobia. *Behaviour Research and Therapy, 30,* 609–617.

Cloitre, M., Heimberg, R. G., Liebowitz, M. R., & Gitow, A. (1992). Perceptions of control in panic disorder and social phobia. *Cognitive Therapy and Research, 16,* 569–577.

Craik, F. I. M., & Tulving, E. (1975). Depth of processing and the retention of words in episodic memory. *Journal of Experimental Psychology: General, 104,* 268–294.

Davison, G. C., Robins, C. & Johnson, M. K. (1983). Articulated thoughts during simulated situations: A paradigm for studying cognition in emotion and behavior. *Cognitive Research and Therapy, 7,* 17–40.

Deffenbacher, J. L., Zwemer, W. A., Whisman, M. A., Hill, R. A., & Sloan, R. D. (1986). Irrational beliefs and anxiety. *Cognitive Therapy and Research, 10,* 281–291.

Dodge, C. S., Heimberg, R. G., Nyman, D., & O'Brien, G. T. (1987). Daily heterosocial interactions of high and low socially anxious college students: A diary study. *Behavior Therapy, 18,* 90–96.

Dodge, C. S., Hope, D. A., Heimberg, R. G., & Becker, R. E. (1988). Evaluation of the Social Interaction Self-Statement Test with a social phobic population. *Cognitive Therapy and Research, 12,* 211–222.

Ellis, A. (1962). *Reason and emotion in psychotherapy.* New York: Lyle Stuart.

Elting, D. T., Hope, D. A., & Heimberg, R. G. (1994). *Logically and empirically defined factors of social phobia.* Manuscript submitted for publication.

Eysenck, M. W. (1992). *Anxiety: The cognitive perspective.* Hove, UK: Erlbaum.

Franklin, M. E., Perry, K. J., Herbert, J. D., & Foa, E. B. (1993, November). *Threat interpretation in generalized social phobia.* Poster presented at the 27th annual convention of the Association for Advancement of Behavior Therapy, Atlanta, GA.

Gelernter, C. S., Uhde, T. W., Cimbolic, P., Arnkoff, D. B., Vittone, B. J., Tancer, M. E., & Bartko, J. J. (1991). Cognitive-behavioral and pharmacological treatments of social phobia: A controlled study. *Archives of General Psychiatry, 48,* 938–945.

Girodo, M., Dotzenroth, S. E., & Stein, S. J. (1981). Causal attribution bias in shy males: Implications for self-esteem and self-confidence. *Cognitive Therapy and Research, 5,* 325–338.

Glass, C. R., Merluzzi, T. V., Biever, J. L., & Larsen, K. H. (1982). Cognitive assessment of social anxiety: Development and validation of a self-statement questionnaire. *Cognitive Therapy and Research, 6,* 37–55.

Gormally, J., Sipps, R., Raphael, R., Edwin, D., & Varvil-Weld, D. (1981). The relationship between maladaptive cognitions and social anxiety. *Journal of Consulting and Clinical Psychology, 49,* 300–301.

Gray, J. A. (1982). *The neuropsychology of anxiety: An enquiry into the functions of the septo-hippocampal system.* Oxford, UK: Oxford University Press.

Hamilton, E. W., & Abramson, L. Y. (1983). Cognitive patterns and major depressive disorders: A longitudinal study in a hospital setting. *Journal of Abnormal Psychology, 92,* 173–184.

Heimberg, R. G. (1991). *A manual for conducting Cognitive-Behavioral Group Therapy for social phobia* (2nd ed.). Unpublished manuscript. (Available from the Center for Stress and Anxiety Disorders, Pine West Plaza, Bldg. 4, Washington Avenue Extension, Albany, NY 12205.)

Heimberg, R. G. (1994). Cognitive assessment strategies and the measurement of outcome of treatment for social phobia. *Behaviour Research and Therapy, 32,* 269–280.

Heimberg, R. E., Becker, R. E., Goldfinger, K., & Vermilyea, J. A. (1985). Treatment of social phobia by exposure, cognitive restructuring, and homework assignments. *Journal of Nervous and Mental Disease, 173,* 236–245.

Heimberg, R. G., Bruch, M. A., Hope, D. A., & Dombeck, M (1990). Evaluating the States of Mind Model: Comparison to an alternative model and effects of method of cognitive assessment. *Cognitive Therapy and Research, 14,* 543–557.

Heimberg, R. G., Chiauzzi, E. J., Becker, R. E., & Madrazo-Peterson, R. (1983). Cognitive mediation of assertive behavior: An analysis of the self-statement patterns of college students, psychiatric patients, and normal adults. *Cognitive Therapy and Research, 7,* 455–464.

Heimberg, R. G., Dodge, C. S., Hope, D. A., Kennedy, C. R., Zollo, L., & Becker, R. E. (1990). Cognitive behavioral group treatment of social phobia: Comparison to a credible placebo control. *Cognitive Therapy and Research, 14,* 1–23.

Heimberg, R. G., Hope, D. A., Rapee, R. M., & Bruch, M. A. (1988). The validity of the Social Avoidance and Distress and the Fear of Negative Evaluation Scales with social phobic patients. *Behaviour Research and Therapy, 26,* 407–410.

Heimberg, R. G., Keller, K. E., & Peca-Baker, T. (1986). Cognitive assessment of social-evaluative anxiety in the job interview: The Job Interview Self-Statement Schedule. *Journal of Counseling Psychology, 33,* 190–195.

Heimberg, R. G., Klosko, J. S., Dodge, C. S., Shadick, R., Becker, R. E., & Barlow, D. H. (1989). Anxiety disorders, depression, and attributional style: A further test of the specificity of depressive attributions. *Cognitive Therapy and Research, 13,* 21–36.

Heimberg, R. G., Mueller, G. P., Holt, C. S., Hope, D. A., & Liebowitz, M. R. (1992). Assessment of anxiety in social interaction and being observed by others: The Social Interaction Anxiety Scale and the Social Phobia Scale. *Behavior Therapy, 23,* 53–73.

Higgins, E. T. (1987). Self-discrepancy: A theory relating self and affect. *Psychological Review, 94,* 319–340.

Higgins, E. T., Klein, R., & Strauman, T. (1985). Self-concept discrepancy theory: A psychological model for distinguishing among different aspects of depression and anxiety. *Social Cognition, 3,* 51–76.

Himle, D. P., Thyer, B. A., & Papsdorf, J. D. (1982). Relationships between rational beliefs and anxiety. *Cognitive Therapy and Research, 6,* 219–225.

Hope, D. A. (1993, March). *Information processing biases in social phobia.* Paper presented at the National Conference on Anxiety Disorders, Charleston, SC.

Hope, D. A., Heimberg, D. A., & Bruch, M. A. (1993). *Cognitive-behavioral group treatment for social phobia: How important is the cognitive component?* Unpublished manuscript.

Hope, D. A., Rapee, R. M., Heimberg, R. G., & Dombeck, M. (1990). Representations of the self in social phobia: Vulnerability to social threat. *Cognitive Therapy and Research, 14,* 177–189.

Ickes, W., Robertson, E., Tooke, W., & Teng, G. (1986). Naturalistic social cognition: Methodology, assessment, and validation. *Journal of Personality and Social Psychology, 51,* 66–82.

Ingram, R. E., & Kendall, P. C. (1987). The cognitive side of anxiety. *Cognitive Therapy and Research, 11,* 523–536.

Ingram, R. E., & Wisnicki, K. (1991). Cognition in depression. In P. A. Magaro (Ed.), *Cognitive bases of mental disorders* (Vol. 1, pp. 187–239). Newbury Park, CA: Sage.

Johnson, R. L., & Glass, C. R. (1989). Heterosocial anxiety and direction of attention in high school boys. *Cognitive Therapy and Research, 13,* 509–526.

Jones, R. G. (1969). A factored measure of Ellis' irrational belief system, with personality and maladjustment correlates (Doctoral dissertation, Texas Technological College, 1968). *Dissertation Abstracts International, 29,* 4739B–4380B. (University Microfilms No. 69–6443)

Kendall, P. C., & Hollon, S. D. (1981). Assessing self-referent speech: Methods in the measurement of self-statements. In P. C. Kendall & S. D. Hollon (Eds.), *Assessment strategies for cognitive-behavioral interventions* (pp. 85–118). New York: Academic Press.

Kendall, P. C., & Ingram, R. E. (1987). The future for cognitive assessment of anxiety: Let's get specific. In L. Michelson & M. Ascher (Eds.), *Anxiety and stress disorders: Cognitive-behavioral assessment and treatment* (pp. 89–104). New York: Guilford Press.

Leary, M. R. (1983). A brief version of the Fear of Negative Evaluation Scale. *Personality and Social Psychology Bulletin, 9*, 371–375.

Levenson, H. (1973). Multidimensional locus of control in psychiatric patients. *Journal of Consulting and Clinical Psychology, 41*, 397–404.

Lohr, J. M., & Bonge, D. (1982). The factorial validity of the Irrational Beliefs Test: A psychometric investigation. *Cognitive Research and Therapy, 6*, 225–230.

MacLeod, C., & Hagan, R. (1992). Individual differences in the selective processing of threatening information, and emotional responses to a stressful life event. *Behaviour Research and Therapy, 30*, 151–161.

MacLeod, C., Mathews, A. M., & Tata, P. (1986). Attentional bias in emotional disorders. *Journal of Abnormal Psychology, 95*, 15–20.

MacLeod, C., & Rutherford, E. M. (1992). Anxiety and the selective processing of emotional information: Mediating roles of awareness, trait and state variables, and personal relevance of stimulus materials. *Behaviour Research and Therapy, 30*, 479–491.

MacLeod, C. M. (1992). Half a century of research on the Stroop effect: An integrative review. *Psychological Bulletin, 109*, 163–203.

Magaro, P. A. (Ed.). (1991). *Cognitive bases of mental disorders* (Vol. 1). Newbury Park, CA: Sage.

Martin, M., Williams, R. M., & Clark, D. M., (1991). Does anxiety lead to selective processing of threat related information? *Behaviour Research and Therapy, 29*, 147–160.

Mathews, A. M., & Klug, F. (1993). Emotionality and interference with color-naming in anxiety. *Behaviour Research and Therapy, 31*, 57–62.

Mathews, A. M., & MacLeod, C. (1985). Selective processing of threat cues in anxiety states. *Behaviour Research and Therapy, 23*, 563–569.

Mattia, J. L., Heimberg, R. G., & Hope, D. A. (1993). The revised Stroop color-naming task in social phobics. *Behaviour Research and Therapy, 31*, 305–315.

Mattick, R. P., & Clarke, J. C. (1989). *Development and validation of measures of social phobia scrutiny, fear and social interaction anxiety.* Unpublished manuscript.

Mattick, R. P., & Peters, L. (1988). Treatment of severe social phobia: Effects of guided exposure with and without cognitive restructuring. *Journal of Consulting and Clinical Psychology, 56*, 251–260.

Mattick, R. P., Peters, L., & Clarke, J. C. (1989). Exposure and cognitive restructuring for social phobia: A controlled study. *Behavior Therapy, 20*, 3–23.

McNally, R. J., Amir, N., Lukach, B. M., Riemann, B. C., Louro, C. E., & Calamari, J. E. (1992, November). Subliminal-processing of threat cues in panic disorder. In B. T. Litz (Chair), *Recent developments in information-processing research in anxiety disorders.* Symposium conducted at the 26th Annual Convention of the Association for Advancement of Behavior Therapy, Boston.

McNally, R. J., Reimann, B. C., & Kim, E. (1990). Selective processing of threat cues in panic disorder. *Behaviour Research and Therapy, 28,* 407–412.

McNeil, D. W., Ries, B. J., Taylor, L. J., Boone, M. L., Carter, L. E., Turk C. L., & Lewin, M. R. (1995). Comparison of social phobia subtypes using Stroop tests. *Journal of Anxiety Disorders, 9,* 47–57.

Moe, K. O., & Zeiss, A. M. (1982). Measuring self-efficacy expectations for social skills: A methodological inquiry. *Cognitive Therapy and Research, 6,* 191–205.

Myszka, M. T., Galassi, J. P., & Ware, W. B. (1986). Comparison of cognitive assessment methods with heterosocially anxious college women. *Journal of Counseling Psychology, 33,* 401–407.

Näätänen, R. (1992). *Attention and brain function.* Hillsdale, NJ: Erlbaum.

Nezu, A. M. (1986). Efficacy of a social problem-solving therapy approach for unipolar depression. *Journal of Consulting and Clinical Psychology, 54,* 196–202.

Obitz, F. W., & Oziel, L. J. (1978). Change in general and specific locus of control in alcoholics as a function of treatment exposure. *International Journal of the Addictions, 13,* 995–1001.

Panksepp, J. (1990). The psychoneurology of fear: Evolutionary perspectives and the role of animal models in understanding human anxiety. In R. Burrows (Ed.), *Handbook of anxiety* (Vol. 3, pp. 3–58), Amsterdam: Elsevier.

Parks, C. W., Jr., & Hollon, S. D, (1988). Cognitive assessment. In A. S. Bellack & M. Hersen (Eds.), *Behavioral assessment: A practical handbook* (3rd ed., pp. 161–212). New York: Pergamon Press.

Persons, J. A., & Rao, P. A. (1985). Longitudinal studies of cognition, life events, and depression in psychiatric inpatients. *Journal of Abnormal Psychology, 94,* 51–63.

Peterson, C., Semmel, A., von Bayer, C., Abramson, L. Y., Metalsky, G. I., & Seligman, M. E. P. (1982). The Attributional Style Questionnaire. *Cognitive Therapy and Research, 6,* 287–300.

Posner, M. L. (Ed.). (1989). *Foundations of cognitive science.* Cambridge, MA: MIT Press.

Rapee, R. M., McCallum, S. L., Melville, L. F., Ravenscroft, H., & Rodney, J. M. (1994). Memory bias in social phobia. *Behaviour Research and Therapy, 32,* 89–99.

Rotter, J. (1966). Generalized expectancies for internal versus external control of reinforcement. *Psychological Monographs, 80*(1, Whole No. 609).

Sanderson, W. C., Di Nardo, P. A., Rapee, R. M., and Barlow, D. H. (1990). Syndrome comorbidity in patients diagnosed with a DSM-III-R anxiety disorder. *Journal of Abnormal Psychology, 99,* 308–312.

Schwartz, R. M., & Garamoni, G. L. (1986). A structural model of positive and negative states of mind: Asymmetry in the internal dialogue. In P. C. Kendall (Ed.), *Advances in cognitive-behavioral research and therapy* (Vol. 5, pp. 1–62). New York: Academic Press.

Shorkey, C. T., Reyes, E., & Whiteman, V. L. (1977). Development of the Rational Behavior Inventory: Initial validity and reliability. *Educational and Psychological Measurement, 37,* 527–534.

Smith, T. W. (1983). Change in irrational beliefs and the outcome of rational-emotive psychotherapy. *Journal of Consulting and Clinical Psychology, 51,* 156–157.

Smith, T. W. (1989). Assessment in rational–emotive therapy. In M. E. Bernard & R. DiGiuseppe (Eds.), *Inside rational–emotive therapy* (pp. 135–153). Orlando, FL: Academic Press.

Smith, T. W., Ingram, R. E., & Brehm, S. S. (1983). Social anxiety, anxious self-preoccupation, and recall of self-relevant information. *Journal of Personality and Social Psychology, 44,* 1276–1283.

Smith, T. W., & Zurawski, R. M. (1983). Assessment of irrational beliefs: The question of discriminant validity. *Journal of Clinical Psychology, 39,* 976–979.

Stopa, L., & Clark, D. M. (1993). Cognitive processes in social phobia. *Behaviour Research and Therapy, 31,* 255–267.

Strauman, T. (1989). Self-discrepancies in clinical depression and social phobia: Cognitive structures that underlie emotional disorders? *Journal of Abnormal Psychology, 98,* 14–22.

Stroop, J. R. (1935). Studies of interference in serial verbal reactions. *Journal of Experimental Psychology, 18,* 643–662.

Trower, P., & Gilbert, P. (1989). New theoretical conceptions of social anxiety and social phobia. *Clinical Psychology Review, 9,* 19–36.

Turner, S. M., Beidel, D. C., Dancu, C. V., & Stanley, M. A. (1989). An empirically derived inventory to measure social fears and anxiety: The Social Phobia and Anxiety Inventory. *Psychological Assessment, 1,* 35–40.

Turner, S. M., Beidel, D. C., & Larkin, K. T. (1986). Situational determinants of social anxiety in clinic and nonclinic samples: Physiological and cognitive correlates. *Journal of Consulting and Clinical Psychology, 54,* 523–527.

Turner, S. M., McCanna, M., & Beidel D. C. (1987). Validity of the Social Avoidance and Distress and Fear of Negative Evaluation Scales. *Behaviour Research and Therapy, 25,* 113– 115.

Watson, D., & Friend, R. (1969). Measurement of social-evaluative anxiety. *Journal of Consulting and Clinical Psychology, 33,* 448–457.

Weilage, M. E., & Hope, D. A. (1993, November). *Self-discrepant cognitions in social phobia and dysthymia.* Poster presented at the 27th annual convention of the Association for Advancement of Behavior Therapy, Atlanta, GA.

Widiger, T. A. (1992). Generalized social phobia versus avoidant personality disorder: A commentary on three studies. *Journal of Abnormal Psychology, 101,* 340–343.

Williams, J. M. G., Watts, F. N., MacLeod, C., & Mathews, A. (1988). *Cognitive psychology and emotional disorders.* NewYork: Wiley.

Zweig, D. R., & Brown, S. D. (1985). Psychometric evaluation of a written stimulus presentation format for the Social Interaction Self-Statement Test. *Cognitive Therapy and Research, 9,* 285–295.

PART IV

Treatment

CHAPTER TWELVE

Cognitive-Behavioral Treatments: Literature Review

RICHARD G. HEIMBERG

HARLAN R. JUSTER

In this chapter, we present a thorough and critical review of the rapidly growing literature on the cognitive-behavioral treatment of social phobia. When we first became involved in the study of social phobia in the early 1980s, there were barely a half-dozen published attempts at cognitive-behavioral treatment. The inclusion of social phobia in the third edition of the *Diagnostic and Statistical Manual of the Mental Disorders* (DSM-III; American Psychiatric Association, 1980) spurred research on cognitive-behavioral interventions, and when Heimberg reviewed the literature in 1989, 17 studies had been conducted. In the brief time since that review was published, 20 additional studies have been conducted, and much more has been learned about the cognitive-behavioral treatment of social phobia.

This chapter updates previous reviews by our research group (Heimberg, 1989; Heimberg & Barlow, 1988, 1991; Hope, Holt, & Heimberg, 1993; Juster, Heimberg, & Holt, in press) and focuses on studies of cognitive-behavioral treatment of social phobia as defined in DSM-III or the revised third edition of DSM (DSM-III-R; American Psychiatric Association, 1987) and on studies of patients who would probably have met the criteria for social phobia had they been applied. Primary categories of treatment are reviewed, including social skills training, relaxation techniques, exposure-based methods, and multicomponent cognitive-behavioral interventions. After review of these areas of research, we address the additional questions of the comparative and combined efficacy of cognitive-behavioral and pharmacological treatment methods, durability of treatment gains, and predictors of successful outcome of cognitive-behavioral treatments for social phobia. Because many of the studies to be reviewed investigate the effectiveness of multiple treatment interventions, evaluative summaries of the various treatments are presented after the review of treatments is complete. We conclude the chapter with a discussion of the state of research on the cognitive-behavioral treatment of social phobia, difficulties posed by this body of research, and directions for future investigation.

Tables 12.1 and 12.2 provide summary information about the studies of cognitive-behavioral treatment of social phobia. Table 12.1 details the characteristics of patient samples in the several studies, and Table 12.2 summarizes the treatments examined in each study and the specifics of treatment outcome.

SOCIAL SKILLS TRAINING

Many early efforts to treat social phobia were based on the presumption that patients' anxiety is related to deficient verbal (e.g., appropriate speech content) and nonverbal (e.g., eye contact, posture, and gestures) social skills. Social skills training (SST) interventions were believed to increase these behavioral skills, thus removing the underlying cause of the anxiety and increasing the probability of successful social outcomes. SST employs modeling, behavioral rehearsal, corrective feedback, social reinforcement, and homework assignments to teach effective social behavior. To date, nine studies of SST as a treatment for social phobia have been conducted.

Marzillier, Lambert, and Kellet (1976) compared SST with systematic desensitization in the treatment of 32 patients who had received diagnoses of personality disorder or neurosis. Since this study predated the publication of DSM-III, no official diagnosis of social phobia could have been assigned. However, inclusion criteria were primary complaints of interpersonal difficulties, anxiety in a wide range of social situations, and deficits in social skills, suggesting that these patients might have met DSM-III-R or DSM-IV (American Psychiatric Association, 1994) criteria for social phobia, generalized type (and possibly avoidant personality disorder as well).

Patients assigned to either SST or systematic desensitization received 15 weekly individual sessions, and their progress was compared to that of a wait-list control group. Patients in both treatments improved on measures of social anxiety and clinical adjustment after treatment, but not significantly more than did waiting-list patients. SST patients increased their range of social activities more than did the waiting-list group, and patients in both SST and systematic desensitization increased their range of social contacts significantly more than did waiting-list patients. No differences were found between the two treatment groups. Although a 6-month follow-up assessment was planned, numerous dropouts in the systematic desensitization group precluded treatment comparisons at this assessment.

TABLE 12.1. Characteristics of Subjects in Studies of the Cognitive-Behavioral Treatment of Social Phobia

Authors	N	n male/ n female	Age (mean, range)	Mean duration of phobia	% married	% employed	Comments
Al-Kubaisy et al. (1992)	28	17/11	35, 18–60	14 yr	42	—	ICD-10 criteria; age data reported only for larger sample, which also included agoraphobics and specific phobics.
Alström et al. (1984)	42	11/31	28, 18–60	7 < 1 yr 9 1–3 yr 26 > 3 yr	29	31	Described as not suited for insight-oriented psychotherapy; most disturbing fear: 20, being in groups; 20, eating with people; 2, being watched while working.
Biran et al. (1981)	3	0/3	42, 37–49	20.3 yr	100	0	All subjects feared writing in public.
Brown et al. (1995)	63	35/28	37	19 yr	40	71	DSM-III-R criteria. Nongeneralized social phobics, generalized social phobics with avoidant personality disorder, generalized social phobics without avoidant personality disorder.
Butler et al. (1984)	45	26/19	28, 18–41	8.2 yr	53	—	DSM-III criteria.
Clark & Agras (1991)	94	40/54	38	22 yr	—	—	DSM-III-R criteria; musicians with performance anxiety. Demographic characteristics reported for sample of 94 musicians who participated in preliminary study. Only 34 subjects participated in treatment study, but they did not differ from the larger sample on any reported characteristic.
DiGiuseppe et al. (1990)	79	43/36	36, 30–50	—	—	—	Community volunteers who responded to newspaper and radio announcements.
Emmelkamp et al. (1985)	34	13/21	31, 21–61	11 yr	—	—	DSM-III criteria.
Falloon et al. (1981)	16	10/6	27, 18–52	—	13	—	DSM-III criteria.
Fava et al. (1989)	7	3/4	33	5.8 yr	71	—	DSM-III-R criteria.
Feske et al. (1994)	48	23/25	34, 19–63	19 yr	43	—	DSM-III-R criteria. Generalized social phobics with or without avoidant personality disorder.
Gelernter et al. (1991)	65	24/41	37, 18–60	—	49	74	DSM-III criteria; 48 subjects reported anxiety and avoidance of specific social situations, 17 had generalized social fears.

(Table continues on p. 264.)

TABLE 12.1. (*Continued*)

Authors	N	n male/ n female	Age (mean, range)	Mean duration of phobia	% married	% employed	Comments
Heimberg et al. (1985)	7	2/5	29, 23–40	—	14	100	DSM-III criteria; most disturbing fear: 2, social interaction; 5, public speaking.
Heimberg et al. (1990)	49	27/22	31, 19–50	12.5 yr	22 yr	80	DSM-III criteria; most disturbing fear: 27, social interaction; 21, public speaking; 1, other.
Heimberg et al. (1994)	133	67/66	35, 19–61	20 yr	30	49	DSM-III-R criteria.
Hope et al. (1990)	43	22/21	34, 18–59	18 yr	35	77	DSM-III-R criteria.
Hope et al. (1995)	23	11/12	36	—	30	—	DSM-III-R criteria. Nongeneralized and generalized social phobics. Also classified by presence or absence of avoidant personality disorder.
Jerremalm et al. (1986)	38	11/27	33, 22–47	17.1 yr	71	74	Anxiety in a wide range of social situations; physiological versus cognitive reactors.
Kanter & Goldfried (1979)	68	18/50	36, 22–52	—	—	—	Socially anxious community volunteers; 40% previously treated for social anxiety.
Lucas & Telch (1993b)	53	19/34	37	—	34	85	DSM-III-R criteria.
Lucock & Salkovskis (1988)	8	5/3	23, 19–30	—	—	—	DSM-III criteria.
Marzillier et al. (1976)	32	24/8	27, 17–43	—	16	—	Socially inadequate psychiatric patients; described as lacking social skills.
Mattick & Peters (1988)	51	24/27	37	15.8 yr	49	—	DSM-III criteria; a variety of specific social fears and avoidance; subjects described as possessing adequate social skills, but several may also have had social interactional anxiety as well.
Mattick et al. (1989)	43	20/23	41	22.1 yr	51	—	DSM-III criteria; a variety of specific social fears and avoidance; subjects described as possessing adequate social skills, but several may also have had social interactional anxiety as well.
Mersch et al. (1989)	74	33/41	32, 18–56	12.6 yr	42	62	DSM-III-R criteria; a subset of 39 patients were classified as either behavioral or cognitive reactors.

Study	n		Age	Duration			Diagnostic criteria/comments
Mersch et al. (1992)	3	2/1	35, 30–38	15 yr	67	67	DSM-III-R criteria; fear of blushing, sweating, or trembling was most prominent fear.
Öst et al. (1981)	32	13/19	34, 21–51	19.7 yr	75	88	Anxiety in a wide range of social situations; physiological versus behavioral reactors.
Scholing & Emmelkamp (1993a)	30	14/16	31	10.4 yr	67	—	DSM-III-R criteria; fear of blushing, sweating, or trembling was most prominent fear.
Scholing & Emmelkamp (1993b)	73	33/40	33, 18–65	17 yr	52	—	DSM-III-R criteria for generalized social phobia; Fear Questionnaire social phobia score greater than 20.
Shaw (1979)	30	19/11	32, 19–51	All > 1 yr	—	—	Severe social anxiety and avoidance; 20 of 30 subjects also included in Trower et al. (1978).
Stravynski (1983)	1	1/0	23	6 yr	0	100	DSM-III criteria; psychogenic vomiter.
Stravynski et al. (1982)	22	17/5	32, 22–57	—	5	—	DSM-III criteria, but also avoidant personality disorder or adjustment disorder.
Trower et al. (1978)	40	29/11	29, 17–51	—	43	—	Patients classified as either social phobic or socially inadequate.
Turner, Beidel, Cooley, et al. (1994)	17	11/6	36, 23–59	23 yr	47	82	DSM-III-R criteria. All met criteria for generalized subtype. One-third had generalized anxiety disorder or dysthymia. Ten also had avoidant or obsessive–compulsive personality disorder.
Turner, Beidel, & Jacob (1994)	72	28/44	35, 18–56	19.2 yr	—	—	DSM-III-R criteria: 55 patients with schizotypal, schizoid, borderline, paranoid, or antisocial personality disorder excluded after structured interview.
Wlazlo et al. (1990)	78	45/33	30	9.3 yr	50	—	DSM-III-R criteria; 30 patients excluded from study because of severe comorbidity; only patients with complete data through 1-yr follow-up included; patients classified as primarily phobic or primarily deficient in social skills.

Note. Dashes (—) indicate information was not presented in published report. % employed, % employed or enrolled in school on a full-time basis. Updated from Heimberg (1989, pp. 110–111). Copyright 1989 by Pergamon Press Ltd. Updated by permission.

TABLE 12.2. Design and Outcome of Studies of the Cognitive-Behavioral Treatment of Social Phobia

Authors	Mode	Treatment conditions	Control conditions	N of sessions	Total treatment time (hr)	Therapists	Length of follow-up (mo)	Outcome	Comments
Al-Kubaisy et al. (1992)	I	1. Clinician-accompanied EX and self-directed EX 2. Self-directed EX 3. RT	None	6	15	MD Nurse-therapist	4.5	Both EX treatments superior to RT on most measures. Clinician-accompanied EX superior to self-exposure, but only on 4 of 27 measures.	6-hr treatment with therapist in all conditions. Patients receiving clinician-accompanied exposure were seen for 9 additional hr. Other patients devoted similar time to self-directed assignments. Unspecified procedures for coping during exposures were included in both EX conditions. Most data reported only for larger sample of mixed phobics.
Alström et al. (1984)	I	1. EX 2. RT 3. Supportive therapy	Basal therapy (information, encouragement, advice on self-exposure; unspecified anxiolytic medications)	4–13 (M = 9)	—	—	9	EX led to more improvement than RT or basal therapy on anxiety, avoidance, and global functioning.	All Ss received basal therapy; groups differed on demographics; some EX patients also received IF; some patients had up to 9 additional sessions during FU.
Biran et al. (1981)	I	1. EX 2. CR	MB across subjects	2 Ss, 10 1 S, 5	2 Ss, 15 1 S, 7.5	DS	9	EX led to improvements in approach behavior and subjective fear. CR was ineffective. Behavioral gains maintained at FU; some increase in subjective fear.	EX and CR were administered in separate 5-session modules. Subject C received exposure only. Others reported CR to be an important element in their overall treatment.

Study	Design	Treatment conditions	Control			Therapist		Results	Comments
Brown et al. (1995)	G (6)	CBGT	None	12	30	2 PhDs DSs	None	Eight Ss dropped out. Full sample improvement on most measures. Nongeneralized social phobics were more likely than generalized social phobics to be classified as responders to treatment. Generalized social phobics with and without APD did not differ on this measure. On most measures, nongeneralized social phobics began treatment less impaired than generalized Ss and remained less impaired after treatment. Generalized social phobics with APD differed from generalized social phobics without APD on only two measures after treatment.	Study examined differences in outcome between nongeneralized social phobics and generalized social phobics and generalized social phobics with and without APD.
Butler et al. (1984)	I	1. EX plus anxiety management training (EX/AMT) 2. EX plus "associative therapy" (placebo)(EX)	WL	7	7.5	2 PhDs 1 MSW	6	Both EX conditions more improved than WL at posttest. EX/AMT Ss showed additional improvement during FU and were generally more improved than Ss in EX.	EX less credible than EX/ AMT. Two booster sessions given between posttest and FU.
Clark & Agras (1991)	CR: G (5–6) Meds: I	1. CR and EX and AR and pill placebo 2. CR and EX and AR and buspirone 3. Buspirone	Pill placebo	5	—	Meds: MD CR: PhD	1	CR subjects had greater reduction in subjective anxiety during musical performance and greater increases in quality of performance than buspirone or placebo subjects. Few differences between buspirone and placebo. CR plus placebo subjects showed more improvement at FU than subjects receiving other treatment combinations.	Small n's per treatment condition. FU brief and included only a single measure. All patients were musicians with performance anxiety. Treatment periods very brief.

(*Table continues on p. 268.*)

TABLE 12.2. (*Continued*)

Authors	Mode	Treatment conditions	Control conditions	N of sessions	Total treatment time (hr)	Therapists	Length of follow-up (mo)	Outcome	Comments
DiGiuseppe et al. (1990)	G (5–8)	1. Beck's cognitive therapy 2. Interpersonal problem-solving skills training 3. RET 4. SIT 5. Assertion training	WL	10	15	DSs	0	Subjects in all active treatments were improved after treatment on self-report and behavioral measures of social anxiety, more so than the WL group. A similar pattern was evident on other measures (e.g., depression), although assertion training was not as likely to surpass WL on these measures. There were no differences among cognitively oriented treatments or between these treatments and assertion training.	Authors state that 3-mo FU was conducted, but no relevant data were presented in published report.
Emmelkamp et al. (1985)	G (4–7)	1. EX *in vivo* and in-group structured exercises 2. RET 3. SIT	None	6	15	2 PhDs 4 DSs	1	Anxiety reduction for all treatments. SIT, RET led to greater reductions in irrational beliefs. EX led to greater reductions in pulse rate during behavioral test.	Most Ss removed from medication before beginning of treatment. Patients in RET and SIT did not receive exposure instructions.
Falloon et al. (1981)	G (16)	1. SST plus propranolol 2. SST plus inert placebo	None	2	12	Us	6	General improvement on most measures. No difference between propranolol and placebo.	SST administered in two intensive 6-hr workshops. Pairs of Ss met for additional rehearsals between sessions.
Fava et al. (1989)	I	1. Self-directed EX	None	8	4	MD	12	Significant improvement on all measures that was maintained at the FU assessment.	Clinical report suggests continued improvement in 6 of 7 patients during FU despite lack of further statistical change.

Study		Treatment	Control					Results/Comments
Feske et al. (1994)	G (4–6)	EX, RT, SD, and SST	None	See comments	17Ss, 32 31 Ss, 42	PhDs Master's	3	Full sample improvement. Generalized social phobics with APD improved with treatment but reported more severe impairment on all measures at posttest and FU than generalized social phobics without APD.	Treatment was delivered workshop-style. Seventeen Ss received 8 hr of treatment on 4 separate days. Others received similar treatment followed by 6 weekly sessions. Study examined whether generalized social phobics without APD might respond more favorably to exposure-based treatment than generalized social phobics with APD. The authors suggest that the poorer outcome of Ss with APD might be accounted for, in part, by their higher levels of depression.
Gelernter et al. (1991)	CBGT: G (10) Meds: I	1. CBGT 2. Phenelzine 3. Alprazolam	Pill placebo	12	CBGT: 24 Meds: 3–6	CBGT: PhDs Meds: MDs	2	Whole sample improvement on most measures. Phenelzine patients more improved than other patients on single anxiety scale. FU maintenance good for phenelzine and CBGT, but not for alprazolam or placebo.	Medication and placebo conditions included instructions for self-exposure. CBGT administered in groups of 10 rather than 6 as recommended. All comparisons that involved all four treatment conditions were based on self-report.
Heimberg et al. (1985)	G (3–4)	Imaginal, simulated, and in vivo EX, CR	MB across groups	14	21	2 PhDs 1 DS	6	Significant reductions on self-report, behavioral, and physiological measures. Gains maintained at FU for 6/7 Ss.	
Heimberg et al. (1990)	G (4–7)	CBGT	ES	12	24	1 PhD 5 DSs	6	Both groups improved on most measures. At posttest, 75% CBGT Ss, 40% ES Ss improved. At FU, CBGT, 81%; ES, 47%.	Treatment conditions equally credible. CBGT patients also improved on cognitive self-statement measures at FU.

(*Table continues on p. 270.*)

269

TABLE 12.2. (*Continued*)

Authors	Mode	Treatment conditions	Control conditions	N of sessions	Total treatment time (hr)	Therapists	Length of follow-up (mo)	Outcome	Comments
Heimberg, Salzman, et al. (1993)	G (4–7)	CBGT	ES	12	24	1 PhD 5 DSs	65	CBGT patients were rated as less phobic and less impaired by independent assessors and reported less social anxiety on questionnaire measures than ES patients. CBGT patients were also rated as less anxious and more skilled during an individualized behavioral test.	FU of Heimberg et al. (1990). FUs ranged from 4.5 to 6.25 years. Nineteen patients participated, and they had been less impaired before treatment than nonparticipants. Therefore, results apply only to less severely impaired social phobics.
Heimberg et al. (1994)	CBGT, ES: G (5–6) Meds: I	1. CBGT 2. Phenelzine	1. ES 2. Pill placebo	12	CBGT, ES: 24 Meds: 6	CBGT, ES: PhDs, DSs Meds: MDs	6	CBGT and phenelzine superior to controls at posttest. Phenelzine superior to CBGT on some measures at posttest despite equivalent overall response rates. CBGT led to better maintenance of gains than phenelzine after treatment termination.	Design: After 12 weeks of treatment, responders to CBGT and phenelzine provided with 6 more months of maintenance treatment, 6-mo FU thereafter. Few differences between treatment sites. Nongeneralized social phobics responded better to treatment than generalized social phobics.
Hope et al. (1990)	G (4–7)	1. CBGT 2. Simulated and *in vivo* EX	WL	12	24	DSs	6	At posttest, CBGT patients reported less anxiety than did other patients during an individualized behavioral test and tended to be rated more positively by therapists. While the EX groups were similar on several measures, EX without CR led to greater improvements on blind assessor ratings of severity and self-ratings of anxiety and fear of negative evaluation. At FU, there were few differences between EX groups with and without CR.	EX without CR replaced the cognitive component of CBGT with lecture and discussion material relevant to a habituation model of exposure. CBGT patients showed less improvement than in studies by Heimberg et al. (1990) or Gelernter et al. (1991). Posttest fear of negative evaluation significantly predicted outcome.

Study	Format	Treatment conditions	Control			Therapist	FU	Results	Comments
Hope et al. (1995)	G (5–7)	CBGT	None	12	24	1 PhD 1 DS	12	Clinically significant gains made by 85% of Ss. Nongeneralized social phobics began treatment less impaired than generalized social phobics and remained less impaired after treatment. Nongeneralized Ss were more likely ($p < .06$) to be classified as fully remitted after treatment. Gains were maintained at FU.	FU assessment consisted of self-report measures only. Study examined differences in outcome between generalized and nongeneralized subtypes of social phobia and between subjects with and without APD. Subtype appeared to affect outcome but APD did not.
Jerremalm et al. (1986)	I	1. AR 2. SIT	WL	10–12	7.5–12	DSs	None	Both treatments more effective than WL but not consistently different from each other; tendency on self-report measures for SIT to fare better than AR.	Treatment conditions equally credible. Authors attempted to match treatment to subject type (cognitive vs. physiological reactor). Less than successful attempt possibly due to unreliability of cognitive measure.
Kanter & Goldfried (1979)	G (8–10)	1. SRR 2. SCD 3. SRR and SCD	WL	7	10.5	DSs	2	All treatment conditions more effective than WL. SRR appeared most effective on basis of self-report measures and resulted in greater generalization to nonsocial situations.	Authors examined impact of anxiety level on treatment response but found no differences.
Lucas & Telch (1993b)	I, G (3–7)	1. CBGT 2. Simulated and *in vivo* EX, CR in individual treatment	ES	12	24	DSs	None	On a conservative measure of reliable change, 61% of CBGT Ss, 50% of individual CBGT Ss, and 24% of ES Ss were judged much or very much improved. Across types of assessments, the cognitive behavioral treatments were generally more effective than ES but there were few differences between them.	Evaluation of Heimberg's CBGT and equivalent protocol administered in individual treatment. Group CBT was substantially more cost-effective than individual CBT. APD and degree of cognitive change were significant predictors of treatment outcome.

(*Table continues on p. 272.*)

271

TABLE 12.2. (*Continued*)

Authors	Mode	Treatment conditions	Control conditions	N of sessions	Total treatment time (hr)	Therapists	Length of follow-up (mo)	Outcome	Comments
Lucock & Salkowskis (1988)	G (8)	1. SST	None	—	—	—	0	SST treatment resulted in reduced social anxiety and avoidance and a lowered estimate of the subjective probability of negative social outcomes.	Authors describe treatment as "cognitively oriented" SST, but no further information is provided.
Marzillier et al. (1976)	I	1. SST 2. SD	WL	15	11.25	PhD	6	Significant within-group changes for SST, SD. Not significantly greater than WL on most measures.	Procedural difficulties and significant dropout in SD; poor attendance at FU.
Mattick & Peters (1988)	G (4–7)	1. EX 2. EX and CR	None	6	12	1 PhD 1 U	3	EX plus CR more improved than EX on measures of behavioral approach, self-rated avoidance, improvement, and end-state functioning.	Changes in fear of negative evaluation significantly predicted end-state functioning.
Mattick et al. (1989)	G (4–7)	1. EX 2. CR 3. EX and CR	WL	6	12	1 PhD 1 U	3	EX plus CR and CR improved on all measures; EX improved on measures of phobia but not on irrational thinking. EX plus CR more improved than EX on two measures of phobia.	Changes in fear of negative evaluation again predicted outcome. CR subjects showed continued improvement during FU; EX subjects showed some deterioration.
Mersch et al. (1989)	G (7–8)	1. SST 2. RET	None	8	20	DSs	1.5	Patients classified as behavioral reactors and cognitive reactors, as in studies by Jerremalm et al. (1986) and Öst et al. (1981). There was general improvement among treated subjects, but behavioral reactors treated with SST and cognitive reactors treated with RET did not show superior response.	From an original sample of 74, 39 participants could be classified. Remaining patients also treated and included in later FU study. No specific exposure instructions were given to patients in either treatment.

Study	Design	Treatments	Control			Measure	FU (weeks)	Results	Comments
Mersch et al. (1991)	G (7–8)	1. SST 2. RET	None	8	20	DSs	14	Patients receiving SST or RET continued to show improvement at the FU assessment. Few differences between behavioral reactors and cognitive reactors in either treatment.	FU of Mersch et al. (1989). Of 62 patients who completed original study, 57 participated. FU included self-report assessment only. Of 57 patients, 25 received additional treatment during FU period. These patients were rated as more anxious and less skilled in a behavioral test before treatment and were less improved after treatment on some measures than were other patients.
Mersch et al. (1992)	I	RET and paradoxical interventions	None	14	14	3 DSs	18	All Ss improved on a broad array of measures. Frequency of feared symptoms was reduced although anxiety experienced on their occurrence remained high. Gains were maintained at FU.	RET given in sessions 2–7. Paradoxical interventions, in sessions 8–14, required Ss to evoke their symptoms in feared situations.
Öst et al. (1981)	I	1. AR 2. SST	None	10–12	7.5–12	DSs	None	Both treatments generally effective. SST more effective for behavioral reactors, AR somewhat more effective for physiological reactors.	Similar design to Jerremalm et al. (1986), more successful attempt at subject treatment matching.
Scholing & Emmelkamp (1993a)	I	1. EX followed by RET 2. RET followed by EX 3. Integrated EX/RET	WL; see comments	16	16	DSs	3	No differences between active treatments and WL after the first 4 weeks although treated subjects showed significant improvement on most measures after treatment was completed. Treated patients were generally improved at posttest and FU with most change occurring during treatment blocks. No significant differences among treatment conditions.	Sessions administered in 2 blocks of 4 weeks with a 4-week period of no treatment in between. One-half of the sample began with an additional 4-week waiting period. No exposure conducted during sessions. Self-report assessment only. Sample included only patients with primary fears of blushing, sweating, or trembling.

(*Table continues on p. 274.*)

TABLE 12.2. (*Continued*)

Authors	Mode	Treatment conditions	Control conditions	N of sessions	Total treatment time (hr)	Therapists	Length of follow-up (mo)	Outcome	Comments
Scholing & Emmelkamp (1993b)	I, G (5–7)	1. EX 2. RET followed by EX 3. Integrated EX/RET	WL; see comments	16	I, 16 G, 37	DSs	3	Treated subjects improved more on target complaints and avoidance behavior than WL subjects after 4 weeks. Treated patients generally improved at posttest and FU with most change occurring during treatment blocks. I-G and treatment condition differences present after 4 weeks on somatic complaints but absent thereafter.	Sessions administered in 2 blocks of 4 weeks with a 4-week period of no treatment in between for two-thirds of sample. Remainder began with an additional 4-week waiting period. Twice weekly sessions. Exposures during G but not I sessions. Self-report assessment only.
Shaw (1979)	I	1. SST 2. SD 3. IF	None	10	10	2 PhDs 4 MDs 1 DS	6	All treatments produced significant within-group change. No differences between treatments.	SST, SD subjects same as in Trower et al. (1978). No control group.
Stravynski (1983)	I	EX, SST, and CR	MB across target behaviors	8	—	PhD	12	Anxiety in several target situations reduced; psychogenic vomiting eliminated.	Informal FU at 2 yr indicated continued positive outcome.
Stravynski et al. (1982)	I, G (3–4)	1. SST 2. SST and CR	None	12	18	PhD	6	Subjects in both conditions improved; no differences between treatments. Gains stable at FU.	No control group; no formal comparison of I, G modes.
Trower et al. (1978)	I	1. SST 2. SD	None	10	SST, 15–17.5 SD, 12.5–15	PhDs MDs	6	Subjects classified as social phobic or socially inadequate. Phobic Ss improved equally with either treatment, socially inadequate Ss improved more with SST.	No control group: SST sessions longer than SD sessions.

274

Study		Treatment	Control	n	Hours	Therapist	FU (mo)	Results	Comments
Turner, Beidel, Cooley, et al. (1994)	I, G (3–4)	Social Effectiveness Therapy (education, SST, *in vivo* and imaginal EX, programmed practice)	None	29	40	PhDs Nurse	None	Four dropouts. Significant improvements in self-reported social phobia and anxiety and performance during two behavioral tests. Significant improvement also noted on clinician ratings and a measure of end-state functioning.	All dropouts had Axis II diagnoses. Promising treatment for a severely impaired group of patients.
Turner, Beidel, & Jacob (1994)	I	1. EX and IF 2. Atenolol	Pill placebo	EX and IF: 20 Meds: 20	EX and IF: 30 Meds: —	EX and IF: PhDs Meds: MDs	6	EX and IF consistently superior to placebo, but atenolol was not. EX and IF superior to atenolol on behavioral measures and composite indices. Improved patients in EX and IF and atenolol remained improved at FU.	FU included only 15 EX and IF patients and 12 atenolol patients.
Wlazlo et al. (1990)	SST: G (6–8) EX: I, G (4–6)	1. SST 2. EX	None	SST: 25 EX: 5	SST: 37.5 EX-I: 12 EX-G: 34	—	30	All treatments led to clinically and statistically significant gains in social phobia and associated complaints (depression, obsessions). Phobic patients reported less posttreatment impairment of functioning than skill deficit patients at FU. Some indication that skill deficit patients did better in group EX than individual EX or SST. Additional improvements noted for several patients during FU.	FUs at 3 mo and at an average of 2.5 yr (range 1.0–5.5). Self-report assessment only. Patients classified as primarily social phobic or primarily deficient in social skills. Patients not randomly assigned to treatments. Large differences in amounts of treatment time. SST and EX both contained components of the other treatment. All assessments self-report.

275

Note. Dashes indicate information was not presented in published report. AMT, anxiety management training; APD, avoidant personality disorder; AR, applied relaxation; CBGT, cognitive-behavioral group therapy; CR, cognitive restructuring; DS, doctoral student; ES, educational–supportive group psychotherapy; EX, exposure; FU, follow-up; G, group treatment; I, individual treatment; IF, imaginal flooding; MB, multiple baseline; RET, rational–emotive therapy; RT, relaxation training; SCD, self-control desensitization; SD, systematic desensitization; SIT, self-instructional training; SSR, systematic rational restructuring; SST, social skills training; U, undergraduate student; WL, waiting list. Updated from Heimberg (1989, pp. 112–116). Copyright 1989 by Pergamon Press Ltd. Updated by permission.

The SST group maintained their increased range of social activities, though they made no additional gains during the follow-up period.

Marzillier et al. (1976) concluded that SST had beneficial effects on limited aspects of patients' social lives, including increased social activities and social contacts. However, treatment did not result in improved social skills or reduced anxiety and had little effect on numerous other clinical measures. Wait-list patients showed improvements on several measures similar to those demonstrated by patients receiving SST or systematic desensitization. These results underscore the importance of including appropriate control conditions in the design of a treatment outcome study but do not reflect well on either SST or systematic desensitization.

Trower, Yardley, Bryant, and Shaw (1978) also examined the comparative efficacy of SST and systematic desensitization for social phobics. Two subgroups of patients were defined by clinical judgment. The first consisted of individuals with deficits in social skills, similar to Marzillier et al.'s (1976) patients. The second group of patients was judged to possess adequate social skills, but because of excessive levels of anxiety, they could not apply those skills appropriately. They experienced excessive anxiety in and avoidance of situations in which they might be evaluated, such as meals, meetings, interviews, making complaints, and being watched while doing something, and appear to match DSM-III-R and DSM-IV definitions of nongeneralized social phobia (Heimberg, Holt, Schneier, Spitzer, & Liebowitz, 1993). It was hypothesized that systematic desensitization, with its emphasis on maintaining a low arousal state while imagining feared situations, would reduce fear for the anxious subgroup, allowing potentially available skills to be more adequately applied. SST was expected to provide the necessary training for patients whose primary problem was deficient social skills.

Patients received 10 individual treatment sessions. Both skill deficit and phobic subgroups evidenced significant reductions in phobic severity, social inadequacy, and general anxiety, regardless of treatment received. Skill deficit patients experienced less difficulty in social situations and a greater frequency of social activities when they were treated with SST. No such interaction occurred for the phobic subgroup, who appeared to benefit equally from either treatment. Gains were maintained at 6-month follow-up.

Shaw (1979) utilized the data for the phobic subgroup treated by Trower et al. (1978) and treated an additional 10 phobic patients with imaginal flooding. Combining the results of these two studies, phobic patients benefited equally when treated with SST, systematic desensitization, or imaginal flooding. Skill deficit patients treated with SST showed some improvement in social functioning not evident in skills deficit patients treated with systematic desensitization, but no differences were found on measures of phobic severity, depression, or general anxiety. Given the results of Marzillier et al. (1976), in which within-group changes were not reflected in differences between control and treatment groups, the omission of a waiting-list group renders the results of Trower et al. (1978) and Shaw (1979) inconclusive. Lucock and Salkovskis (1988) also reported positive effects of SST, but their study was similarly uncontrolled.

Öst, Jerremalm, and Johansson (1981) attempted to match treatment to specific patterns of phobic response, although their methods were quite different from those of Trower et al. (1978). By examining cardiac response and overt behavioral signs of anxiety during a role-played social interaction, Öst et al. (1981) classified 32 social phobics as either "behavioral reactors" or "physiological reactors." Behavioral reactors demonstrated relatively poorer behavioral performance, while physiological reactors showed relatively larger differences between baseline and mean heart rate during the interaction. Half the patients in each group were treated with SST, and the other half received a physiologically focused method, applied relaxation (AR). (AR techniques are described below under "Relaxation Strategies.") The authors hypothesized that patients treated with the method matching their particular response pattern would achieve better results than would the group treated with the mismatched method.

Behavioral reactors receiving SST exhibited significantly greater improvements than did behavioral reactors receiving AR on several self-report measures. Specifically, SST-treated behavioral reactors reported less social fear, less difficulty in and avoidance of previously troublesome social situations, and reduced anxiety during the behavioral test. They also reported increased social activities and social contacts. Physiological reactors receiving AR participated in more social activities, made more social contacts, and evidenced fewer visible signs of anxiety during the behavioral test than did SST-treated physiological reactors. Thus, patients appear to have achieved better outcomes when they received the treatment matched to their specific pattern of difficulties. However, the overall findings are mixed. Behavioral reactors appeared to respond better to SST, but only on self-report measures. Physiological reactors showed greater response to AR, but only on two questionnaires and one behavioral measure. Most analyses resulted in no differences between groups. Patients were excluded if they were high or low in both behavioral and physiological reactivity, thus limiting generalizability of the findings to patients with relatively pure response patterns. As in previous studies, there was no control condition to test for changes in responses due to time, repeated testing, or other non-specific factors.

Mersch, Emmelkamp, Bögels, and van der Sleen (1989) used a similar strategy to extend the results of Öst et al. (1981) to behavioral reactors and cognitive reactors. Behavioral reactors were identified using the procedures of Öst et al. Cognitive reactors, first studied by Jerremalm, Jansson, and Öst (1986) in a study to be reviewed later, scored lower on a measure of rational thinking. As in Öst et al. (1981), patients scoring high or low in both domains were excluded. SST was provided to half the behavioral reactors and half the cognitive reactors, and rational–emotive therapy (RET; Ellis, 1962) was provided to the remaining patients. All four treatment groups showed reductions in social anxiety. Behavioral and cognitive reactors receiving SST, for example, reported more positive self-statements and were rated as being less anxious and more skillful on a behavior test from pretreatment to posttreatment assessment. Behavioral and cognitive reactors receiving RET rated themselves as more skillful and less anxious from pretreatment to posttreatment and from posttreatment to 6-week follow-up. There were virtually no differences between behavioral and cognitive reactors treated either with SST or RET.

Wlazlo, Schroeder-Hartwig, Hand, Kaiser, and Münchau (1990) compared a semistructured, individually tailored SST program to individual and group exposure as treatments for social phobia. Seventy-eight patients were retrospectively classified as having "primary social skills deficits" or "primary social phobia" by a team of clinical raters. Like several of the studies described above, Wlazlo et al. examined the hypothesis that patients with social skills deficits would fare better with SST while patients with primary phobia would demonstrate greater improvement with one of the exposure programs. However, the treatment-matching effort was largely compromised because patients were not randomly assigned to treatments, total amount of time devoted to treatment differed across conditions, exposure instructions were given to patients receiving SST, and exposure conditions included modeling, prompting, and coaching of desired social behaviors for patients judged to have social skills deficits. Despite these methodological problems, the majority of patients demonstrated significant improvements. Improvements were noted in self-reported social skills, social anxiety, avoidance, interference of symptoms in daily life activities, and the associated symptoms of depression and obsessive rumination. However, there were few differences among treatments at either the posttreatment or 3-month follow-up assessment.

Stravynski, Marks, and Yule (1982) compared SST alone with SST plus cognitive restructuring (based on RET) in the treatment of 22 social phobic patients diagnosed by DSM-III criteria. No changes occurred during a control waiting period in which patients were repeatedly assessed. Treatment consisted of 12, 1.5-hour weekly individual or group sessions. Patients in both conditions improved significantly, reporting increases in social interaction, reduced levels of depression, and reduced irrational beliefs regarding social situations. Group and individual treatment produced very similar results, but assignment to group versus individual treatment was not made randomly. At 6-month follow-up, improvement was maintained in both conditions with no apparent benefit from the addition of cognitive restructuring procedures to SST.

In a similarly designed study, Falloon, Lloyd, and Harpin (1981) treated 16 patients meeting DSM-III criteria for social phobia with either SST plus propranolol (Inderal), a beta blocker, or SST plus placebo in a double-blind trial. Treatments began after a 4-week waiting period. SST began with a 6-hour session in which each patient met with another patient and a nonprofessional "therapist" to practice the skills required for use in targeted social situations. For the next 2 weeks, the patient and therapist practiced these skills in the first of two targeted situations. A second 2-week period was devoted to the second situation. Assessments before and after the waiting period revealed no changes on self-report measures. Pre-to-posttreatment analyses showed reductions in social anxiety and increases in positive self-image. Gains were maintained in the 81% of patients who responded to the follow-up 6 months later. Propranolol did not enhance the effects of SST at either posttest or follow-up.

RELAXATION STRATEGIES

The application of relaxation techniques to social phobia is based on the straightforward notion that they should provide the person with a means of coping with the physiological manifestations of anxiety. Studies reviewed above by Marzillier et al. (1976), Trower et al. (1978), and Shaw (1979) examined the effectiveness of systematic desensitization in social phobics (also see the discussion of Kanter & Goldfried, 1979, below). Despite their intuitive appeal, however, only four other studies have examined the effect of relaxation strategies on social phobia (Al-Kubaisy et al., 1992; Alström, Nordlund, Persson, Härding, & Ljungqvist, 1984; Jerremalm et al., 1986; Öst et al., 1981). There is some support for their efficacy if the person is given the opportunity to practice relaxation skills when he or she experiences anxiety in problematic social situations, that is, when relaxation strategies are combined with exposure techniques. Al-Kubaisy et al. (1992) and Alström et al. (1984) did not follow this guideline and reported minimal improvement in social phobics treated with relaxation techniques. Öst et al. (1981) and Jerremalm et al. (1986) reported greater success with AR (Öst, 1987).

According to Öst (1987), AR patients are taught to (1) recognize early signs of their anxiety (i.e., physiological arousal) and (2) cope with their anxiety rather than be overwhelmed by it. The procedural goal of AR is to learn to relax in 20–30 seconds and to use this skill to counteract physical symptoms encountered in problematic situations. In early AR sessions, patients examine their own specific early signs of anxiety through self-monitoring exercises. They are next taught the skills of progressive muscle relaxation, a widely used procedure that involves the alternating tensing and relaxing of specific muscle groups. As they become proficient with these procedures through repeated practice, they learn to relax without first tensing their muscles and then to relax in response to the cue word "relax." The next task is to maintain a state of relaxation while engaged in a variety of physical activities (initially these are simple movements; later they are specific tasks of daily living that are not in themselves anxiety evoking). The final phase of AR, application training, involves the utilization of relaxation skills during role-plays of anxiety-evoking social situations and during exposure to targeted situations that occur between sessions.

The study by Öst et al. (1981) was described above. In that study, physiological reactors who received AR participated in more social activities, made more social contacts, and showed fewer behavioral signs of anxiety during the social interaction test than did physiological reactors who received SST. Jerremalm et al. (1986) conducted a similar study in which AR and self-instructional training (SIT; a highly structured cognitive-behavioral technique; see Meichenbaum, 1985) were compared to a waiting-list condition. AR was more effective than the waiting-list across the board and as effective as SIT on a number of measures. The results of this study are described in greater detail in the section "Cognitive Behavioral Interventions" below.

EXPOSURE

Exposure to real-life feared situations has long been acknowledged as a central component of effective fear reduction (Barlow & Beck, 1984). In fact, the effective component of other techniques such as SST or AR may be the exposure to feared situations that is inherent within them (Heimberg, Dodge, & Becker, 1987). Several studies have now examined exposure protocols for social phobia (e.g., Al-Kubaisy et al., 1992; Alström et al., 1984; Biran, Augusto, & Wilson, 1981; Butler, Cullington, Munby, Amies, & Gelder, 1984; Emmelkamp, Mersch, Vissia, & van der Helm, 1985; Fava, Grandi, & Canestrari, 1989; Hope, Heimberg, & Bruch, 1990; Mattick & Peters, 1988; Mattick, Peters, & Clarke, 1989; Turner, Beidel, & Jacob, 1994; Wlazlo et al., 1990). These protocols typically involve (1) the collaborative development by therapist and patient of a list of anxiety-evoking situations and (2) confrontation of these situations by the patient, working from the least to the most anxiety-evoking. However, they differ rather dramatically in the amount of therapist involvement, the amount of time devoted to exposure per session and in total, the spacing of practice sessions, the inclusion of imaginal exposure, and whether patients are expected to remain in the situation until anxiety is substantially reduced. Few of these parameters of exposure treatment have been examined in the context of treatment of social phobia, although Al-Kubaisy et al. (1992)

found that therapist-directed exposure added little to the effectiveness of patients' own self-directed exposure efforts. Below, we review studies that evaluate exposure as a sole treatment for social phobia, often in comparison to other cognitive-behavioral techniques. Later in this chapter, we examine the question of whether the effects of exposure are enhanced by the addition of cognitive techniques.

Fava et al. (1989) treated 10 social phobics with self-directed exposure in an uncontrolled study. The 7 patients who completed treatment showed significant reductions in both self-report and observer-rated measures of anxiety after eight sessions. Al-Kubaisy et al. (1992) treated 28 social phobics as part of a larger series that also included agoraphobics and specific phobics. Exposure was effective in reducing anxiety and increasing approach behavior on a number of indices, much more so than relaxation training. However, patients receiving nine hours of therapist-directed exposure fared better than did patients receiving only instructions for self-directed exposure on just 4 of 27 measures.

Alström et al. (1984) randomly assigned 42 social phobics to exposure, dynamically oriented supportive therapy, relaxation therapy, or "basal therapy" (unspecified anxiolytic medication and encouragement to practice self-exposure). Patients in the first three groups also received basal therapy as a component of their treatment. Exposure patients received prolonged therapist-directed exposure to moderately difficult but common situations and were instructed to remain in feared situations until anxiety decreased. Situation difficulty was gradually increased, and therapist assistance was gradually withdrawn. Exposure in imagination supplemented this procedure for some patients.

Reductions in anticipatory anxiety and anxiety in difficult situations were most evident for exposure patients, who avoided less when faced with difficult situations and showed greater improvement on a global rating scale of disturbance than did patients treated with relaxation or basal therapy alone. At 9-month follow-up, most differences between exposure, relaxation therapy and supportive therapy were no longer evident, to some extent a result of deterioration among exposure patients. However, exposure patients did maintain their advantage over patients receiving basal therapy at follow-up on measures of situational and anticipatory anxiety.

Several aspects of this study make its findings difficult to interpret. For example, patients selected for participation were described as unsuitable for insight-oriented psychotherapy. In other reports by these researchers, unsuitability was reported to be associated with lower dominance, higher neuroticism, greater impairment, and poorer treatment outcome in a predominantly agoraphobic sample (Persson & Alström, 1983, 1984). It is unclear how this exclusion impacts on outcome of social phobia treatment since no patients deemed suitable for insight-oriented psychotherapy were included. Other concerns include gender, demographic, and pretreatment impairment differences across groups, unsystematic administration of treatments within and across groups (imaginal flooding in the exposure condition and medication across conditions), and the inclusion of self-exposure instructions in basal therapy.

Emmelkamp et al. (1985) compared exposure with RET and SIT in the treatment of 34 social phobics meeting DSM-III criteria. Treatments were conducted in groups of four to seven patients with each session 2.5 hours in length. Exposure consisted of role-plays within the group (e.g., public speaking) and specific exercises completed between sessions (e.g., asking questions in shops, speaking to strangers). Cognitive treatments are described in a later section.

Exposure resulted in reductions in social anxiety and general psychopathology at posttreatment assessment and additional improvements at 1-month follow-up. At posttest, exposure patients evidenced significantly greater reduction in heart rate before and after a behavior test than did patients treated with SIT or RET. No other differences favored exposure at posttest or follow-up. Patients receiving cognitive treatments reported fewer irrational beliefs than did exposure patients.

As reported earlier, Wlazlo et al. (1990) compared SST with individual- and group-administered exposure in the treatment of patients classified as having primary social skills deficits or primary social phobia. All treatments produced significant within-group changes on most measures. Phobic patients receiving group exposure reported less fear of social contact and greater ability to refuse requests than did patients with social skills deficits treated with group exposure. However, problems with this study, noted previously, reduce our ability to determine the relative benefits of these treatments.

The study of combined imaginal and *in vivo* exposure treatment of social phobia conducted by Turner, Beidel, and Jacob (1994) is described in the section "Comparison to Pharmacological Treatments for Social Phobia" below. However, Turner, Beidel, Cooley, Woody, and Messer (1994) have reported preliminary data on a new multicomponent treatment package they have labeled Social Effectiveness Therapy (SET). SET consists of patient education, SST, imaginal and *in vivo* exposure, and programmed practice. It is administered in a combination of individual and group treatment sessions for a total of 40 treatment hours. It is an intensive protocol that may hold promise for the treatment of severe social phobia. In their pilot study, Turner, Beidel, Cooley, et al. (1994) administered SET to 17 generalized social phobics, several of whom also carried diagnoses of avoidant or obsessive–compulsive personality disorder according to DSM-III-R criteria. The 13 treatment completers showed improvement on a number of indices, including self-reported social anxiety, anxiety and performance during behavioral tests, clinician ratings, and a measure of end-state functioning.

COGNITIVE-BEHAVIORAL INTERVENTIONS

Butler (1985) and Emmelkamp (1982) assert that cognitive factors are more central to the development and maintenance of social phobia than is the case for other anxiety disorders (see also Clark & Wells, Chapter 4, and Leary & Kowalski, Chapter 5, this volume). At its very base, fear of scrutiny or negative evaluation by others is a problem of the *perception* of other peoples' motives and behavior. These authors further suggest that interventions that address distorted thoughts and perceptions may be especially important components of the treatment of social phobia. In fact, Butler (1985) concludes that "social phobia might be resistant to treatment . . . which does not include a cognitive element" (p. 655). In this section, we review studies in which cognitive interventions have been studied, either as singular treatments or as part of multicomponent treatment strategies that may include other techniques such as exposure. In the following section, we address the question of combining exposure and cognitive techniques.

Kanter and Goldfried (1979) examined a variation of RET in the first test of a cognitive treatment for 68 volunteers who appear to have met diagnostic criteria for social phobia. In systematic rational restructuring (SRR; Goldfried, Decenteceo, & Weinberg, 1974), patients utilize imagery of anxiety-provoking situations to identify unrealistic thoughts, challenge these thoughts, and substitute more adaptive ones in their place. Patients use their experience of anxiety during the imagery process as a cue to begin identifying maladaptive thoughts. SRR was compared to self-control desensitization (SCD; Goldfried, 1971), in which patients respond to anxiety experienced during imagery procedures with progressive relaxation, the combination of SRR and SCD, and to a waiting-list control. Patients were treated in groups of 8–10 for seven weekly 1.5-hour sessions.

Patients in the three active treatments improved significantly more than did waiting-list patients. Patients in SRR and the combined treatment showed significant improvement on 16 of 19 measures, including measures of social anxiety, trait anxiety, and irrational beliefs. SCD patients improved on 10 of 19 measures. However, SRR patients reported lower trait anxiety, fewer irrational beliefs, and lower anxiety during a behavior test than did SCD patients, and combined treatment patients reported less anxiety about the prospect of giving a speech and less anxiety during a behavior test than did SCD patients. The behavior test was not administered at a 9-week follow-up assessment, limiting this assessment to self-report. While patients in all active treatments showed significant improvement from pretreatment to follow-up, SRR patients had significantly greater reductions in trait anxiety, fear of negative evaluation, and irrational beliefs than did SCD patients.

In a study described earlier, Emmelkamp et al. (1985) compared RET and self-instructional training (SIT) with exposure. RET focused on disputing irrational beliefs commonly held by social phobic patients. SIT was a modified version of Meichenbaum's (1985) stress-inoculation training (minus relaxation procedures). SIT patients were trained to identify and record negative thoughts and feelings that occurred in social situations. Using imaginal rehearsal, patient and therapist developed and practiced realistic thoughts designed to increase coping with the anticipatory phase of social situations, the situation itself, and the postsituation phase in which negative bias regarding performance is common among social phobics. Neither cognitive treatment included instruction for exposure. Nevertheless, patients in both cognitive treatments reported reductions in social anxiety, general psychopathology, and irrational beliefs. RET patients reported less social anxiety on one measure than did SIT patients, but there were few other differences between the cognitive treatments. Exposure was superior to both cognitive treatments on the pulse rate measure at posttest. At follow-up, RET patients showed additional improvement on social anxiety and irrational beliefs, while SIT patients reported less general psychopathology. RET patients continued to report less social anxiety than did SIT patients, and patients in both cognitive treatments reported fewer irrational beliefs than did patients in the exposure treatment.

In another study of 79 socially anxious volunteers, DiGiuseppe, McGowan, Sutton-Simon, and Gardner (1990) examined the relative effectiveness of four cognitive-behavioral treatments: (1) cognitive therapy, modeled on the program developed for depression by Beck, Rush, Shaw, and Emery (1979), (2) interpersonal cognitive problem-solving skills training (Spivack, Platt, & Shure, 1976), (3) RET, and (4) SIT. These cognitive-behavioral interventions were compared to a behavioral treatment without the cognitive component, assertion training (essentially SST with a specific focus on the development of assertiveness skills; Heimberg, Montgomery, Madsen, & Heimberg, 1977) and a waiting-list control. On self-report and behavioral measures of social anxiety, the four cognitive-behavioral treatments and assertion training were equally effective and superior to the waiting-list control. On measures of related states (e.g., depression), the cognitive-behavioral treatments were more likely than was assertion training to surpass the waiting-list in effectiveness. There were no differences among the cognitive-behavioral treatments on any measure.

Using a design similar to Öst et al. (1981), Jerremalm et al. (1986) classified 38 social phobics as physiological reactors (based on relatively large heart rate increases during a role-played social interaction) or cognitive reactors (based on a relatively higher frequency of negative thoughts during the interaction). Patients of each type were randomly assigned to either AR, SIT, or a waiting-list condition. Physiological reactors receiving either AR or SIT were more improved than were waiting-list patients on measures of anxiety and heart rate during the behavioral test. Physiological reactors receiving SIT reported more positive thoughts and fewer negative thoughts than did the control group. Cognitive reactors receiving either treatment evidenced significant improvement in thought index scores, with SIT resulting in improvement beyond that seen in patients treated with AR. Cognitive reactors treated with SIT improved significantly more than did those treated with AR on three of seven self-report measures. No advantage was found for the physiological reactors treated with AR, and on two measures, SIT was actually more effective than AR.

These results did not strongly support Jerremalm et al.'s (1986) treatment-matching hypothesis, and the authors offered several possible explanations for their results. Classification of cognitive reactors may not have been successful, since the instrument used for this purpose was found to have low test–retest reliability. The authors also questioned the adequacy of their classification of physiological reactors, but this same methodology was employed successfully by Öst et al. (1981). Finally, they suggest that the cognitive treatment may have offered a more robust method of coping with social fears, regardless of patients' individual response patterns.

Mersch et al. (1989), in a study described above, further tested the treatment-matching hypothesis, comparing RET with SST in the treatment of social phobic patients classified as cognitive or behavioral reactors. While there were numerous improvements among patients receiving either RET or SST, there was virtually no support for the matching of treatment to individual response pattern.

Heimberg, Becker, Goldfinger, and Vermilyea (1985) treated seven social phobic patients in small groups with a combination of imaginal exposure, exposure to role-played social situations, cognitive restructuring, and homework assignments. During sessions, cognitive restructuring followed each exposure and focused on identifying thoughts that occurred during the role-play, repeatedly questioning the meaning of these thoughts (especially their long-range consequences), and revealing their faulty logic. As homework assignments, patients were instructed to engage in exposure and cognitive restructuring in the natural environment. Significant reductions in social anxiety, general anxiety, and fear of negative evaluation were evident from pretreatment to posttreatment and from pretreatment to 6-month follow-up. Attributions for negative outcomes became less internal and stable, and patients took less responsibility for negative outcomes. After treatment, patients reported less anxiety, rated their own behavioral performance as higher in quality, and were rated by observers as exhibiting fewer signs of anxiety during a behavioral test. Gains were maintained at 6-month follow-up for all but one patient, whose anxiety returned to baseline levels.

Heimberg et al. (1990) removed imaginal exposure from the above protocol and expanded the range of cognitive restructuring activities. The new protocol, Cognitive-Behavioral Group Therapy for Social Phobia (CBGT), attempts to maximize the integration of cognitive and behavioral procedures. The program is administered by two cotherapists to six patients in 12 weekly sessions and is comprised of several components: (1) development of a cognitive-behavioral explanation of social phobia; (2) training of patients in the skills of identification, analysis, and disputation of problematic cognitions through the use of structured exercises; (3) exposure of patients to simulations of anxiety-provoking situations during group sessions; (4) use of cognitive restructuring procedures to teach patients to control their maladaptive thinking before, during, and after simulated exposures; (5) homework assignments for *in vivo* exposure to situations already confronted during exposure simulations; and (6) self-administered cognitive restructuring activities for use before and after completion of behavioral homework assignments. CBGT was compared to a placebo-therapy group developed to control for therapist attention, treatment credibility, and outcome expectancy (Educational–Supportive Group Psychotherapy, ES). ES sessions combined educational presentations on topics relevant to problems generally reported by social phobics and time for members to share ideas, insights, and advice with each other in a supportive environment. Ratings of treatment credibility and outcome expectations for CBGT and ES were virtually equivalent.

Forty-nine social phobics were randomly assigned to either CBGT or ES. At posttest, CBGT patients, compared to ES patients, reported less anxiety during an individualized behavior test and were rated as less severely impaired by clinical assessors. At 6-month follow-up, CBGT patients maintained their gains and also reported more positive and fewer negative thoughts during the behavior test than did ES patients. Clinically significant improvement was defined as a 2-point decrease from pretreatment assessment on the assessor's 0-to-8 rating of phobic severity and a score below the clinically significant level (3 or less). Using these criteria, 75% of CBGT patients were improved at posttest, and 40% of ES patients improved. At 6-month follow-up, 81% and 47% of CBGT and ES patients, respectively, were improved using this index.

In a reanalysis of a subset of the data from this study, Bruch, Heimberg, and Hope (1991) examined the relationship between CBGT outcome and cognitive change. Schwartz and Garamoni (1986) have suggested that the ratio of positive thoughts to the sum of positive plus negative thoughts (P / [P + N]), termed the "states of mind ratio," is linked to varying levels of psychopathology. States of mind ratios of .00 to .31 (termed *negative monologue*), .32 to .44 (*negative dialogue*), and .45 to .55 (*internal dialogue of conflict*) are linked to severe, moderate, and mild psychopathology, respectively. A shift from any of these ranges to a *positive dialogue* (ratio of

.56 to .68) is hypothesized to be a primary mechanism by which cognitive treatments produce change. This range is hypothesized to be associated with healthy adjustment, since it combines an optimistically positive view of one's circumstances (i.e., a majority of positive thoughts) with a sufficient awareness of environmental threat (i.e., a nontrivial, but smaller, percentage of negative thoughts). Higher ratios (termed *positive monologues*) are also said to be associated with dysfunction because they represent insufficient attention to threat.

After patients participated in their individualized behavioral test, they were asked to record all the thoughts that had occurred to them in anticipation of or during the test situation. Thoughts for 14 CBGT patients and 16 ES patients who provided complete data at the pretreatment, posttreatment, and 6-month follow-up assessments were then categorized as positive (facilitative of performance), negative (disruptive to performance), or neutral by independent judges. The states of mind ratio for the entire sample before treatment was .29, within the range of negative monologue and, according to Schwartz and Garamoni, indicative of severe psychopathology. At posttest, patients in both treatments exhibited similar ratios, indicative of internal dialogue of conflict. At 6-month follow-up, however, CBGT patients exhibited a ratio within the theoretical ideal range (.67) while the ratio for ES patients returned to baseline levels. In a further analysis of the role of state of mind, Bruch et al. (1991) examined the association between improvement status and the states of mind ratio, regardless of treatment condition. Using the same index of improvement as Heimberg et al. (1990), improvers had higher average ratios than did nonimprovers at both posttest and follow-up assessment.

Lucas and Telch (1993b) conducted a replication of Heimberg et al.'s (1990) comparison of CBGT and ES, with the addition of an individually administered version of the cognitive-behavioral treatment. The individual treatment was faithful to the group approach described above. Patients receiving CBGT were more improved than were ES patients on a number of indices, substantially replicating the previous trial. However, beyond measures of cost-effectiveness, the group treatment did not lead to significantly better outcomes than did individual treatment. On a conservative measure of reliable change, 61% of CBGT patients, 50% of individual cognitive-behavioral treatment patients, and 24% of ES patients achieved clinically significant change. The difference between CBGT and ES on this measure was significant.

COMBINING COGNITIVE AND EXPOSURE TREATMENTS

As reviewed above, several studies have examined the effectiveness of cognitive-behavioral treatment packages with social phobics. These treatments employed multiple techniques to teach patients cognitive coping skills while also engaging patients in behavioral pursuits such as graduated exposure to feared social situations. While these multicomponent packages resulted in positive treatment response, it is not clear whether the cognitive techniques contributed to outcome or whether positive results could be attributed solely to the behavioral treatment components. Since cognitive techniques are unlikely to be employed clinically without the use of behavioral assignments, a more relevant analysis is one that examines whether the effectiveness of the behavioral technique is enhanced by the utilization of cognitive procedures. Six studies have examined this question. Three support the utility of cognitive techniques and three do not.

Biran et al. (1981) used a multiple-baseline design to examine the effectiveness of exposure and cognitive restructuring for three female patients with fears of writing in public. Five sessions of cognitive restructuring were followed by five sessions of exposure for two patients while the third received exposure only. Exposure was conducted according to a standard hierarchy of feared writing situations. During cognitive restructuring, patients were trained to identify maladaptive ideas while imagining phobic situations. Through discussion and modeling, a realistic appraisal of the situation was developed, presumably displacing maladaptive thinking and reducing anxiety.

Patients evidenced no change in the number of tasks completed on a behavior test during baseline assessment or following cognitive restructuring. They attained maximal levels of approach after exposure and maintained these changes through the 9-month follow-up. While increases in approach behavior were directly related to exposure, patterns of change in subjective fear differed across patients, with one showing reductions during baseline assessment, the second showing reductions following cognitive restructuring, and the third showing no change until the 1-month follow-up. Avoidance was low at the 9-month follow-up, but fear returned to pretreatment levels. At least for avoidance behavior, exposure led to significant change and was not facilitated by cognitive restructuring. This finding is similar to that reported by Stravynski et al. (1982), who found that cognitive restructuring did not enhance the effectiveness of SST in a sample of 22 social phobics.

Hope et al. (1990) compared exposure to exposure plus cognitive restructuring and a waiting-list condition. The combined treatment was the CBGT protocol described above, while the exposure alone condition replaced cognitive restructuring activities with content relevant to a habituation model of exposure. Both active treatments were more effective than was the waiting-list condition at the end of 12 weeks. CBGT patients also reported less anxiety during an individualized behavioral test and tended to be rated more positively by therapists than were exposure-alone patients, but exposure alone led to significantly greater improvements on blind assessor ratings and self-ratings of anxiety and fear of negative evaluation. At follow-up, CBGT and exposure alone were equally effective. However, CBGT in this study was less effective than in other studies of this protocol by Heimberg et al. (1990), Gelernter et al. (1991), and Lucas and Telch (1993b), making these results difficult to interpret.

Butler et al. (1984) randomly assigned 45 patients who met DSM-III criteria for social phobia to exposure, exposure plus anxiety management training (EX/AMT) or a waiting-list control group. Patients received seven weekly individual sessions, and booster sessions were provided 2 weeks and 6 weeks after treatment concluded. In the exposure conditions, patients were encouraged to engage in approximately 1 hour of exposure each day, focusing on graded tasks that were clearly defined, repeatable, and had previously resulted in anxiety or avoidance. AMT consisted of relaxation, distraction, and rational self-talk, and Butler et al. (1984) hypothesized that the addition of these techniques would enhance the effects of exposure by reducing psychological disengagement. In order to equalize the amount of exposure and therapist attention that each patient received, a filler treatment ("associative therapy") was provided as part of the exposure condition. Associative therapy occupied the same amount of time as AMT, included discussion about exposure, but excluded discussion of specific coping strategies.

At posttest, patients in the two exposure treatments demonstrated significant change on patient-rated and assessor-rated measures of phobic severity and on anxiety during a behavioral test. They also appeared less generally anxious and depressed. These changes were significantly greater than those demonstrated by the waiting-list group. On the Fear of Negative Evaluation Scale and the Social Avoidance and Distress Scale (Watson & Friend, 1969), the EX/AMT group showed significantly greater posttreatment changes than did either the exposure or waiting-list subjects, who did not differ. At 6-month follow-up, EX/AMT proved superior to exposure on several measures of phobic anxiety and avoidance, general anxiety, and depression, as well as the two scales mentioned above. In the year after treatment, 40% of exposure patients sought additional treatment, whereas no patients receiving EX/AMT did so.

AMT appeared to facilitate exposure in the Butler et al. (1984) study, but the study's design does not allow us to determine which components of AMT were responsible for this effect. However, the authors conducted a post hoc analysis of patients' use of AMT coping strategies. Before treatment, most patients reported using one or more of these techniques, most commonly distraction. After treatment, use of distraction and relaxation techniques had doubled, but use of rational self-talk had increased fivefold. Eleven of 14 EX/AMT patients used rational self-talk. Thus, rational self-talk may have been the key ingredient in AMT.

One complicating factor in the interpretation of Butler et al. (1984) concerns treatment credibility. Credibility ratings for the exposure condition were significantly lower than were ratings for EX/AMT by the fourth week of treatment, and this may have accounted for differences in outcome between the two treatment variations.

Mattick and Peters (1988) compared therapist-assisted guided exposure with and without cognitive restructuring. Therapists accompanied groups to locations where they could engage their feared situation (e.g., eating or drinking at a café). Difficulty level was gradually increased while direct assistance was gradually withdrawn. The therapist remained available and provided feedback and support, despite providing less direct aid. Cognitive restructuring focused on irrational beliefs regarding social phobics' concerns that others have negative opinions of them, that they are being observed, and that signs of anxiety are public and can be seen by others. Thoughts related to these beliefs were identified in the context of past and hypothetical feared situations, and their logic and adaptiveness was evaluated. Development of rational and adaptive thoughts was followed by encouragement to actively use these thoughts in feared situations.

The 51 participants in this study were described as having circumscribed fears. However, a substantial subset might have met criteria for the DSM-III-R generalized type, since two-thirds of the sample in another study by this group (Mattick et al., 1989) did so. Treatment was administered in groups of four to seven patients, for 6 weeks, 2 hours each week. Both exposure alone and exposure combined with cognitive restructuring led to significant improvements, but combined treatment surpassed exposure alone on measures of behavioral approach, self-rated avoidance, and end-state functioning. While both treatments were effective at follow-up, the combined treatment was superior to exposure alone, especially on percentage of tasks completed during a behavioral test, phobic avoidance, and composite measures of improvement and end-state functioning. At follow-up, 48% of exposure-alone patients continued to report definite avoidance, compared to only 14% of combined treatment patients.

Mattick et al. (1989) compared exposure, cognitive restructuring, and exposure plus cognitive restructuring to a waiting-list control group in an attempt to disentangle the effects found in the previous study. Forty-three social phobic patients participated. All three treatments produced posttreatment improvement when compared with the waiting-list condition on percentage of tasks completed during a behavior test and self-report of phobic severity and avoidance. At posttreatment assessment, exposure alone and the combined treatment were more effective than was cognitive restructuring alone in increasing the number of tasks completed on a behavior test. At follow-up assessment, patients in the cognitive restructuring condition and the combined treatment had continued to improve while patients in the exposure-alone condition had deteriorated slightly. Overall, combined treatment patients completed a higher percentage of behavioral tasks than did patients in the exposure and cognitive restructuring treatments.

COMPARISON TO PHARMACOLOGICAL TREATMENTS FOR SOCIAL PHOBIA

Five studies have now been completed that examine the relative or combined efficacy of cognitive-behavioral and pharmacological interventions for social phobia. These studies compare diverse cognitive and behavioral interventions with a range of medications, including the monoamine oxidase inhibitor phenelzine sulfate (Nardil), the triazolobenzodiazepine alprazolam (Xanax), the beta-adrenergic blockers propranolol (Inderal) and atenolol (Tenormin), and the nonbenzodiazepine anxiolytic buspirone (BuSpar).

Turner, Beidel, and Jacob (1994) compared the efficacy of a combination of imaginal and *in vivo* exposure to feared situations to that of the cardioselective beta blocker atenolol and placebo in 72 social phobics. Atenolol and placebo were administered double-blind on an escalating dosage schedule, increasing from 25 mg per day of atenolol (or the equivalent amount of placebo) the 1st week to 100 mg per day the 4th week of a 3-month treatment period. Dosage was adjusted as needed for side effects or if blood pressure or pulse rate fell below predetermined criteria. Exposure patients received 20 sessions during the treatment period, meeting twice weekly in the first 2 months and weekly in the third. The first nine sessions were devoted to imaginal exposure, the next seven sessions alternated between imaginal exposure and therapist-assisted in vivo exposure, and the last four sessions were devoted to self-directed exposure.

Assessment in Turner, Beidel, and Jacob (1994) was broadly based, including self-report, independent assessment, response to a public speaking behavioral test, and indices of improvement and end-state functioning that were composites of measures from each of the other domains. On most self-report and independent assessment measures, exposure was significantly more effective than placebo. Mean scores of atenolol patients fell between those of exposure and placebo patients, not significantly different from either one. Analysis of behavioral test measures and composite indices showed a preference for exposure over either atenolol or placebo. Exposure patients reported less anxiety, more positive self-statements, and fewer negative self-statements during the behavioral test than did atenolol or placebo patients, who did not differ from each other. On the composite measures, exposure patients were significantly more improved and showed better end-state functioning than did patients receiving atenolol or placebo. On the improvement index, 55.6% of exposure patients were classified as greatly improved, compared to 13.3% of atenolol patients and 6.3% of placebo patients.

Only 12 of 21 atenolol patients and 15 of 21 exposure patients participated in the 6-month follow-up, so statements about follow-up status must be made with caution. Most analyses suggested that patients who were improved at posttest maintained their gains, regardless of which treatment they had received. However, exposure patients outperformed atenolol patients at the 6-month follow-up on two self-report measures and the length of time they engaged in their speech task before asking that it be terminated. Although they made substantial improvements, treated patients remained significantly inferior to a comparison group of normal subjects.

Gelernter et al. (1991) compared Heimberg's CBGT protocol to treatment with phenelzine, alprazolam, and pill placebo in a sample of 65 patients with social phobia. Patients receiving phenelzine began treatment at a dosage of 10 mg per day and increased to a maximum dose of 90 mg per day (mean daily dose = 55 mg, range = 30–90 mg). Patients receiving alprazolam began treatment at a dosage of 0.7 mg per day and increased to a maximum dose of 6.3 mg per day (mean daily dose = 4.2 mg, range = 2.1–6.3 mg). Patients took medications (or placebo tablets) four times daily on a fixed dosage schedule, and all treatments lasted 12 weeks. In the pharmacotherapy conditions, physicians "firmly encouraged patients to push themselves into phobic situations" (p. 940), and these treatments may best be conceptualized as combinations of medications (or placebo) and instructions for self-exposure. CBGT was administered according to the procedures described in Heimberg (1990), but each group consisted of 10 patients, rather than 6 as recommended by Heimberg.

Assessments in the Gelernter et al. (1991) study were limited to several self-report measures of social phobia, anxiety, depression, work and social disability, and positive and negative self-statements experienced during a behavioral test. Additional ratings of work and social disability were completed by physicians, but these ratings were not completed for CBGT patients and are not discussed here. All treatment conditions, including the combination of placebo plus self-exposure instructions, led to significant improvements on all measures, with few differential treatment effects. Patients treated with phenelzine were more improved than were other patients on a measure of trait anxiety at posttest and 2-month follow-up, but similarities far outweighed differences. Patients were classified as "unequivocal responders" if they achieved a posttreatment score below the general population mean on the social phobia subscale of the Fear Questionnaire (Marks & Mathews, 1979). While the highest percentage of unequivocal responders was found in the phenelzine group, this difference did not achieve statistical significance. During follow-up, patients receiving CBGT or phenelzine maintained their gains, but alprazolam patients did not.

The findings of Gelernter et al. (1991) are difficult to interpret for several reasons, including sole reliance on self-report assessment, inclusion of self-exposure instructions as part of all medication treatments, and deviation from recommended CBGT procedure. The finding of equivalent change in the placebo condition further complicates matters, but placebo response is an unlikely rival hypothesis since the placebo group did not do as well as the phenelzine or alprazolam groups on blind physician ratings of work and social disability.

Heimberg et al. (1994), in a recently completed study, also examined the relative efficacy of CBGT and phenelzine. The 133 patients from the two sites of this collaborative study (59 from the State University of New York at Albany Center for Stress and Anxiety Disorders, 74 from the New York State Psychiatric Institute) were randomly assigned to CBGT, phenelzine, pill placebo, or ES (the comparison treatment employed by Heimberg et al., 1990). All patients (other than dropouts) received 12 weeks of treatment. Thereafter, ES and placebo patients and those who failed to respond to CBGT or phenelzine (as determined by independent assessor interview) were removed from the study. Responders to CBGT and phenelzine then received 6 additional months of maintenance treatment (i.e., reduced frequency of contact) and were then repeatedly assessed over a 6-month treatment-free follow-up period. Repeated assessments included independent assessment interviews, self-report questionnaires, and individualized behavioral tests. Detailed presentation of results await the published report. However, preliminary analyses suggest that (1) phenelzine produced more rapid response than did CBGT, with positive effects noted after 6 weeks of treatment, (2) CBGT and phenelzine produced equivalent response rates after 12 weeks of treatment, and both were superior to ES and placebo, (3) phenelzine was more effective than was CBGT on some measures after 12 weeks, but (4) during untreated follow-up, CBGT patients maintained their gains while a number of phenelzine patients relapsed.

Two studies have evaluated the utility of combining cognitive-behavioral and pharmacologic interventions. In a study described earlier, Falloon et al. (1981) found no enhancement of the effects of SST with the addition of the beta blocker propranolol. In the other combined treatment study, Clark and Agras (1991) examined the effects of brief cognitive-behavioral intervention and buspirone on performance anxiety among 34 musicians who met DSM-III-R criteria for social phobia. Four treatment conditions were compared: cognitive-behavioral treatment with buspirone, cognitive-behavioral treatment with placebo, buspirone alone, and placebo alone. Buspirone was initially administered in 5-mg doses three times daily and was increased as tolerated to a maximum daily dose of 60 mg. After 6 weeks of treatment, buspirone patients received a mean daily dose of 32 ± 11 mg. Cognitive-behavioral treatment was administered in 5 sessions to groups of five to six patients. Treatment consisted of identifying maladaptive self-statements and replacing them with more adaptive alternatives, provision of coping models, applied relaxation training, and *in vivo* exposure.

Assessments consisted of self-report questionnaires, heart rate and self-rated anxiety during a laboratory musical performance and a speech task, and blind observer ratings of the quality of the musical performance. Buspirone was not effective in this study, failing to outperform placebo on a single measure. In contrast, cognitive-behavioral treatment (with or without buspirone) resulted in significant reductions in subjective anxiety during the musical performance and speech and increased quality of musical performances. At 1-month follow-up, cognitive-behavioral treatment with placebo surpassed all other treatment combinations (including cognitive-behavioral treatment with buspirone) on patients' report of their confidence as performers. No other measures were administered at this brief follow-up.

LONG-TERM DURABILITY
OF ANXIETY REDUCTION

When Heimberg reviewed the literature in 1989, little was known about the posttreatment course of patients who had received cognitive-behavioral treatments. In most cases, immediate posttreatment outcome was favorable, and there was maintenance of gains at the follow-up assessment. Several studies (e.g., Mattick et al., 1989) suggested that there might be further modest improvements from the end of treatment to the follow-up assessment. However, the average length of follow-up for the 17 studies was only 5.12 months, and only one report (of the treatment of a single case; Stravynski, 1983) included a follow-up period as long as 1 year. The majority of studies conducted since that time have done little to improve this situation (see Table 12.2). However, five additional reports are now available with follow-up intervals of a year or greater.

Fava et al. (1989) report an uncontrolled trial of exposure treatment of 10 social phobic patients. Seven patients completed the trial and showed substantial improvements on self-report and assessor-rated measures of social phobia. All 7 patients were reassessed after a 1-year follow-up and maintained their posttreatment gains. Fava et al. report that 6 of 7 patients showed further improvements during the follow-up period, although this assertion was not supported by their statistical analyses.

Mersch, Hildebrand, Lavy, Wessel, and van Hout (1992) present a series of three patients with fears that their physiological symptoms (e.g., blushing, sweating, trembling) would cause public embarrassment. All patients improved on a broad array of measures after treatment with a combination of RET and paradoxical interventions. Frequency of feared symptoms was reduced, although anxiety experienced on occurrence of these symptoms remained high. These gains were maintained at an 18-month follow-up.

Mersch, Emmelkamp, and Lips (1991) assessed 57 of 62 patients 14 months after they had completed treatment with either RET or SST in the study originally reported by Mersch et al. (1989). As noted earlier, patients were prospectively classified as either cognitive or behavioral reactors. At the conclusion of treatment, patients receiving SST reported significant changes on measures of social skill, positive self-statements, and anxiety, while patients receiving RET demonstrated improvements on measures of anxiety and social skill. However, there were virtually no posttreatment differences between patients treated with SST and RET.

Assessment at the 14-month follow-up was restricted to a battery of self-report questionnaires. Patients appear to have maintained their improvement at follow-up, regardless of the specific treatment received or the specific locus of their deficits. However, 25 of 57 patients (43.9%) sought and received additional treatment during the follow-up period, suggesting that there was substantial room for further improvement. Patients who sought additional treatment had been rated before treatment as less skilled and more anxious during the behavioral test than patients who did not. Thus, these patients may have been more impaired and less responsive to the treatment interventions.

Wlazlo et al. (1990) compared SST and group and individual exposure for social phobic patients. Posttreatment and 3-month follow-up findings were discussed above. These investigators also reported a longer-term follow-up assessment, with follow-up lengths varying from 1.0 to 5.5 years (mean = 2.5 years). There was additional improvement on several measures between the 3-month and 2.5-year follow-ups. At the latter follow-up, patients with primary phobia reported less interference with daily activities than did skill deficit patients. Surprisingly, skill deficit patients showed their best long-term response to treatment with group exposure. However, the meaningfulness of this finding is open to question, since the treatment conditions were not as different as they might ideally have been (Juster et al., in press).

Heimberg, Salzman, Holt, and Blendell (1993) report a long-term follow-up of the evaluation of CBGT and ES (the credible placebo-control) originally reported by Heimberg et al. (1990). Of the 40 patients who completed treatment in Heimberg et al. (1990), 32 were recontacted, and

19 agreed to participate in the follow-up study. Follow-up intervals varied from 4.5 to 6.25 years (mean = 5.5 years). Patients who participated in this long-term follow-up had been less impaired before treatment than were nonparticipating patients. However, CBGT and ES were equivalent in terms of participant–nonparticipant differences.

At the long-term follow-up, patients who had received CBGT several years earlier were functioning better on a number of indices than were patients who had received ES. CBGT and ES patients did not differ in the amount of treatment they received during the follow-up period. Nevertheless, independent assessors rated CBGT patients' social phobias as less severe and their symptoms as interfering less with work, social activities, and family life than comparison patients. Eighty-nine percent of CBGT patients and 44% of ES patients were judged to be clinically improved by independent assessors. CBGT patients were rated as having few remaining symptoms, while ES patients were rated as requiring further treatment. On self-report measures, CBGT patients rated their phobias as less severe and reported less social avoidance. Finally, judges who were also blind to treatment condition viewed videotapes of individualized behavioral test performances and rated CBGT patients as significantly less anxious and more socially skilled than ES patients.

PREDICTORS OF OUTCOME OF COGNITIVE-BEHAVIORAL TREATMENTS FOR SOCIAL PHOBIA

There has not been much research conducted on this important topic. Studies that have been conducted fall into three basic areas: (1) studies that attempt to match treatments to patients' specific areas of difficulty, (2) studies of the impact of subtype of social phobia or the presence or absence of avoidant personality disorder on treatment outcome, and (3) studies that examine the relationship of change in fear of negative evaluation or other cognitive characteristics to treatment outcome.

The first group of studies (Jerremalm et al., 1986; Mersch et al., 1989; Öst et al., 1981; Trower et al., 1978; Wlazlo et al., 1990) has been reviewed above. Trower et al. (1978) found that skills deficit patients do somewhat better with SST than with systematic desensitization. Öst et al. (1981) found that their behavioral reactors fare somewhat better with SST than with AR and that physiological reactors fare somewhat better with AR than with SST. However, in both these studies, similarities in treatment response were larger than differences. Mersch et al. (1989) reported no difference in the response of behavioral reactors to SST or RET. Although Jerremalm et al. (1986) found some support for the idea that cognitive reactors fare better with a cognitive treatment than with a mismatched treatment, Mersch et al. (1989) did not.

Furthermore, against their hypothesis, Jerremalm et al. (1986) report a tendency for physiological reactors to do better with SIT than with AR. Wlazlo et al.'s (1990) study adds little to this confusing mix, since their treatments (SST, exposure) each contained important aspects of the other.

Four studies examine the impact of subtype of social phobia on outcome of CBGT (Brown, Heimberg, & Juster, 1995; Heimberg 1986; Holt, Heimberg, & Hope, 1990; Hope, Herbert, & White, 1995). Heimberg (1986) and Holt et al. (1990) both reported that subtype was a significant predictor of CBGT outcome, although Holt et al. noted that this was no longer the case when the severity of social phobic symptoms was controlled. Brown et al. (1995) and Hope et al. (1995) conducted similar studies of samples of 63 and 23 social phobic patients, respectively. In each study, patients were prospectively classified as meeting criteria for generalized versus nongeneralized social phobia. In both studies, a similar pattern of results emerged. Patients with generalized social phobia were more severely anxious and more broadly impaired than were patients with nongeneralized social phobia before the beginning of treatment. Both subtype groups showed significant and generally equivalent improvement over the course of treatment. However, at the end of treatment, generalized social phobics continued to exhibit greater impairment. In the Brown et al. (1995) study, nongeneralized social phobics were more likely to be classified as treatment responders by independent assessors than were generalized social phobics. Hope et al. (1995) reported a similar trend.

Brown et al. (1995) also subclassified generalized social phobics into groups with and without comorbid avoidant personality disorder. Presence of avoidant personality disorder had little impact on degree of change or classification of generalized social phobics as responders or nonresponders to treatment. Hope et al. (1995) also found no effect for avoidant personality disorder. However, Lucas and Telch (1993b) did find avoidant personality disorder to be significantly (and negatively) associated with CBGT outcome.

Feske, Perry, Chambless, Renneberg, and Goldstein (1994) examined the effect of avoidant personality disorder on the treatment response of 48 patients with generalized social phobia. Treatment in this study consisted of 32−42 hours of group exposure, relaxation training, systematic desensitization, and SST, and there was improvement for the sample as a whole. In a pattern similar to that reported above for subtypes of social phobia, generalized social phobics with avoidant personality disorder began treatment more impaired than did generalized social phobics without avoidant personality disorder and remained that way, despite significant improvement, at posttest and 3-month follow-up assessments.

Butler (1985) suggests that fear of negative evaluation (FNE) is especially important in the treatment of social phobia, and there is some research to support this claim. Mattick and Peters (1988) and Mattick et al. (1989) examined change in FNE, irrational beliefs, and locus of control as predictors of outcome in cognitive-behavioral treatment of social phobia. In both studies, change in fear of negative evaluation was most strongly associated with improvement, suggesting that interventions that can effectively alter this fear will more likely result in improvement in the functioning of social phobic individuals. Hope et al. (1990) performed a similar analysis, regressing independent assessor classification of responder versus nonresponder on posttest FNE scores, fear and avoidance hierarchy ratings, and reduction in self-reported anxiety during an individualized behavioral test. Once again, FNE was the strongest predictor of treatment response. Similarly, Lucas and Telch (1993b) examined the ability of several variables, including residualized change on the appraisal of social concerns (ASC), a measure of social phobics' concern about visibility of anxiety symptoms, impaired performance, and negative responses from others (Lucas & Telch, 1993a), to predict improvement in cognitive-behavioral and educational–supportive treatment. ASC change accounted for 32% of the variance in posttreatment social anxiety scores.

CONCLUDING COMMENTS

In this closing section, we look back on each of the major treatment methods and summarize the state of knowledge and research on cognitive-behavioral treatments for social phobia.

SST, at first glance, appears to produce significant improvements in social anxiety and other clinically relevant measures of functioning in social phobic clients. Upon closer inspection, however, methodologic shortcomings limit the extent to which generalizations regarding the efficacy of this treatment can be made. In the only controlled study (Marzillier et al., 1976), 15 weeks of SST produced clinical outcomes no better than did a waiting-list control. Only mild increases were noted in social activities and social contacts. In contrast, in several other studies, SST resulted in significant improvements in various aspects of social phobia, such as reductions in self-reported anxiety, depression, and difficulty in social situations (Falloon et al., 1981; Lucock & Salkovskis, 1988; Stravynski et al., 1982; Trower et al., 1978; Wlazlo et al., 1990). Furthermore, SST produced improvements roughly equivalent to those produced by systematic desensitization (Marzillier et al., 1976; Trower et al., 1978), AR (Öst et al., 1981), imaginal flooding (Shaw, 1979), RET (Mersch et al., 1989), and group and individual exposure (Wlazlo et al., 1990). However, with the sole exception of Marzillier et al. (1976), these studies failed to include adequate control conditions, and it is not possible to state with confidence that treatments were responsible for successful outcomes or that training in social skills was the aspect of SST that led to these outcomes. The utility of SST as a treatment for social phobia remains unproven, at best. A need for well-controlled outcome studies using credible comparison groups still exists. The combination of SST and exposure (Turner, Beidel, Cooley, et al., 1994) appears to merit further examination.

In reviewing the literature on SST, we have been concerned about the use of the term "social skills deficit." In our understanding of this term, a social skills deficit is a conclusion about a person's capacity. If a person has a social skills deficit, then he or she cannot perform the behavior in question or perform it up to some sort of standard because he or she does not know how. Social skills deficits are *inferred* from inadequate social behavior, not defined by it, since poor social behavior can occur for any number of reasons. Unfortunately, social skills deficits are often confused with (or the term is incorrectly used to reflect) *performance deficits*. There has been little demonstration that social phobics have social skills deficits (i.e., that they lack the capacity to execute a behavior), while there are ample data indicating that some social phobics do exhibit performance deficits (i.e., for whatever reasons, including but not limited to social skills deficits, they may not execute a behavior or execute it well). In our experience, many social phobics possess adequate social skills but are inhibited when it comes to applying them in social situations. When asked to engage in social interaction or performance situations as part of a behavior test or exposure exercise during treatment, they are typically capable of such behavior. Furthermore, their self-reports are often marked by negative bias regarding their own social skills (Rapee & Lim, 1992), and self-ratings of social skills are therefore best considered as measures of biased self-perception rather than as veridical indices of social skill. See Rapee (Chapter 3, this volume) for further discussion of this issue.

The efficacy of relaxation training and other anxiety-reduction strategies for social phobia has not been sufficiently evaluated. Systematic desensitization and self-control desensitization have served as comparison treatments in tests of other techniques, such as SST (Marzillier et al., 1976; Trower et al., 1978) and systematic rational restructuring (Kanter & Goldfried, 1979). Interestingly, patients in those studies benefited from these anxiety-reduction strategies. Studies comparing systematic desensitization to SST suggest equivalent outcomes with these treatments, except for the possibility that more impaired patients showed somewhat greater improvements with SST. Self-control desensitization was also effective on a number of measures, but somewhat less so than systematic rational restructuring. Studies by Alström et al. (1984) and Al-Kubaisy et al. (1992) suggest that progressive muscle relaxation by itself is of little value in the treatment of social phobia. However, AR, with its strong exposure component, appears promising. AR has been evaluated in only two studies, both by the same team of investigators. Only one study (Jerremalm et al., 1986) included a control condition, and neither evaluated follow-up outcome. Like SST, AR requires much further evaluation as a treatment for social phobia, both as a primary treatment modality and in combination with other treatment techniques.

Exposure has clearly produced positive effects in the treatment of social phobia. Every study of exposure treatment reported significant reductions in social phobia and related impairments, in comparison to baseline levels or to the response of various control groups. However, response of social phobic patients to exposure therapy may be less than complete, as is often the case in the exposure treatment of agoraphobia (Barlow, 1988). Exposure as a sole treatment for social phobia may not produce desired long-term maintenance of gains, as evidenced by posttreatment deterioration (Alström et al., 1984; Mattick et al., 1989) and a high frequency of treatment-seeking during the follow-up period (Butler et al., 1984).

Butler (1985) outlined several difficulties in devising exposure tasks for social phobics that may not be encountered during exposure for other phobias. First, it is difficult to specify graduated and repeatable tasks that allow social phobics to practice in incrementally more difficult situations. This is especially true in naturally occurring social situations, which do not lend themselves well to imposed control. Second, actual social situations are difficult to prolong for sufficient periods that individuals will experience the decreasing anxiety or habituation that would naturally occur over time. Third, many social phobics continue to enter feared situations despite high levels of anxiety. Despite their self-initiated exposure, anxiety often persists, leading Butler (1985) to conclude that social phobics may fail to become psychologically engaged in exposure treatment. Butler described patients who report disengaging from external cues when in feared situations. Others often report pretending to be somewhere else, and depersonalization or dissociation is common. Butler calls these examples of "internal avoidance," which may limit the effectiveness of exposure should they occur during treatment.

Butler (1985) offers suggestions for each of the concerns noted above. In order to manipulate the physical qualities of the exposure situation (e.g., length, content), exposures are best conducted within the treatment setting before moving to the world beyond. In this controlled environment, role-players can be active or passive and can alter their behavior in order to gradually increase difficulty level. Length of exposure can be predetermined or adjusted "on the fly" to maximize gains. An example of the latter situation might be when an exposure is artificially extended to provide additional time for habituation to occur. To counter the effects of internal avoidance, Butler suggests that social phobics engage in specific behaviors (e.g., making eye contact), be an active participant (e.g., ask questions) in situations in which reticence might make the situation more difficult, and provoke anxiety symptoms (e.g., wearing a sweater when concerned about perspiring), especially during periods of improvement.

Butler (1985) also advocates the combination of exposure and cognitive restructuring techniques. While several treatment packages that prominently feature cognitive restructuring techniques (e.g., cognitive-behavioral group therapy, systematic rational restructuring, rational–emotive therapy, self-instructional training) have demonstrated efficacy for social phobia, it is less clear whether the cognitive aspects of these packages are responsible for, or contribute to, these positive outcomes. As reviewed earlier, of the six studies that address this question, three support the combination of cognitive and behavioral techniques (Butler et al., 1984; Mattick & Peters, 1988; Mattick et al., 1989), while three do not (Biran et al., 1981; Hope et al., 1990; Stravynski et al., 1982).

It has been argued (Heimberg, 1989; Heimberg et al., 1987) that the Biran et al. (1981) and Stravynski et al. (1982) studies were methodologically flawed in several ways. In Stravynski et al. (1982), the two treatment groups (SST with and without cognitive modification) produced equivalent results. However, the failure to include a control condition (waiting-list or placebo group) prohibits us from attributing change to the specific treatments. In Biran et al.'s (1981) multiple baseline design, only two measures (subjective fear and behavioral approach) were collected, and one of these (changes in subjective fear) appeared to be unrelated to the active treatment. In both studies, questions have been raised about the appropriateness of the patient sample (Heimberg et al., 1987). Stravynski et al. (1982) describe their patients as having both social phobia and avoidant personality disorder. These patients are described in ways that suggest substantial impairment. However, mean scores on self-report measures of social anxiety for Stravynski et al. (1982) and for one of the three patients in Biran et al. (1981) were lower than those reported in other studies of social phobia. In fact, these scores were in the normative range of scores originally reported for these measures (Watson & Friend, 1969).

Neither Biran et al. (1981) nor Stravynski et al. (1982) may have administered cognitive techniques in a way that would maximize their effectiveness. Specifically, cognitive restructuring was administered in isolation (in different sessions or different parts of sessions) from SST or exposure. For instance, in the Biran et al. study, two patients received five sessions of cognitive treatment before five exposure sessions. By design, no exposure was offered during cognitive restructuring sessions, so no truly combined treatment was utilized. While therapists instructed patients to notice and attempt to refute irrational thinking when it occurred between sessions, behavioral practice outside of sessions was not specifically encouraged. Since all subjects reported substantial avoidance of problematic situations, there may have been little to notice! In this situation, it is difficult to envision how patients could learn to adequately apply their cognitive skills in real-life situations. While Stravynski et al. employed SST and cognitive techniques in the same session, these techniques were never employed in an integrated fashion; that is, patients could not rehearse new social behaviors and discuss their negative predictions or fears about entering these same situations. Nor was there any description of the use of cognitive techniques during behavioral homework assignments. In contrast, Heimberg (1989) called for the integration of cognitive and behavioral techniques. For example, cognitive restructuring could immediately precede and follow exposures during sessions or as part of homework assignments making cognition more readily available for modification. In fact, studies conducted in this fashion support the combination of cognitive and behavioral techniques in three of four cases, the lone exception being Hope et al. (1990).

While we believe that integrated cognitive-behavioral treatments will ultimately be demonstrated to be among the most effective, there are additional data that do not support this conclusion. Specifically, two recent studies by Scholing and Emmelkamp (1993a, 1993b) compare integrated packages of RET and exposure to exposure only and "nonintegrated" cognitive-behavioral treatments. These two studies delivered treatment in two 4-week blocks sandwiched around a 4-week waiting period. A portion of patients also started treatment after an initial 4-week waiting period. Scholing and Emmelkamp (1993a) treated 30 social phobics with primary fears of blushing, sweating, or trembling in front of others. Integrated RET and exposure was compared to RET followed by exposure and exposure followed by RET. All treatments produced substantial improvements, but there were few differences between them. Scholing and Emmelkamp (1993b) conducted a similar study with 73 generalized social phobics, comparing integrated RET and exposure to exposure only to RET followed by exposure. Again, substantial improvements were noted, both within groups and in comparison to the initial waiting list. Few differences between treatments occurred, although the integrated treatment made the *worst* showing on a measure of somatic symptoms after the first treatment block. An assessment of additional treatment-seeking in the year after termination revealed that 37% of exposure-only patients and 30% of RET-followed-by-exposure patients sought additional treatment, compared to only 15% of integrated-treatment patients. While the authors reported no statistical analysis of this finding, it is similar to that reported by Butler et al. (1984).

A few additional comments on this issue are in order. First, if cognitive techniques are useful adjuncts to behavioral treatment, their advocates cannot make the unequivocal statement that it is their cognitive nature that makes them so. It may be that other noncognitive coping techniques can be used effectively in exposure situations (e.g., AR) or that some noncognitive aspect of the cognitive techniques is the active ingredient. Second, cognitive techniques may be important, but not for all patients with social phobia. Patients differ in how "cognitive" they are, that is, how receptive they are to cognitive interventions, how much control they can exert over their thinking processes when in phobic situations, and so on. Others may make meaningful cognitive changes when treated with non-cognitive techniques. An important area of investigation is the examination of how treatment techniques and individual difference variables, such as cognitive styles or personality traits, interact with each other. The question of the utility of cognitive techniques in the treatment of social phobia is a long way from resolved.

Comparison of cognitive-behavioral and pharmacological treatments for any disorder is a long and difficult process, one that is just beginning for social phobia. Few studies have been conducted, and few different cognitive-behavioral interventions and medications have been examined. Therefore, these studies cannot provide a definitive answer regarding the relative or combined effectiveness of cognitive-behavioral and pharmacological treatments. The above notwithstanding, these studies suggest that cognitive-behavioral treatments may be as effective as some pharmacological treatments. CBGT compared well to phenelzine in the Gelernter et al. (1991) and Heimberg et al. (1994) studies. Although it may be somewhat less effective after 12 weeks of treatment, CBGT may be associated with greater protection from relapse than is phenelzine. CBGT may also have been more effective than was alprazolam during follow-up in the Gelernter et al. study. A brief cognitive-behavioral intervention was more effective than was buspirone for musicians with social phobia in the study by Clark and Agras (1991), but the brevity of the treatment period, the ineffectiveness of buspirone relative to placebo, and the specific nature of the patients' concerns suggest that further study is necessary. The combination of imaginal and *in vivo* exposure was more effective than was atenolol in the controlled trial by Turner, Beidel, and Jacob (1994). However, in a comparison of phenelzine, atenolol, and placebo conducted by Liebowitz et al. (1992), atenolol was also less effective than was phenelzine. A post hoc comparison by Turner, Beidel, and Jacob (1994) of their results and those of Liebowitz et al. suggests that atenolol was equally effective in the two studies, and that the behavioral intervention of Turner, Beidel, and Jacob (1994) was similar in effectiveness to phenelzine in the Liebowitz et al. study. Thus, behavioral treatment was more effective than was atenolol, but atenolol may not be a particularly effective pharmacological treatment for social phobia.

The issue of combined cognitive-behavioral-pharmacological intervention has received insufficient attention. The studies by Falloon et al. (1981)

and Clark and Agras (1991) suggest that propranolol does not add to the effectiveness of SST and that buspirone may actually detract from the effectiveness of cognitive-behavioral treatment. However, these were very small studies, one of which lacked adequate experimental controls (Falloon et al., 1981) and the other of which treated a very special group of social phobics (musicians; Clark & Agras, 1991). Neither included the medications that might be most effective when compared with placebo, that is, phenelzine or the benzodiazepine clonazepam (Klonopin) (see Potts & Davidson, Chapter 14, this volume).

Follow-up assessments of less than a year have been commonplace in studies of the cognitive-behavioral treatment of social phobia and have shown that treated patients are likely to maintain (or even expand upon) their gains in the short run. Six studies now report follow-ups of 1 year to 5.5 years and suggest that gains realized in cognitive-behavioral treatment are, in fact, durable over extended periods of time. The studies by Mersch et al. (1991) and Wlazlo et al. (1990) tentatively suggest that successfully treated patients may show additional progress over an extended follow-up period. However, blanket acceptance of these statements does not appear to be warranted, given the small number of studies, the small number of interventions examined, the lack of effort devoted to examination of variables that may influence long-term posttreatment course, and the problem of follow-up attrition reported in some of these studies. Heimberg, Salzman, et al. (1993) assessed only 19 of 40 treatment completers, and these patients were less impaired than those who did not participate in the long-term follow-up. Wlazlo et al. examined 78 patients but excluded 25 patients whose data were not complete for all assessment points and 30 patients who showed severe comorbidity, and the differences between the patients whose data were included and those whose data were excluded is unknown. Mersch et al. (1991) reported that almost half of their patients sought additional treatment during the follow-up period, and these patients appeared to have been more impaired before treatment. The conclusion that long-term maintenance seems to be the case for moderately impaired patients but that it is inadequately addressed for more severely impaired patients appears to be justified at this time.

Attempts to match specific treatment techniques to specific deficits of social phobic patients have produced few replicated and consistent results. Intuitively, the design of these studies is logical, yet the outcome is sometimes contrary to expectations. One problem may lie within the methods used to classify subgroups. This has been done using either subjective means (e.g., Trower et al., 1978) or objective means that sometimes proved unreliable (Jerremalm et al., 1986). It is also possible that attempts to match treatment to subgroup may overemphasize differences among patients that are less critical to treatment outcome than are their similarities. Fear of negative evaluation may be a common underlying theme among social phobics whether they respond to specific phobic situations primarily with physiological symptoms, with cognitive symptoms, or with overt signs of anxiety. This may account for the robust findings for cognitive-behavioral treatments, regardless of patients' response tendencies. Further work is necessary to fully understand the findings of studies examining the effect of subtypes of social phobia and avoidant personality disorder on the outcomes of cognitive-behavioral treatments.

Finally, the degree of improvement experienced by patients in cognitive-behavioral treatment is satisfying but not necessarily sufficient. Much more work is needed to examine the parameters of effective treatment, develop new interventions, and investigate the possible potentiating effects of cognitive-behavioral and pharmacological treatment for social phobia.

ACKNOWLEDGMENTS

Preparation of this chapter was supported in part by Grant No. 44119 to Richard G. Heimberg from the National Institute of Mental Health, and the views expressed herein are those of the authors.

REFERENCES

Al-Kubaisy, T., Marks, I. M., Logsdail, S., Marks, M. P., Lovell, K., Sungur, M., & Araya, R. (1992). Role of exposure homework in phobia reduction: A controlled study. *Behavior Therapy, 23,* 599–621.

Alström, J. E., Nordlund, C. L., Persson, G., Hårding, M., & Ljungqvist, C. (1984). Effects of four treatment methods on social phobic patients not suitable for insight-oriented psychotherapy. *Acta Psychiatrica Scandinavica, 70,* 97–110.

American Psychiatric Association. (1980). *Diagnostic and statistical manual of mental disorders* (3rd ed.). Washington, DC: Author.

American Psychiatric Association. (1987). *Diagnostic and statistical manual of mental disorders* (3rd ed., rev.). Washington, DC: Author.

American Psychiatric Association. (1994). *Diagnostic and statistical manual of mental disorders* (4th ed.). Washington, DC: Author.

Barlow, D. H. (1988). *Anxiety and its disorders: The nature and treatment of anxiety and panic.* New York: Guilford Press.

Barlow, D. H., & Beck, J. G. (1984). The psychosocial treatment of anxiety disorders: Current status, future directions. In J. B. W. Williams & R. L. Spitzer (Eds.), *Psychotherapy research: Where are we and where should we go?* (pp. 29–66). New York: Guilford Press.

Beck, A. T., Rush, A. J., Shaw, B. F., & Emery, G. (1979). *Cognitive therapy of depression.* New York: Guilford Press.

Biran, M., Augusto, F., & Wilson, G. T. (1981). *In vivo* exposure vs. cognitive restructuring in the treatment of scriptophobia. *Behaviour Research and Therapy, 19*, 525–532.

Brown, E. J., Heimberg, R. G., & Juster, H. R. (1995). Social phobia subtype and avoidant personality disorder: Effect on severity of social phobia, impairment, and outcome of cognitive-behavioral treatment. *Behavior Therapy, 26*, 467–486.

Bruch, M. A., Heimberg, R. G., & Hope, D. A. (1991). States of mind model and cognitive change in treated social phobics. *Cognitive Therapy and Research, 15*, 429–441.

Butler, G. (1985). Exposure as a treatment for social phobia: Some instructive difficulties. *Behaviour Research and Therapy, 23*, 651–657.

Butler, G., Cullington, A., Munby, M., Amies, P., & Gelder, M. (1984). Exposure and anxiety management in the treatment of social phobia. *Journal of Consulting and Clinical Psychology, 52*, 642–650.

Clark, D. B., & Agras, W. S. (1991). The assessment and treatment of performance anxiety in musicians. *American Journal of Psychiatry, 148*, 598–605.

DiGiuseppe, R., McGowan, L., Sutton-Simon, K., & Gardner, F. (1990). A comparative outcome study of four cognitive therapies in the treatment of social anxiety. *Journal of Rational–Emotive and Cognitive-Behavior Therapy, 8*, 129–146.

Ellis, A. (1962). *Reason and emotion in psychotherapy.* New York: Lyle Stuart.

Emmelkamp, P. M. G. (1982). *Phobic and obsessive–compulsive disorders: Theory, research, and practice.* New York: Plenum Press.

Emmelkamp, P. M. G., Mersch, P. P. A., Vissia, E., & van der Helm, M. (1985). Social phobia: A comparative evaluation of cognitive and behavioral interventions. *Behaviour Research and Therapy, 23*, 365–369.

Falloon, I. R. H., Lloyd, G. G., & Harpin, R. E. (1981). The treatment of social phobia: Real-life rehearsal with nonprofessional therapists. *Journal of Nervous and Mental Disease, 169*, 180–184.

Fava, G. A., Grandi, S., & Canestrari, R. (1989). Treatment of social phobia by homework exposure. *Psychotherapy and Psychosomatics, 52*, 209–213.

Feske, U., Perry, K. J., Chambless, D. L., Renneberg, B., & Goldstein, A. J. (1994). *Avoidant personality disorder as a predictor for severity and treatment outcome among generalized social phobics.* Manuscript submitted for publication.

Gelernter, C. S., Uhde, T. W., Cimbolic, P., Arnkoff, D. B., Vittone, B. J., Tancer, M. E., & Bartko, J. J. (1991). Cognitive-behavioral and pharmacological treatments for social phobia: A controlled study. *Archives of General Psychiatry, 48*, 938–945.

Goldfried, M. R. (1971). Systematic desensitization as training in self-control. *Journal of Consulting and Clinical Psychology, 37*, 228–235.

Goldfried, M. R., Decenteceo, E. T., & Weinberg, L. (1974). Systematic rational restructuring as a self-control technique. *Behavior Therapy, 5*, 247–254.

Heimberg, R. G. (1986, June). *Predicting the outcome of cognitive-behavioral treatment of social phobia.* Paper presented at the annual meeting of the Society for Psychotherapy Research, Wellesley, MA.

Heimberg, R. G. (1989). Cognitive and behavioral treatments for social phobia: A critical analysis. *Clinical Psychology Review, 9*, 107–128.

Heimberg, R. G. (1990). Cognitive behavior therapy (for social phobia). In A. S. Bellack & M. Hersen (Eds.), *Comparative handbook of treatments for adult disorders* (pp. 203–218). New York: Wiley.

Heimberg, R. G., & Barlow, D. H. (1988). Psychosocial treatments for social phobia. *Psychosomatics, 29,* 27–37.

Heimberg, R. G., & Barlow, D. H. (1991). New developments in cognitive-behavioral therapy for social phobia. *Journal of Clinical Psychiatry, 52*(11 Suppl.), 21–30.

Heimberg, R. G., Becker, R. E., Goldfinger, K., & Vermilyea, J. A. (1985). Treatment of social phobia by exposure, cognitive restructuring, and homework assignments. *Journal of Nervous and Mental Disease, 173,* 236–245.

Heimberg, R. G., Dodge, C. S., & Becker, R. E. (1987). Social phobia. In L. Michelson & M. Ascher (Eds.), *Cognitive behavioral assessment and treatment of anxiety disorders* (pp. 280–309). New York: Plenum Press.

Heimberg, R. G., Dodge, C. S., Hope, D. A., Kennedy, C. R., Zollo, L., & Becker, R. E. (1990). Cognitive-behavioral group treatment of social phobia: Comparison to a credible placebo control. *Cognitive Therapy and Research, 14,* 1–23.

Heimberg, R. G., Holt, C. S., Schneier, F. R., Spitzer, R. L., & Liebowitz, M. R. (1993). The issue of subtypes in the diagnosis of social phobia. *Journal of Anxiety Disorders, 7,* 249–269.

Heimberg, R. G., Juster, H. R., Brown, E. J., Holle, C., Makris, G. S., Leung, A. W., Schneier, F. R., Gitow, A., & Liebowitz, M. R. (1994, November). *Cognitive-behavioral versus pharmacological treatment of social phobia: Posttreatment and follow-up effects.* Paper presented at the annual meeting of the Association for Advancement of Behavior Therapy, San Diego, CA.

Heimberg, R. G., Montgomery, D., Madsen, C. H., Jr., & Heimberg, J. S. (1977). Assertion training: A review of the literature. *Behavior Therapy, 8,* 953–971.

Heimberg, R. G., Salzman, D. G., Holt, C. S., & Blendell, K. A. (1993). Cognitive-behavioral group treatment for social phobia: Effectiveness at five-year followup. *Cognitive Therapy and Research, 17,* 325–339.

Holt, C. S., Heimberg, R. G., & Hope, D. A. (1990, November). *Success from the outset: Predictors of cognitive-behavioral therapy outcome among social phobics.* Paper presented at the annual meeting of the Association for Advancement of Behavior Therapy, San Francisco.

Hope, D. A., Heimberg, R. G., & Bruch, M. A. (1990, March). *The importance of cognitive interventions in behavioral group therapy for social phobia.* Paper presented at the 10th National Conference on Phobias and Related Anxiety Disorders, Bethesda, MD.

Hope, D. A., Herbert, J. D., & White, C. (1995). Diagnostic subtype, avoidant personality disorder, and efficacy of cognitive behavioral group therapy for social phobia. *Cognitive Therapy and Research, 19,* 285–303.

Hope, D. A., Holt, C. S., & Heimberg, R. G. (1993). Social phobia. In T. R. Giles (Ed.), *Handbook of effective psychotherapy* (pp. 227–251). New York: Plenum Press.

Jerremalm, A., Jansson, L., & Öst, L.-G. (1986). Cognitive and physiological reactivity and the effects of different behavioral methods in the treatment of social phobia. *Behaviour Research and Therapy, 24,* 171–180.

Juster, H. R., Heimberg, R. G., & Holt, C. S. (in press). Social phobia: Diagnostic issues and review of cognitive-behavioral treatment strategies. In M. Hersen, R. Eisler, & P. Miller (Eds.), *Progress in behavior modification*. Pacific Grove, CA: Brooks/Cole.

Kanter, N. J., & Goldfried, M. R. (1979). Relative effectiveness of rational restructuring and self-control desensitization in the reduction of interpersonal anxiety. *Behavior Therapy, 10,* 472–490.

Liebowitz, M. R, Schneier, F., Campeas, R., Hollander, E., Hatterer, J., Fyer, A., Gorman, J., Papp, L., Davies, S., Gully, R., & Klein, D. F. (1992). Phenelzine vs. atenolol in social phobia: A placebo-controlled comparison. *Archives of General Psychiatry, 49,* 290–300.

Lucas, R. A., & Telch, M. J. (1993a, November). *A new cognitive assessment measure for social phobia.* Paper presented at the annual meeting of the Association for Advancement of Behavior Therapy, Atlanta, GA.

Lucas, R. A., & Telch, M. J. (1993b, November). *Group versus individual treatment of social phobia.* Paper presented at the annual meeting of the Association for Advancement of Behavior Therapy, Atlanta, GA.

Lucock, M. P., & Salkovskis, P. M. (1988). Cognitive factors in social anxiety and its treatment. *Behaviour Research and Therapy, 26,* 297–302.

Marks, I. M., & Mathews, A. M. (1979). Brief standard self-rating for phobic patients. *Behaviour Research and Therapy, 17,* 263–267.

Marzillier, J. S., Lambert, C., & Kellet, J. (1976). A controlled evaluation of systematic desensitization and social skills training for socially inadequate psychiatric patients. *Behaviour Research and Therapy, 14,* 225–238.

Mattick, R. P., & Peters, L. (1988). Treatment of severe social phobia: Effects of guided exposure with and without cognitive restructuring. *Journal of Consulting and Clinical Psychology, 56,* 251–260.

Mattick, R. P., Peters, L., & Clarke, J. C. (1989). Exposure and cognitive restructuring for social phobia: A controlled study. *Behavior Therapy, 20,* 3–23.

Meichenbaum, D. (1985). *Stress inoculation training.* New York: Pergamon Press.

Mersch, P. P. A., Emmelkamp, P. M. G., Bögels, S. M., & van der Sleen, J. (1989). Social phobia: Individual response patterns and the effects of behavioral and cognitive interventions. *Behaviour Research and Therapy, 27,* 421–434.

Mersch, P. P. A., Emmelkamp, P. M. G., & Lips, C. (1991). Social phobia: Individual response patterns and the long-term effects of behavioral and cognitive interventions. A follow-up study. *Behaviour Research and Therapy, 29,* 357–362.

Mersch, P. P. A., Hildebrand, M., Lavy, E. H., Wessel, I., & van Hout, W. J. P. J. (1992). Somatic symptoms in social phobia: A treatment method based on rational emotive therapy and paradoxical interventions. *Journal of Behavior Therapy and Experimental Psychiatry, 23,* 199–211.

Öst, L.-G. (1987). Applied relaxation: Description of a coping technique and review of controlled studies. *Behaviour Research and Therapy, 25,* 397–409.

Öst, L.-G., Jerremalm, A., & Johansson, J. (1981). Individual response patterns and the effects of different behavioral methods in the treatment of social phobia. *Behaviour Research and Therapy, 19,* 1–16.

Persson, G., & Alström, J. E. (1983). A scale for rating suitability for insight-oriented psychotherapy. *Acta Psychiatrica Scandinavica, 68,* 117–125.

Persson, G., & Alström, J. E. (1984). Suitability for insight-oriented psychotherapy as a prognostic factor in treatment of phobic women. *Acta Psychiatrica Scandinavica, 69,* 318–326.

Rapee, R. M., & Lim, L. (1992). Discrepancy between self- and observer ratings of performance in social phobics. *Journal of Abnormal Psychology, 101,* 727–731.

Scholing, A., & Emmelkamp, P. M. G. (1993a). Cognitive and behavioural treatments of fear of blushing, sweating or trembling. *Behaviour Research and Therapy, 31,* 155–170.

Scholing, A., & Emmelkamp, P. M. G. (1993b). Exposure with and without cognitive therapy for generalized social phobia: Effects of individual and group treatment. *Behaviour Research and Therapy, 31,* 667–681.

Schwartz, R. M., & Garamoni, G. L. (1986). A structural model of positive and negative states of mind: Asymmetry in the internal dialogue. In P. C. Kendall (Ed.), *Advances in cognitive-behavioral research and therapy* (Vol. 5, pp. 1–62). New York: Academic Press.

Shaw, P.M. (1979). A comparison of three behaviour therapies in the treatment of social phobia. *British Journal of Psychiatry, 134,* 620–623.

Spivack, G., Platt, J. J., & Shure, M. B. (1976). *The problem-solving approach to adjustment.* San Francisco: Jossey-Bass.

Stravynski, A. (1983). Behavioral treatment of psychogenic vomiting in the context of social phobia. *Journal of Nervous and Mental Disease, 171,* 448–451.

Stravynski, A., Marks, I., & Yule, W. (1982). Social skills problems in neurotic outpatients: Social skills training with and without cognitive modification. *Archives of General Psychiatry, 39,* 1378–1385.

Trower, P., Yardley, K., Bryant, B., & Shaw, P. (1978). The treatment of social failure: A comparison of anxiety-reduction and skills-acquisition procedures on two social problems. *Behavior Modification, 2,* 41–60.

Turner, S. M., Beidel, D. C., Cooley, M. R., Woody, S. R., & Messer, S. C. (1994). A multicomponent behavioral treatment for social phobia: Social Effectiveness Therapy. *Behaviour Research and Therapy, 32,* 381–390.

Turner, S. M., Beidel, D. C., & Jacob, R. G. (1994). Social phobia: A comparison of behavior therapy and atenolol. *Journal of Consulting and Clinical Psychology, 62,* 350–358.

Watson, D., & Friend, R. (1969). Measurement of social-evaluative anxiety. *Journal of Consulting and Clinical Psychology, 33,* 448–457.

Wlazlo, Z., Schroeder-Hartwig, K., Hand, I., Kaiser, G., & Münchau, N. (1990). Exposure *in vivo* vs. social skills training for social phobia: Long-term outcome and differential effects. *Behaviour Research and Therapy, 28,* 181–193.

CHAPTER THIRTEEN

Cognitive-Behavioral Treatments: Clinical Applications

GILLIAN BUTLER
ADRIAN WELLS

THE LINK BETWEEN THEORY AND PRACTICE

Social phobia is not easy to treat. It may be relatively easy to describe and to recognize, but the complexity of the problem and its heterogeneity pose many problems for the practicing clinician. This chapter provides some ideas about how to solve some of these problems based on the principle that successful treatment relies on the development and use of a coherent formulation. A formulation is the tool that provides the link between theory and practice, helping both patient and therapist to understand the particular manifestation of the problem and draw from that understanding specific implications for how it can be solved (Persons, 1989; Butler & Booth, 1991). We will argue here that the most productive model on which to base a clinical formulation at present is the cognitive model. Cognitions play a central part both in the definition of social phobia and in its secondary aspects, and treatments based on a cognitive model have been shown to be at least as effective as other methods (Heimberg et al., 1990; Heimberg, Salzman, Holt, & Blendell, 1993; Mattick & Peters, 1988; Mattick, Peters, & Clarke, 1989). The generic cognitive model of anxiety (e.g., Beck, Emery, & Greenberg, 1985) provides the therapist with a useful initial framework, and Clark and Wells (Chapter 4, this volume) present a more detailed model that they have developed specifically for the treatment of social phobia. For a discussion of other models, see Schlenker and Leary (1982); Heimberg and Barlow (1988); Trower and Gilbert (1989); and Leary and Kowalski (Chapter 5, this volume). Our aim here is to explain and to illustrate the advantages of using a cognitive formulation to guide treatment for social phobia.

Working without such a formulation, for example, using well-established, traditional psychological methods such as exposure, relaxation, and anxiety management, can at times be very successful (e.g., Butler, Cullington, Munby, Amies, & Gelder, 1984; see the review by Heimberg & Juster, Chapter 12, this volume), and therapists can easily be seduced into persisting with such methods. However if treatment is not successful or if improvement is elusive and the therapist runs out of strategies to suggest, it is difficult to overcome the problem without recourse to a coherent formulation.

We start this chapter by describing the general diagnostic criteria for social phobia, and we then examine some of the cognitive and affective characteristics and concomitants of the problem. In particular, we emphasize some of the difficulties that can be encountered in engaging these patients in treatment. The structure of the rest of the chapter follows developments over the last decade, focusing in turn on the ways in which behavioral methods have to be adapted for use with social phobia, on the advantages of combining behavioral and cognitive methods of treatment, and on integrating cognitive and behavior therapy. As well as showing how treatment has developed over the last decade, this allows us to pinpoint a succession of difficulties posed for the therapist by this group of patients and in the end to speculate about likely future directions and developments.

Social Phobia: Beyond the Definition

The bare bones of the definition of social phobia on which the rest hangs are persistent and irrational fear and a desire to avoid interpersonal situations in which the person is concerned about being humiliated or embarrassed (American Psychiatric Association, 1994). The definition focuses attention on the fear of being negatively evaluated by others as a consequence of perceived inadequacies in social performance. Social phobics tend to perceive their own performance as poor, may think of themselves as being in some way inadequate, and believe that others both notice these deficiencies and judge them negatively as a result. Cognitive aspects of the problem play a central role in the definition.

Other important aspects of social phobia, which are given less emphasis in the definition, become familiar with increased clinical practice. These include the frequent occurrence of symptoms that others might be expected to notice, such as blushing, trembling, or sweating, and the disruptive influence of social anxiety on others. For example, when someone finds it difficult both to think of what to say and to make eye contact, their social awkwardness interferes with the interaction and influences the behavior of both participants in the interaction. This makes it hard for social phobics to gain other kinds of experience.

Social phobia is often long-standing and may be associated with an early history of shyness exacerbated by the interpersonal demands and turbulence of adolescence. However, social phobics relatively rarely ask for treatment at this stage, and by the time such a request is made, they have often developed secondary problems such as poor self-confidence, low self-esteem, loss of motivation for change, social isolation, a degree of depression, and more generalized forms of anxiety, including worry and apprehension. For trained clinicians, it is relatively easy to make the distinction between the primary aspects of the problem, focused on the fear of negative evaluation, and its secondary aspects. For patients, this is a great deal harder, and they may feel hopelessly confused by what is happening to them and by its creeping pervasiveness. In addition, social anxiety makes it hard to come for treatment and to make use of the opportunity, if it is available. Treatment involves both interacting with someone else and disclosing to them the fears and vulnerabilities that could provoke negative evaluation. Thus, the first challenge to therapists is to think carefully about how to help the patient become engaged in treatment.

There are many reasons why social phobics may not come for treatment. Their tendency to avoid social interactions may mean that they have little experience of shared problem solving, and they may not think of therapy as a valuable option. They often avoid provoking their anxiety, for example by increased social withdrawal, not accepting engagements and opportunities to interact with others, and so on; thus, they may experience little anxiety on a daily basis even though the social phobia interferes considerably with the way they lead their lives. Social phobia makes it hard to talk to someone else, especially concerning emotionally salient matters, so therapy may seem to be an alarming possibility. They may also attempt to cope with social anxiety by drinking alcohol or using tranquilizers and may not come to the attention of therapists unless these behaviors create additional problems.

Social phobics have much in common with patients suffering from generalized anxiety disorder. In both cases, patients feel especially at risk because the conditions that provoke their symptoms are not under obvious external control. They cannot protect themselves by avoiding difficult situations, in the way that simple phobics can, because the problem is partly internal or cognitive and because other people, the "cause" of the problem, may do unpredictable, anxiety-provoking things. In social phobia, it is harder than in other phobias to control the level of symptoms by controlling the level of exposure. As anxiety interferes with performance and produces a spreading awkwardness, it interferes with, or contaminates, social interactions. With each patient, therapists need to become aware both of the specific way in which the social phobia manifests itself and of the effect the social phobia has on other people, including themselves.

The population of social phobics is extremely heterogeneous, to the extent that for the inexperienced therapist it can be difficult to recognize commonalities between two people with the same condition. This diversity was acknowledged in the revised third edition of the *Diagnostic and Statistical Manual of Mental Disorders* (DSM-III-R; American Psychiatric Association, 1987) by defining subtypes according to whether the problem is generalized or has a specific focus such as eating, writing, or speaking in public. However, in clinical practice the diversity is greater and more confusing than this and reflects a parallel diversity in social behaviors, conventions, and interactions, which is equally hard to separate into distinct categories. Most relatively specific social phobias have some generalized aspect, though often this only becomes apparent when the patient starts to improve.

It is helpful, therefore, during assessment and when developing a preliminary formulation, to explore both specific and more general aspects of the problem. Differentiating between different types of social vulnerability clarifies the nature of the presenting problem. Broad groupings of symptoms appear to cluster (see, e.g., Holt, Heimberg, Hope, & Liebowitz, 1992), and knowing about these provides therapists with some initial hypotheses to guide their questions and elicit the patient's central fears. For example, if the problem focuses on a particular activity such as eating with others, it is useful to ask about reactions to other performance activities such as handling money or writing in front of others. The aim is to determine what the patient thinks in situations that provoke symptoms and whether other types of situation elicit similar fears.

Basic Themes in Social Phobia

If the social phobia is more generalized, the two most obvious possibilities are (1) that increasing degrees of intimacy will exacerbate the problem, which may make it hard for the patient to develop stable intimate relationships, or (2) that their anxiety increases with the potential for attracting attention and therefore with the size or "threat value" of the audience. If it is predominantly the attention of others that provokes anxiety, then situations such as going to the hairdresser or being asked a question in a meeting may also provoke symptoms. When patients report that they have always been shy, they often have difficulty with assertiveness, which interferes when dealing with people in authority, asking for help, making and refusing requests, accepting positions of responsibility, and so on. The point is that the general theme, the fear of "being found wanting," can be associated with many other themes, and these should be differentiated in order to develop a formulation. Common subthemes include those about general acceptability, self-worth, likeability, intimacy and its consequences, responsibility for social success, and the need to conform or to perform adequately.

Underlying these themes there is an assumption that there is a "right" and therefore also a "wrong" way of doing things—an assumption that leads to rigidity in social behavior. Most social phobics appear not to be socially unskilled but, rather, to be inhibited in the use of their skills. They may also have a narrower range of experience than do others and start to become more confident and to respond more flexibly to different situations as the range of their experience increases. Therefore, it may not be necessary to teach social skills, although it may be helpful to address matters such as self-presentation if these could interfere with social acceptability, as in the case of personal cleanliness or inappropriate dress.

General Implications for Therapy

Therapists treating social phobics should constantly be aware of, and use, their own social skills, or they too will be caught up in the contaminating effects of the problem. They should develop their sensitivity to the ways in which social phobia can interfere with the process of treatment and develop ways of overcoming the ensuing difficulties. Three illustrative examples follow.

First, the social awkwardness that springs from the anxiety about being evaluated will almost certainly occur during therapy. When this happens, patients often become increasingly self-aware. Their attention may be distracted by self-denigratory thoughts or by sensations associated with embarrassment. This makes it hard for them to concentrate on what is being said or to remain fully engaged in the process of therapy. Therapists should watch out for this, for when it occurs it may be necessary to repeat key ideas more than once, to make use of frequent summaries, and to encourage patients to give feedback and to write down the points they wish to remember. These shifts in affect and processing can also be used to illustrate linkages in the cognitive model, such as the role of self-focused processing in constructing the self-image (see Clark & Wells, Chapter 4, this volume).

Second, the process of cognitive therapy involves asking many questions, which are intended to help patients to look for new perspectives and new ways of seeing things. But sometimes this questioning method can provoke sufficient anxiety to inhibit, rather than facilitate, disclosure. The less the patient is able to say, the more questions the therapists asks and the more the therapist is inclined to talk instead. The vicious cycle that maintains anxiety outside the session may therefore exert its influence inside the session as well. In this situation, the most important skill the therapist needs is flexibility so as to find other ways of collecting the same information. If the patient discloses very little, it can help to use more statements and reflections than questions: for example "It must have been difficult for you"; "I would like to know more about that"; "I wonder if . . ."; "You thought you were making an idiot of yourself . . ."; and so on. These problems also can provide an opportunity to explain the cognitive model and to socialize the patient.

Third, there are many different sources of social discomfort, any of which may be present in therapy. Some people find that conventional degrees of interpersonal proximity provoke anxiety and that they respond better if given more physical space. Some need extra time to think about what they want to say, and their anxiety increases if they feel rushed. Others feel more awkward if faced with a silence and become more comfortable if the therapist bridges gaps and keeps the interaction moving. Skilled therapists can adapt their use of nonverbal aspects of the interaction, such as posture, use of gestures, eye contact, and so on, to set the patient at ease. These aspects of the therapeutic interaction, if sensitively used, can facilitate the process of therapy, which may otherwise suffer from the same kind of social contamination and awkwardness that occurs elsewhere. It is important, however, that the therapist does not make therapy "completely safe," for this will remove vital opportunities for exploring fears and challenging beliefs.

Of course it would not be helpful to reinforce behaviors that are likely to continue to interfere with social interactions, but by adapting their own social behavior, therapists can facilitate disclosure, help the patient give attention to the matters being discussed, and arrive at a better understanding of how the social phobia interferes with the patient's life. Appropriate behavioral changes can then be suggested and practiced outside the session.

When patients' difficulties are exacerbated by disclosing self-relevant information, or by talking to strangers, a mastery of basic psychotherapeutic skills is especially important. The same applies if patients have difficulty conversing with members of the opposite sex and the therapist falls into this category. In these circumstances, greater sensitivity is needed when obtaining details of relevant affective responses, thoughts, and beliefs. It is important not to shy away from discussing painful material, but, rather, to use this opportunity to find out more about the precise nature of the thoughts and feelings, because these "hot" cognitions (thoughts identified during the heat of the emotion) usually mirror those central to social interaction in general.

DEVELOPMENT OF EFFECTIVE TREATMENTS
SINCE THE MID-1980s

Literature on the development of effective treatments for social phobia since the mid-1980s reveals four main types of psychological treatment: (1) social skills training, (2) exposure, (3) anxiety management, including relaxation, and (4) cognitive techniques. All can make some claim to effectiveness, but their relative value is hard to evaluate given differences in measures, methodology, patient selection, comparisons made, and so on. The more wide-ranging reviews are strikingly inconclusive (e.g., Edelmann, 1992; Heimberg, 1989; Heimberg & Barlow, 1991; Hollon & Beck, 1994). The processes of change remain unclear, so therapists are left wondering how their treatments work when they do and what went wrong when they do not. Looking to the clinical outcome literature for clues as to how to proceed provides many ideas but no clear answers, possibly because each of the treatments listed above has face validity, and all of them use a mixture of strategies. The following account is not meant to be a review (see Heimberg & Juster, Chapter 12, this volume), but an illustrative argument based both on the evidence available and on our extensive clinical experience with this group of patients.

Social skills training is based on the assumption that patients with social phobia suffer from skills deficits and would benefit from learning and practicing such skills. It therefore involves exposure to feared situations and probably also involves cognitive reappraisal as anxiety decreases and social performance improves. However, because social skills training is a multicomponent approach, successful treatment does not demonstrate that patients needed to learn new skills. Social skills training could free them up so that they are able to respond more flexibly to the changing demands of social interactions (or work in other ways). Breaking down social performance into its separate skills (observational, listening, meshing, nonverbal skills, etc.) can be helpful when devising practice tasks or helping a patient find a way out of a social difficulty (Butler, 1985, 1989). It may be a useful way of redirecting attention away from internal, distressing sensations and stimulating cognitive reappraisal. But socially appropriate behavior does not have to be learned in the piecemeal fashion assumed during social skills training, nor is socially appropriate behavior a guarantee of social success or social comfort.

Exposure has consistently received better press, and it seems that optimal conditions for its general effectiveness can be specified: It should be graduated, repeated, and prolonged. These conditions, however, are not easy to achieve in the case of social phobia (see Butler, 1985, 1989). Social situations are often time limited; they have a disturbing degree of unpredictability, so they cannot easily be graduated or repeated; and avoidance appears to be more subtle and inconsistent than in other phobias. When exposure is adapted for use in social phobia, for example by explaining the rationale and involving the patient in thinking about how to become fully engaged while carrying out exposures and making use of brief or ungraduated opportunities for exposure as they arise, then it is beneficial even when not combined with other procedures (Butler et al., 1984; Emmelkamp, Mersch, Vissia, & van der Helm, 1985; Mattick & Peters, 1988). However, it has consistently been found that while measures of anxiety and avoidance show significant change, measures of cognitions (beliefs as well as the fear of negative evaluation) do not change, and this failure may leave the patient vulnerable to relapse. It would be hard to treat social phobia without using exposure, but exposure is difficult to plan and may need to be supplemented with something else.

Adding anxiety management to exposure appears to provide added value (Butler et al., 1984), but anxiety management contains many components (in the study by Butler et al., it consisted of a combination of relaxation, distraction, and individualized but brief cognitive procedures). The cognitive component of anxiety management appears to be particularly useful, though the added value of relaxation has not been evaluated. In the Butler et al. study, patients reported a fivefold increase in the frequency with which they used cognitive techniques over the course of treatment, compared with a twofold increase in the use of relaxation or distraction. Subsequently, two studies (Mattick & Peters, 1988; Mattick et al., 1989) reported that the best predictor of long-term outcome was change in the cognitive component of social anxiety, the fear of negative evaluation, which supports the conclusion that cognitive change is important.

Various techniques have been used to achieve cognitive change, including self-instructional training, rational–emotive therapy, and varieties of cognitive-behavioral therapy (e.g., Emmelkamp et al., 1985; Mattick & Peters, 1988; Scholing & Emmelkamp, 1993), and a number of these studies have tried to estimate the value of matching the treatment more precisely to characteristics of the presenting patients. So far, these studies have been inconclusive (e.g., Jerremalm, Jannson & Öst, 1986; Mersch, Emmelkamp, Bögels, & van der Sleen, 1989; Mersch, Emmelkamp & Lips, 1991), but the idea behind them remains extremely important and has clinical implications that should not be ignored: namely, that when faced with a heterogeneous group of patients such as social phobics, the response to standardized treatments will be variable.

The implication for cognitive therapy is that it is important to identify the precise form and idiosyncratic content of each person's cognitions. A cognitive treatment that attends insufficiently to the individualized nature of thoughts and beliefs may lose much of its potential and fail to help patients develop a new way of thinking about social interactions and the risks or threats that they perceive in them.

The theory behind cognitive treatments is relatively straightforward and accessible, but their application is difficult, and therapists can fall into many traps along the way. The most common are probably labeling the patients' thoughts as irrational (and necessarily wrong), providing alternative suggestions instead of encouraging patients to come up with and evaluate their own ideas, and asking patients simply to replace one kind of thought with another. In practice cognitive therapists need to listen to, elucidate, and join in the reexamination of each patient's internal dialogue without giving the impression that there is a right and a wrong way of thinking. If at the same time they can combine the cognitive work with relevant behavioral exposure tasks (see also Heimberg, Becker, Goldfinger, & Vermilyea, 1985; Hope & Heimberg, 1993), the outcome is likely to be better. While the evidence on the added value of combining cognitive with exposure techniques is mixed, it is likely that cognitive procedures have not always been delivered in an optimal way. They may have been combined without being fully integrated. When the two are integrated, exposure tasks can be presented within the context of a cognitive formulation and their outcome evaluated in such a way as to facilitate relevant belief change (Wells, 1992; Wells et al., 1995).

It is clear that the literature so far does not provide conclusive reasons for choosing one method of treatment rather than another, but it does provide the clinician with many useful clues. Behavioral, cognitive, and affective change are not equally well achieved by all methods, and the variability in social situations combines with the variability in social phobias to make it hard to derive hard-and-fast rules. Different methods of treatment may work in the same or in different ways and may be more or less efficient ways of engaging the necessary processes of change. In this state of affairs, the best policy to adopt seems to be an experimental one based on hypothesis testing. Hypotheses about individual cases of social phobia, and the maintaining factors involved, are most productively based on adequate case formulations that have direct and specific implications for treatment. In the next section we consider a potentially more informative and integrative cognitive perspective.

APPLYING A COGNITIVE PERSPECTIVE

A cognitive model of social phobia has been presented elsewhere in this volume (Clark & Wells, Chapter 4, this volume). In general terms, the cognitive approach assumes that therapies are effective when they modify both the dysfunctional thoughts and beliefs that underlie distress and the behaviors and biases in information processing that maintain those dysfunctional beliefs.

The cognitive approach suggests that exposure is effective when it modifies the negative beliefs underlying patients' problems (e.g., Wells et al., 1995). However, as already mentioned, traditional methods of applying exposure may not provide the best means of producing this effect, particularly in social phobics. The brevity of many social situations means that exposure provides insufficient time for patients to experience a decline in their anxiety. Social situations also tend to be highly specific (every encounter has a specific description) and highly variable (each one changes as it unfolds), so that it may be difficult to repeat or to grade exposure. According to the cognitive view, change no longer depends on the duration, frequency, or graduated nature of exposure but on activating patients' fears in each situation (evidenced by heightened belief in catastrophic or other negative appraisals). Exposure should be followed by maneuvers that (potentially) disconfirm the belief.

One of the features of social phobia that is difficult to account for in learning theory terms is that social phobics frequently encounter their feared situations but their anxiety does not extinguish. The cognitive account proposes that this occurs because patients fail to process disconfirmatory information. Failures of this type could occur for several reasons:

1. Patients engage in safety behaviors during exposure that they believe prevent feared catastrophes (e.g., they avoid pauses in speech, or try to relax). Therefore the nonoccurrence of catastrophes such as loss of control is attributed to the behavior which kept them safe and re-appraisal is unlikely (e.g., Salkovskis, 1991).
2. Patients may fail to process disconfirmatory information because of the attentional strategies adopted in the feared situation. They may not notice, or they may discount, others' positive reactions to them. Processing is often predominantly self-focused, and this may reduce the processing of external interpersonal feedback capable of facilitating disconfirmation (e.g. Wells & Mathews, 1994; Clark & Wells, Chapter 4, this volume).
3. Social phobics may repeatedly reprocess information that is consistent with their fears, engaging in the postmortem described by Clark and Wells. They do notice, and do not discount, information that to them suggests they are being evaluated negatively.

Wells et al. (1995) tested the hypothesis that brief exposure (typically 5 minutes) presented with a cognitive rationale (emphasizing the modification of behavior to challenge belief in negative appraisals) and in conjunction with decreasing safety behaviors (see Clark & Wells, Chapter 4, this volume) was effective in reducing both anxiety and belief in negative appraisals during exposure. The data supported their hypothesis, and in addition, this was significantly more effective than was brief exposure presented with a learning theory rationale (emphasizing habituation of anxiety through planned exposure). These data suggest that optimal combinations of cognitive procedures and exposure, i.e., those presented within a framework that facilitates belief change, can be particularly effective.

The primary aims of cognitive therapy for social phobia may be summarized as follows:

1. The formulation of each patient's problem in terms of the interaction between *cognitive, affective,* and *behavioral* systems;
2. Modification of behaviors (e.g., safety behaviors and avoidance) and cognitive responses (e.g., attentional bias) that interfere with the effects of exposure and with the processing of disconfirmatory information;
3. Reexamination of dysfunctional thoughts and beliefs, identification of more realistic or functional ones, and accumulation of relevant evidence in suport of functional beliefs.

The Specific Cognitive Content of Social Phobia

The common theme in the negative automatic thoughts of social phobics concerns the fear of being the center of attention and of being judged negatively by other people (Beck et al., 1985). As would be expected, social phobics also evaluate their own social behavior negatively (Stopa & Clark, 1993). At least three types of cognition can be distinguished in conceptualizing the social phobic patient: specific situational appraisals expressed in the form of negative automatic thoughts, assumptions expressed as conditional rules or statements that guide behavior, and underlying beliefs that are unconditional and relate more closely to the self-concept. It may be difficult to elicit beliefs underlying negative appraisals, particularly if the problem is long-standing, but assumptions are relatively easy to identify and to challenge. Assumptions typically concern the predicted reactions of people or other consequences of "failed" social performance. Table 13.1 presents a range of typical negative automatic thoughts, assumptions, and core beliefs of social phobics.

Illustrative Case Formulation

The first step in formulating a case using this cognitive model is to elicit the specific content of the patient's situational appraisals and their idiosyncratic

TABLE 13.1. Cognitive Content of Social Phobia: Typical Examples

Automatic thoughts

I'll look foolish.	I'm losing it.
They think I'm stupid.	I'm being boring.
I'll get my words wrong.	I'll lose control of my hands.
They don't like me.	This is terrible.
Everyone is looking at me.	They can see how nervous I am.
I don't belong.	I've got nothing to contribute.

Assumptions

Unless I appear calm and collected people will reject me.
I must be witty and interesting or people won't like me.
Everyone will stare at me if I don't act normally.
I can't be happy unless everyone likes me.
If it goes badly it's my fault.
Nobody I like would like me.
If I am alone I'm bound to be unhappy.
I have to do things right in order to be acceptable.
If others want to know me they'll let me know.

Beliefs

I'm vulnerable.	I'm unlikable.
I'm inferior.	I'm stupid.
I'm weird.	I'm boring.
I'm ugly.	I'm inadequate.
I'm different.	I'm unacceptable.
I can't change.	

negative implications. The next step is to identify the processes that maintain belief in these appraisals, including overt avoidance and safety behaviors as well as thoughts, assumptions, and beliefs. Typically, this information can be obtained by asking the patient slowly to recount the details of a recent episode in which he or she was anxious, with the aim of eliciting his or her thoughts and appraisals. Thoughts are often readily accessible even though their significance may not be understood, and they can often be reported without direct exposure.

To illustrate how the cognitive model may be implemented, the cognitive formulation for a 36-year-old male patient recently treated by one of us (A.W.) is presented in Figure 13.1. This patient presented with "anxiety attacks," which occurred when he was required to make formal presentations at work. He had experienced intermittent social anxiety since age 13, consisting predominantly of difficulty talking in groups. Over the past 5 years, the problem had escalated until he dreaded many aspects of his work. Initially he stated that he feared "making a fool" of himself. When asked how this would happen he said, "I'll lose control" and "I'll be paralyzed and unable to speak." His fear was accompanied by a range of bodily sensations: palpitations, sweating, shortness of breath, and trembling. On recounting a recent episode, the following in-situation and preparatory safety behaviors were identified:

In-situation behaviors	*Preparatory behaviors*
Try and distract myself	Plan the talk in fine detail
Take deep breaths	Rehearse what I'm going to say
Try and relax	Try and imagine the situation
Say less	
Think ahead of myself	
Get the audience to focus on overheads instead of on me	
Move around more	

It is important to note that these may be exactly the kind of strategies used during behavioral treatments for social phobia. They *may* disconfirm beliefs, but not necessarily. The danger is that they may also augment confirmatory negative processing (e.g., "I have to keep control or something will go dreadfully wrong"). Therefore, they should be backed up and supplemented with specific cognitive interventions to check out and reexamine cognitive factors that may otherwise maintain social anxiety. In this case, using a safety behavior, such as distraction, impeded the processing of feedback from others and compromised mental efficiency when making presentations at work. Saying less also reduced the opportunity for disconfirming beliefs in negative appraisals such as "I can't do this."

Aside from the role of safety behaviors in maintaining his catastrophic beliefs, a number of cognitive factors, including misinterpretation of anxiety symptoms, also contributed to the maintenance of this problem. These are displayed in Figure 13.1. An initial understanding of the interplay between these cognitive and behavioral factors in maintaining anxiety was followed by conceptualization of the role of the patient's self-focused processing as advocated by Clark and Wells (Chapter 4, this volume).

Socializing the Patient

After developing an initial formulation, the next stage of treatment consists of socializing the patient into the cognitive model of social phobia. This serves both to provide a framework for the content of treatment and to generate a cognitive set that, in conjunction with the procedures employed in treatment, facilitates belief change. Socialization consists of sharing the formulation with the patient, checking for "goodness of fit" between the formulation and the patient's presenting problem, discussing any doubts or reservations expressed by the patient, and also educating the patient

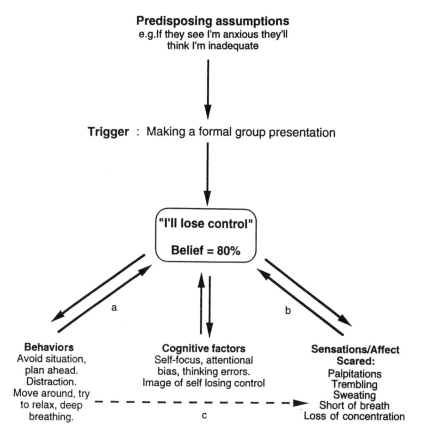

FIGURE 13.1. Example of an initial cognitive-behavioral case formulation (adapted from Clark & Wells, Chapter 4, this volume). a, prevention of disconfirmation; b, misinterpretation of bodily sensations as evidence for belief; c, exacerbation effects of behaviors on some of the sensations.

about the nature and content of cognitive therapy. Particular emphasis is placed on the part played in treatment by collaboration and homework, as is standard in cognitive therapy (Beck et al., 1985). Illustration of the linkages expressed in the formulation forms an important component of socialization. For example, the patient can be asked to engage in an interaction with a confederate while engaging in safety behaviors so as to examine the effect of these behaviors on performance.

COMBINING COGNITIVE AND BEHAVIORAL TECHNIQUES

Using the cognitive model to derive an individual formulation changes the emphasis of treatments for social phobia and suggests particular adaptations of traditional behavioral treatment strategies. The main point is that both verbal and behavioral strategies can be used so as to facilitate the process of reattribution: "These symptoms need not interfere . . . "; "It's only natural to be anxious"; "Anxiety does not lead to loss of control"; "People tend not to think badly about anxious behavior"; "Anxious behavior is rarely obvious." In the case presented above, both verbal and behavioral strategies were used to challenge the patient's belief that he would lose control, and the two categories of technique are typically employed together to modify belief in negative appraisals. For example, this patient was encouraged to stop using safety behaviors, and eventually, paradoxically to lose control by dropping things and making errors during presentations. This behavioral exercise provided an opportunity to test his predictions that others would react badly toward him and that his symptoms would escalate until he was totally paralyzed and unable to speak.

Standard verbal techniques (see, e.g., Beck et al., 1985; Burns, 1989; Hawton, Salkovskis, Kirk, & Clark, 1989) involve (1) questioning the patient's evidence for believing specific appraisals (e.g., "I've got nothing interesting to say"; "No one is interested in me"; "I don't really belong"); (2) collecting contrary evidence; (3) generating rational responses with relevant evidence; (4) labeling thinking errors: *mind-reading* (assuming one knows what another person is thinking), *personalization* (attaching personal meaning to events or the behavior of others when there is none), *catastrophizing* (predicting and dwelling on the worst possible outcome of a situation), *mental filtering* (selectively processing negative information); and (5) identifying and challenging thoughts using the dysfunctional thoughts record, or similar adaptation (see below).

Within this integrated approach, behavioral strategies are most usefully presented as "mini-experiments" designed to test belief in the salient appraisals. These experiments often involve exposure to the feared situation in combination with other maneuvers aimed at disconfirming dysfunctional beliefs. Exposure is thus a useful strategy because it provokes anxiety and activates dysfunctional beliefs, which then become amenable to modification. Activating beliefs provides optimal conditions for disconfirming them, and such disconfirmation is then more likely to generalize (Foa & Kozak, 1986; Wells & Matthews, 1994). Exposure as used with social phobics may also involve techniques that provoke interoceptive responses. For example, if the patient misinterprets bodily sensations (e.g., dizziness or sweating) as a sign of an imminent psychosocial "catastrophe," treatment can be geared toward actively provoking these sensations in order to illustrate that nothing actually catastrophic does occur. Detailed examination of the outcome of such experiments can then be carried out within a framework that increases the likelihood of belief change.

Exposure used in a cognitive way can be explicitly targeted at challenging the patient's beliefs, for example in catastrophic or other biased appraisals (Butler, 1989; Wells, 1992). Three maneuvers that can be combined with exposure to facilitate this are (1) preventing the patient from adopting safety behaviors which are conceptually linked to the maintenance of key negative appraisals, (2) paradoxical strategies, and (3) attentional strategies.

Safety Behaviors

Safety behaviors can be identified through detailed analysis of the particular behaviors that are logically linked to preventing specific "catastrophes." (Detailed examples are given in Clark & Wells, Chapter 4, this volume.) The role of such behaviors in preventing disconfirmation and maintaining symptoms can be illustrated using examples and by evoking target behaviors in the therapy session. Vicious circle models like the one presented in Figure 13.1 are shared with the patient in order to create a cognitive set for belief change. The patient is then instructed to enter feared situations without using safety behaviors. For example, someone who fears being unable to swallow when eating in public will select soft foods, drink repeatedly, and eat slowly in the belief that this prevents humiliation from choking. This stage can be difficult for the patient to implement alone, as a first homework assignment, and therapist-assisted exposure can provide useful preparation.

Paradoxical Strategies

These involve engaging in behaviors that make the feared outcome seem more likely. For example, a patient who feared that people would react negatively if he made a "mistake" in speech was instructed to make such errors deliberately. Similarly, a patient who misinterpreted certain bodily sensations and feared collapsing or losing control when they occurred was instructed to induce and exacerbate precisely those body sensations that she believed would lead to this catastrophe. Paradoxical procedures can also be applied in situations in which patients fear that they have no control, either to illustrate the extent of the control that they do have or to elucidate the exaggerated perceived need for control. For example, a social phobic may be instructed to practice making "errors" in social situations (e.g., dropping something; forgetting someone's name) and then recovering from the ensuing difficulties. Patients fearful of blushing may be asked to try to blush deliberately. Usually they are unable to do this, and even if they can, the outcome can be used as an opportunity to observe and manipulate the reactions of others, or to test other negative beliefs about the feared outcome.

Attention Modification

Experiments can be used to increase the patients' processing of interpersonal feedback so that fear-incongruent information may be processed. This typically requires the patient to actively monitor and analyze aspects of the environment, such as other people's facial expressions, dress, and behaviors (see also Butler, 1989; Clark & Wells, Chapter 4, this volume). For example, a social phobic who was fearful of shopping alone because he assumed that this would attract negative evaluation from others was asked to observe the number of other lone shoppers and the reactions of others to them. This required a shift from self-attentive and self-evaluative processing to processing of external information. The previous emphasis on self-focused processing may have precluded the processing of corrective information in the environment (in this case, the number of lone shoppers of all ages and sexes). It is also important to check how any new information is interpreted in order to ensure that it is not discounted or distorted (e.g., "everyone else has good reason to be alone"). If heightened self-consciousness remains a problem, other specific distraction and attention modification techniques may be used. Wells (1990) has developed an auditory attentional training procedure that can be effective in reducing the degree of self-focus and increasing flexibility of attention in anxious patients, and Hartmann (1986) has developed an "other-centered" therapy involving externally focused mental operations during social situations. It is important, however, that such strategies do not become new safety behaviors. Modification of attention is necessary to facilitate disconfirmatory processing, that is, to shift away from processing the self and toward processing external information that is inconsistent with negative beliefs.

FUTURE DIRECTIONS

Using the cognitive model as an integrating, guiding principle in the treatment of social phobia has made it much easier for the clinician to tackle these complex problems with clarity and confidence. These methods can also be extended for use with those social phobics who present with long-standing problems such as low self-esteem and who also fulfill criteria for one of the personality disorders. Frequently, social phobia overlaps with avoidant personality disorder. Liebowitz et al. (1992) suggest that "at least substantial aspects of avoidant personaliy disorder are best viewed as manifestations of a chronic anxiety disorder" (p. 299). Social phobia and avoidant personality disorder share many characteristics, but differ in the degree to which dysfunctional core self-schemata contribute to low self-esteem. Social phobics without an avoidant personality sometimes have an exaggerated need for acceptance and approval concerning social performance, but this still has limited implications for the self as a whole. Social phobics with a concurrent diagnosis of avoidant personality disorder are likely to have more pervasive beliefs concerning the potentially hazardous nature of social interaction as well as profoundly negative beliefs about the self. Both of these contribute to poor self-concept. Further research is required to establish cognitive-behavioral antecedents and modulators of social phobia and its relationship to avoidant personality disorder.

In cases where relatively stable negative self-concepts are involved, treatment approaches may adopt schema-focused cognitive therapy procedures (e.g. Beck, Freeman, & Associates, 1990; Young, 1990), as is illustrated in the example presented below.

ILLUSTRATIVE CASE: TREATING LONG-STANDING, CHRONIC SOCIAL ANXIETY

Jane started cognitive therapy with one of us (G.B.) at the age of 29 after three attempts over the preceding 10 years to find a therapy that would reduce her distress. At interview she was extremely tense, unable to make appropriate eye contact, and spoke in brief staccato sentences, displaying an apparent concern that she express each thought correctly. Her anxiety in social situations focused on the fear that her symptoms would attract attention and make people think that she was "weird," largely because they would notice a mismatch between her superficially acceptable appearance and her "obvious" personal inadequacy. Jane was elegantly dressed and looked like a casual but well-dressed business woman. She was extremely socially isolated, worked washing up in a canteen, avoided social contact with anyone she respected or admired (young, attractive, or intelligent) and associated only with a few well-known women friends. She was unable to travel by bus, to shop locally, or to go into town with Tom, with whom she had been living for 3 years and about whom she expressed much ambivalence. He was neither attractive nor intelligent, so being seen with him would be embarrassing and would reflect badly on her ("People judge me by who I'm with"). She said she was fond of him, that he was supportive and the only friend to whom she had spoken about her fears, but that if she were "better" she would leave him at once. The formulation on which her treatment was based is described below.

Early experience

No experience of physical closeness with parents; frequent parental-arguments

Overweight and clumsy as an adolescent

Teased by father; ignored or "leaned on" by mother
Academic interests at variance with those of sporting family

Beliefs

I'm a complete failure.
I'm not acceptable as I am.
Anybody I like wouldn't like me.
When I lose my looks I'll lose everything.

Main assumption

If I keep up appearances, I might manage all right (scrape by).

Critical incidents (incidents linked to beliefs and remembered by Jane with
   a high degree of painful emotion)

Age 6: hid from visitors to the house, her distress ignored by mother
Age 11: Father laughed at her appearance when dressed in new clothes
Age 16: Had to cope for her mother when her father suddenly died
Present: Traveling on a bus, catching the eye of the driver. He looks away
   and she thinks "he must think I'm odd." He continues looking and
   she thinks "he must be able to see how inadequate I am."

Maintenance cycles

1. *A belief cycle*: If she made herself look "acceptable" by dressing well,
   any successes were discounted as superficial. If she made herself look
   "unacceptable" (e.g., wearing revealing clothes), any successes were
   unacceptable. Both behaviors confirmed the belief in her unacceptability.
2. *A behavioral cycle*: Jane never left the house without wearing her "mask"
   (make-up and smart clothes). Feeling good confirmed that she needed
   the mask. Feeling bad increased the desire to hide behind the mask.

The maintenance cycles worked in two ways, trapping Jane in a "no win"
situation (a combination of schema maintenance and schema compensa-
tion in Young's terms). It is immediately clear that purely behavioral ways
of breaking these cycles were unlikely to be effective in the absence of
simultaneous work on the underlying beliefs.

Summary of Treatment Strategies Used

Sharing the formulation and discussing its implications, including expectations about therapy, helped Jane realize that it was unlikely that the problem would resolve itself and that it was more likely that change would be
a slow process involving hard work. Her main reaction to the formulation

was that her social anxiety had so far prevented her developing skills and talents. She expressed the wish to enroll in further education classes once she felt sufficiently confident. This became a goal of treatment.

Treatment thereafter focused on four main interlocking areas of work: her perceived unacceptability, her tendency toward self-blame both for early experiences and for current social failures, associated behavioral exercises, and confidence building. Frequent reference was made to the formulation and various modifications were made to it as treatment progressed.

The belief that she was unacceptable was reexamined using standard cognitive procedures (see, e.g., Hawton et al., 1989), with special attention being paid to Jane's tendency to discount evidence contrary to her belief. She learned how to identify and reexamine her thoughts in particular situations, first within the treatment session, then in written form as a homework assignment, and finally in her head. She chose to do the written exercise using a three-column technique, the three columns being labeled "The incident," "What I think people think," and "Other possibilities?" Some examples of her homework using this method are shown in Table 13.2. She adapted these methods both to work on specific distressing incidents (e.g., trembling visibly when serving in the canteen) and to work on more pervasive attitudes (e.g., "The better people know you the more likely they are to reject you").

The second area of work related to her low self-esteem and her tendency to blame herself for the distressing aspects of her childhood and involved integrating cognitive and behavioral strategies in the ways described earlier in this chapter. Behavioral work was initiated as soon as the main themes had become clear and increased in variety as treatment progressed. She allowed Tom to meet the friends she had kept from him and went out with him to the local pub, with the aim of finding out

TABLE 13.2. Examples of Jane's Written Homework

The incident	What I think people think	Other possibilities?
Took brother to airport and cried in public.	Strangers can see me for what I am, which is weak.	It's a natural reaction in an airport.
Reaching up to fill machine with coffee beans.	She looks nervous. She's got wet armpits.	Maybe they just observe me without judging me.
Bus driver catches my eye.	He thinks that I'm a weirdo and regrets saying good morning to me.	Maybe he is indifferent. He says the same to everyone.
In pub, with friends, eating to keep my hands busy.	Why can't she learn to relax with us? She's known us for three years.	They know my quirks and still like me.

whether people really did "judge me by who I'm living with." She experi-
mented with different ways of "dropping the mask" and being herself. We
made a videotape of Jane in conversation and viewed it together when
examining sources of information about her public self-concept and working on modifying thoughts about the self-evident nature of her social awkwardness. The work on confidence building was designed to help her to
develop a more accurate and functional sense of herself and of her talents,
preferences, and skills. The specific tasks chosen were selected to help her
find out what she liked doing and what she was good at. She kept a diary
in which she recorded positive interactions with others and activities that
she enjoyed. She collected information about possible training courses,
work opportunities, and evening classes. She went out with a friend and
did some dressmaking for Tom's sister.

Each behavioral step was difficult for Jane, and she regularly faced
the common conflict between the wish to wait until she felt better before
doing something new and the wish to behave differently. She quickly
realized that one of the best ways to build her confidence was by doing
things. Referring back to the formulation helped her both to understand
why the conflict occurred and to plan an attack on the beliefs and behaviors
that constantly tempted her to hide behind the mask again for fear of being
found to be unacceptable and inadequate.

In general, the procedures used to treat patients with long-standing,
chronic social phobia are very similar to those used in more straightforward
cases. However, the treatment process is more difficult, and it is helpful to
keep a (relatively simple) formulation clearly in mind, which guides the
selection of treatment interventions and enables understanding of the difficulties that arise in treatment. Behavioral experiments provide one of the
best ways to change beliefs when the two aspects of treatment are properly
integrated. That means that the tasks should be carefully devised in the
ways outlined previously and then interpreted with reference to the original
beliefs, without discounting successful experiences. If at the same time,
links can be made between episodes of distress in the present and past
experiences, it seems gradually to become easier for patients to make sense
of their distress. Making such links helps patients to ask themselves questions like "How does this fit with what happened to me earlier on?"; "How
are things different today?"; and "What can I now do to find out whether
they really are different?" The issue for the therapist becomes one of refram-
ing the responsibility for what might have happened in the past (e.g., "It's
not that 'I'm bad,' but that I found myself in a 'bad situation,' for which
someone else was responsible"). This helps to counteract the external evidence, for example of poor social performance, that patients mistakenly
use to confirm their beliefs.

Before treatment started, Jane was moderately anxious (Beck Anxiety
Inventory [BAI; Beck, Brown, Epstein, & Steer, 1988] score = 22) and

also moderately depressed (Beck Depression Inventory [BDI; Beck, Ward, Mendelson, Mock, & Erbaugh, 1961] score = 21). At that stage, she rated her general satisfaction with her life (considering work, relationships, leisure etc.) at − 3 on a scale that ranged from − 5 to + 5. After treatment, she had clearly changed: BAI = 13; BDI = 5; General Satisfaction = + 2. Six months later, she had maintained these gains, was slightly less anxious, and had also taken the first steps toward starting a new career.

CONCLUSION

In this chapter, we have illustrated how a specific cognitive approach to the treatment of social phobia, in which the individual case formulation plays a central role, can integrate cognitive and behavioral (largely exposure-based) strategies within a single framework.

While a variety of cognitive and eclectic approaches to the problem have been used in the past, we believe that advances in the treatment of social phobia will depend on the development and implementation of a detailed cognitive model, together with a consideration of practical treatment issues such as the ones outlined here. The emphasis in treatment should be on the development of a comprehensive and coherent cognitive formulation that can account for the maintenance of the problem, and from which hypotheses concerning potentially effective intervention strategies can be derived and tested.

REFERENCES

American Psychiatric Association. (1987). *Diagnostic and statistical manual of mental disorders* (3rd ed., rev.). Washington, DC: Author.

American Psychiatric Association. (1994). *Diagnostic and statistical manual of mental disorders* (4th ed.). Washington, DC: Author.

Beck, A. T., Brown, G., Epstein, N., & Steer, R. A. (1988). An inventory for measuring clinical anxiety: Psychometric properties. *Journal of Consulting and Clinical Psychology, 56*, 893−897.

Beck, A. T., Emery, G., & Greenberg, R. (1985). *Anxiety disorders and phobias: A cognitive perspective.* New York: Basic Books.

Beck A. T., Freeman, A., & Associates. (1990). *Cognitive therapy of personality disorders.* New York: Guilford Press.

Beck, A. T., Ward, C. H., Mendelson, M., Mock, J., & Erbaugh, J. (1961). An inventory for measuring depression. *Archives of General Psychiatry, 4*, 561−571.

Burns, D. (1989). *The feeling good handbook.* New York: Penguin Books USA, Inc.

Butler, G. (1985). Exposure as a treatment for social anxiety: Some instructive difficulties. *Behaviour Research and Therapy, 23*, 651−657.

Butler, G. (1989). Issues in the application of cognitive and behavioral strategies for the treatment of social phobia. *Clinical Psychology Review, 9*, 91−106.

Butler, G., & Booth, R. (1991). Developing psychological treatments for generalized anxiety disorder. In R. M. Rapee & D. H. Barlow, (Eds.), *Chronic anxiety: Generalized anxiety disorder and mixed anxiety–depression* (pp. 187–209). New York: Guilford Press.

Butler, G., Cullington, A., Munby, M., Amies, P., & Gelder, M. (1984). Exposure and anxiety management in the treatment of social phobia. *Journal of Consulting and Clinical Psychology, 2,* 642–650.

Edelmann, R. J. (1992). *Anxiety: Theory, research and intervention in clinical and health psychology.* Chichester, UK: Wiley.

Emmelkamp, P. M. G., Mersch, P. P. A., Vissia, E., & van der Helm, M. (1985). Social phobia: A comparative evaluation of cognitive and behavioural interventions. *Behaviour Research and Therapy, 23,* 365–369.

Foa, E. B., & Kozak, M. J. (1986). Emotional processing and fear: Exposure to corrective information. *Psychological Bulletin, 99,* 20–35.

Hartmann, L. M. (1986). Social anxiety, problem drinking and self-awareness. In L. M. Hartmann & K. R. Blankstein (Eds.), *Perception of self in emotional disorder and psychotherapy* (pp. 265–281). New York: Plenum Press.

Hawton, K., Salkovskis, P., Kirk, J., & Clark, D. (1989). *Cognitive behavioural therapy for psychiatric problems: A practical guide.* Oxford: Oxford University Press.

Heimberg, R. G. (1989). Cognitive and behavioral treatments for social phobia: A critical analysis. *Clinical Psychology Review, 9,* 107–128.

Heimberg, R. G., & Barlow D. H. (1988). Psychosocial treatments for social phobia. *Psychosomatics, 29,* 27–37.

Heimberg, R. G., & Barlow, D. H. (1991). New developments in cognitive-behavioral treatments for social phobia. *Journal of Clinical Psychiatry, 52* (11, Suppl.), 21–30.

Heimberg, R. G., Becker, R. E., Goldfinger, K., & Vermilyea, J. A. (1985). Treatment of social phobia by exposure, cognitive restructuring, and homework assignments. *Journal of Nervous and Mental Disease, 173,* 236–245.

Heimberg, R. G., Dodge, C. S., Hope, D. A., Kennedy, C. R., Zollo, L. J., & Becker, R. E. (1990). Cognitive behvioral treatment for social phobia: Comparison with a credible placebo control. *Cognitive Therapy and Research, 14,* 1–23.

Heimberg, R. G., Salzman, D. G., Holt, C. S., & Blendell, K. A. (1993). Cognitive behavioral group treatment for social phobia: Effectiveness at five-year followup. *Cognitive Therapy and Research, 17,* 325–339.

Hollon, S. D., & Beck, A. T. (1994). Cognitive and cognitive-behavior therapies. In E. A. Bergin & S. L. Garfield (Eds.), *Handbook of psychotherapy and behavior change: An empirical analysis* (4th ed., pp. 428–466). New York: Wiley.

Holt, C. S., Heimberg, R. G., Hope, D. A., & Liebowitz, M. R. (1992). Situational domains of social phobia. *Journal of Anxiety Disorders, 6,* 63–77.

Hope, D. A., & Heimberg, R. G. (1993). Social phobia and social anxiety. In D. H. Barlow (Ed.), *Clinical handbook of psychological disorders: A step-by-step treatment manual* (2nd ed., pp. 99–136). New York: Guilford Press.

Jerramalm, A., Jansson, L., & Öst, L.-G. (1986). Cognitive and physiological reactivity and the effects of different behavioral methods in the treatment of social phobia. *Behaviour Research and Therapy, 24,* 171–180.

Liebowitz, M. R., Schneier, F., Campas, R., Hollander, E., Hatterer, J., Fyer, A., Gorman, J., Papp, L., Davies, S., Gully, R., & Klein, D. F. (1992). Phenelzine vs atenolol in social phobia: A placebo-controlled comparison. *Archives of General Psychiatry, 49*, 290–300.

Mattick, R. G., & Peters, L. (1988). Treatment of severe social phobia: Effects of guided exposure with and without cognitive restructuring. *Journal of Consulting and Clinical Psychology. 56*, 251–260.

Mattick, R. P., Peters, L., & Clarke, J. C. (1989). Exposure and cognitive restructuring for social phobia: A controlled study. *Behavior Therapy, 20*, 3–23.

Mersch, P. P. A., Emmelkamp, P. M. G., Bögels, S. M., & van der Sleen, J. (1989). Social phobia: Individual response patterns and the effects of behavioural and cognitive interventions. *Behaviour Research and Therapy, 27*, 421–434.

Mersch, P. P. A., Emmelkamp, P. M. G., & Lips, C. (1991). Social phobia: Individual response patterns and the long-term effects of cognitive and behavioral interventions. A follow-up study. *Behaviour Research and Therapy, 29*, 357–362.

Persons, J. B. (1989). *Cognitive therapy in practice: A case formulation approach.* New York: Norton.

Salkovskis, P. M. S. (1991). The importance of behaviour in the maintenance of anxiety and panic. *Behavioural Psychotherapy, 19*, 6–19.

Schlenker, B. R., & Leary, M. R. (1982). Social anxiety and self-presentation: A conceptualization and model. *Psychological Bulletin, 92*, 641–669.

Scholing, A., & Emmelkamp, P. M. G. (1993). Cognitive and behavioural treatments of fear of blushing, sweating or trembling. *Behaviour Research and Therapy, 31*, 155–170.

Stopa, L., & Clark, D. M. (1993). Cognitive processes in social phobia. *Behaviour Research and Therapy, 31*, 255–268.

Trower, P., & Gilbert, P. (1989). New theoretical conceptions of social anxiety and social phobia. *Clinical Psychology Review, 9*, 19–35.

Wells, A. (1990). Panic disorder in association with relaxation induced anxiety: An attentional training approach to treatment. *Behavior Therapy, 21*, 273–280.

Wells, A. (1992). Cognitive therapy for anxiety and cognitive theories of causation. In G. D. Burrows, M. Roth & R. Noyes (Eds.), *Handbook of anxiety* (Vol. 5, pp. 233–254). Amsterdam: Elsevier.

Wells, A., Clark, D. M., Salkovskis, P, M. S., Ludgate, J., Hackmann, A., & Gelder, M. (1995). Social phobia: The role of in-situation safety behaviors in maintaining anxiety and negative beliefs. *Behavior Therapy, 26*, 153–161.

Wells, A., & Mathews, D. (1994). *Attention and emotion: a clinical perspective.* Hove, UK: Erlbaum.

Young, J. (1990). *Cognitive therapy for personality disorders.* Sarasota, FL: Professional Resource Exchange.

CHAPTER FOURTEEN

Pharmacological Treatments: Literature Review

NICHOLAS L. S. POTTS
JONATHAN R. T. DAVIDSON

As with most other anxiety disorders, social phobia is now known to be a medication-responsive condition. Performing artists, students taking examinations, and many others have tried beta blocker drugs in order to lessen performance anxiety. In the mid-1970s, investigators began to look at this class of drugs in the context of performance situations. The rationale for using beta blockers was related to their ability to reduce some of the sympathetically mediated peripheral manifestations of anxiety. In one survey, 27% of professional musicians admitted to daily or as-needed use of beta blockers (Clark & Agras, 1991).

Following a series of studies that investigated beta blockers during the 1970s and 1980s, and that are reviewed below, attention turned to other drug categories, most notably the monoamine oxidase inhibitors (MAOIs) and, more recently, benzodiazepines and selective serotonin reuptake inhibitors (SSRIs). In this chapter, we review the published literature on all major drug categories that have been investigated in the treatment of social phobia and related forms of anxiety.

MONOAMINE OXIDASE INHIBITORS

Irreversible, Nonselective MAOIs

The older-generation MAOIs phenelzine (Nardil) and tranylcypromine (Parnate) inhibit the enzyme monoamine oxidase (MAO), a widespread degradative enzyme that regulates the breakdown of catecholamines and indoleamines. Because the drug binds irreversibly to the enzyme, this inhibition is long-lasting, and it is only by synthesis of new enzyme that MAO activity can return. Each of these irreversible MAOIs is also nonselective, in that they inhibit both the A and B forms of MAO. This means that the effects of a variety of substrates will be potentiated when ingested or taken in association with drug. These substrates include tyramine, dopamine, tryptophan, and other amines. As a result, dietary and medication restrictions are essential to maximize the safety of treatment.

Phenelzine (Nardil)

There have been a number of clinical reports on the efficacy of phenelzine in social phobia. A few early controlled studies documented its effects in mixed populations of social phobia and agoraphobia, without separating the two groups (Mountjoy, Roth, Garside, & Leitch, 1977; Solyom et al., 1973; Solyom, Solyom, LaPierre, Pecknold, & Morton, 1981; Tyrer, Candy, & Kelly, 1973).

Liebowitz, Fyer, Gorman, Campeas, and Levin (1986) conducted an open pilot study of phenelzine in 11 patients who met the criteria for social phobia of the third edition of the *Diagnostic and Statistical Manual of Mental Disorders* (DSM-III; American Psychiatric Association, 1980). The dose was started at 30 mg per day and increased up to a possible maximum of 90 mg per day. Seven patients (64%) exhibited marked improvement, and 4 (36%) showed moderate improvement to the drug. Improvement was usually observed within the first 4 weeks, and the optimal drug dose was 45 mg per day or less in 6 of 11 patients. Side effects included insomnia, memory problems, irritability, sexual dysfunction, overstimulation, and edema at higher doses, all being well-recognized side effects of the drug.

Subsequently, Liebowitz et al. (1992) reported the results of a large double-blind clinical trial evaluating phenelzine, the cardioselective beta blocker atenolol (Tenormin), and placebo. This study had four phases. An initial 2-week drug-free period was followed by a 1-week single-blind placebo lead-in. Nonresponding patients were then randomly assigned to receive 8 weeks of treatment with phenelzine, atenolol, or placebo. At the end of that time, patients who had achieved at least minimum improvement on the Clinical Global Impressions (CGI) Scale (Guy, 1976) were enrolled into 8 further weeks of maintenance treatment in order to examine the durability of improvement and to see if additional gains took place. In the final phase, patients who showed either much or very much improvement on the CGI and who were receiving one of the two active drugs were then either switched to placebo following taper or continued for another 8 weeks on active drug, double-blind. This study used DSM-III criteria but included subjects with avoidant personality disorder and with social phobia secondary to some other medical problem. Patients were excluded from the study if they had previously received phenelzine at doses of 45 mg per day or greater or atenolol at doses of 50 mg per day or greater. Patients were prospectively assigned to either discrete or generalized types of social phobia. The Liebowitz Social Anxiety Scale (LSAS; Liebowitz, 1987), the Social Phobic Disorders Severity and Change Form (SPDSC; Liebowitz et al., 1986), and the Hamilton Depression and Anxiety Scales (Hamilton, 1959, 1960) were completed by an independent evaluator, blind to dose and side effects. Self-ratings consisted of the Symptom Check List—90 (SCL-90; Derogatis, Lipman, & Covi, 1973), the Social Avoidance and Distress Scale (SAD; Watson & Friend, 1969), the Fear of Negative Evaluation Scale (FNE; Watson & Friend, 1969), the Fear Questionnaire (FQ; Marks & Mathews, 1979), the Willoughby Personality Inventory (Willoughby, 1932), and the Sheehan Disability Scale (SDS; Sheehan, 1984).

In this study, of 117 subjects who received single-blind placebo, 85 were randomized into one of the three treatment cells. Seventy-four patients completed at least 4 weeks of treatment, with 2 weeks of therapeutic dose. At week 8, the following response rates were observed: phenelzine, 64% (16 of 25), atenolol, 30% (7 of 23) and placebo, 23% (6 of 26). There was a reduction in both social and performance anxiety and an improvement in social and work function. Greater changes were noted on clinician scales than on self-ratings. A mean dose of 75.7 mg per day (*SD* = 16.0) phenelzine was administered and of 97.6 mg per day (*SD* = 10.9) for atenolol.

In generalized social phobia, response rates were as follows: 68% (13 of 19), 28% (5 of 18), and 21% (4 of 19) for phenelzine, atenolol, and placebo, respectively. In the discrete subtype, response rates were 50% (3 of 6), 40% (2 of 5), and 29% (2 of 7) for phenelzine, atenolol, and placebo, respectively.

Among patients who entered the maintenance phase, there was no real change in status, and numbers were quite small in each treatment group. In the discontinuation phase, there were 11 phenelzine patients and 5 atenolol patients. Of the 11 phenelzine subjects, 6 were switched to placebo, and 2 (33%) of these subjects relapsed. Among the 5 who stayed on phenelzine, 1 (20%) dropped out, and 4 (80%) remained well. Of the 5 atenolol patients, 3 were switched to placebo, and 1 (33%) of these subjects relapsed. Of the 2 who remained on atenolol, 1 (50%) relapsed. These sample sizes are very small, and maintenance and discontinuation studies with larger samples are needed.

A second double-blind study was conducted by Gelernter et al. (1991), in which patients with social phobia, diagnosed according to the criteria of the revised third edition of the *Diagnostic and Statistical Manual of Mental*

Disorders (DSM-III-R; American Psychiatric Association, 1987), were randomly assigned to one of the following four treatment groups: cognitive-behavioral therapy (CBT) as described by Heimberg et al. (1990), phenelzine, alprazolam (Xanax), or placebo. All pharmacotherapy patients were also given exposure instructions. The only clinician-rated outcome measure was the physician's rating of work and social disability, and the major self-rating outcome measures were the FQ, FNE, SAD, Beck Depression Inventory (BDI; Beck, Ward, Mendelson, Mock, & Erbaugh, 1961), and State–Trait Anxiety Inventory (STAI; Spielberger, Gorsuch, & Lushene, 1970). Patients were considered to be responders if their final FQ social phobia score was equal to, or below, that obtained in normative samples by Mizes and Crawford (1986) and Kendall and Grove (1988).

The medication was given to the following maximum doses: phenelzine up to 90 mg per day and alprazolam up to 6.3 mg per day. Actual mean doses were phenelzine 55 mg per day $(SD = 16)$, and alprazolam 4.2 mg per day $(SD = 1.3)$. Dose ranges were 30–90 mg per day for phenelzine and 2.1–6.3 mg per day for alprazolam.

At 12 weeks, there was only one statistically significant difference between groups on the self-rating scales, although significant within-group changes took place on all measures. Phenelzine was superior to the other groups on the STAI. On the physician-rated scale, phenelzine and alprazolam were both significantly more effective than was placebo at posttreatment (week 12). At the 2 month follow-up, phenelzine was more effective than were either alprazolam or placebo. When results were expressed in terms of improvement rates on the FQ, the following outcome rates were obtained: phenelzine 69%, alprazolam 38%, CBT 24%, and placebo 20%. When patients were seen 2 months after active treatment had ceased, phenelzine was significantly superior to placebo, whereas alprazolam patients had relapsed.

Although phenelzine was effective on the physician-rated scales and a weak effect was seen for alprazolam, the results are difficult to interpret because an exceptionally conservative response criterion was chosen (i.e., patients' scores had to be *better* than that of the average normative subject). Moreover, the normative groups against which the scores were compared achieved lower scores than did the original normative group included in Marks and Mathews (1979). In addition, the study was not a specific test of pharmacotherapy alone, since all subjects received self-exposure instructions. Blind physician ratings were completed only for the medication groups, therefore introducing another confound in the way in which treatments were assessed.

In a third major study of phenelzine, Versiani et al. (1992) reported a three-phase, double-blind evaluation of phenelzine, moclobemide (a reversible MAOI, see below), and placebo in social phobia. The first phase was an 8-week evaluation of all three treatments. At the end of that time, responders continued on double-blind maintenance treatment for another 8 weeks. At week 16, responders were then randomized to receive either placebo or continued treatment with active drug for 8 further weeks. Tapering took place between weeks 17 and 19 in those patients who were switched from active drug to placebo.

Doses of phenelzine were increased gradually up to a maximum possible dose of 90 mg per day, and doses of moclobemide were raised up to 600 mg per day. Lowering of dose, or halting of the increase, took place only if significant side effects developed.

Ratings were based upon clinician and patient measures. Clinician-rated scales included the LSAS, CGI, and Hamilton Scales for Depression and Anxiety. The following self-rating measures were used: the Willoughby Personality Inventory, the SAD, the FNE, the SCL-90, and the SDS.

By week 8, mean doses of phenelzine and moclobemide were 67.5 mg per day and 580.7 mg per day, respectively. By week 16, mean doses of phenelzine and moclobemide in the remaining (i.e., week 8 responder) group were 69.3 mg per day and 583.2 mg per day, respectively.

Results of the week 8 comparisons showed that phenelzine was superior to placebo on all global and social phobia measures, but that no differences were found with regard to disability, SCL-90, or Hamilton Scale scores. Phenelzine was superior to moclobemide on a few measures at week 4, but by week 8, it was superior only on the social avoidance subscale of the LSAS. However, symptom scores were uniformly lower in the phenelzine group than in the moclobemide group at week 8. Responder status was defined by scores of 1 or 2 on the CGI Improvement scale and SDS, as well as a 70% drop on the LSAS. Of patients who were classified as responders at week 8, 91% of phenelzine patients remained responsive at week 16.

Side effects of phenelzine between weeks 1 and 8 consisted of sleepiness (50%), orthostatic hypotension (42%), dry mouth (38%), constipation (38%), reduced libido (27%), impaired ejaculation (19%), insomnia (15%), vertigo (11%), and headache (10%). At week 16, five of these side effects had increased whereas four had decreased in frequency.

Side effects were associated with placebo during weeks 1 to 8 as follows: sleepiness (11%), dry mouth (8%), constipation (8%), headache (4%), orthostatic hypotension (4%), and vertigo (4%).

In a recent report, Oberlander, Schneier, and Liebowitz (1994) described 11 patients who met all DSM-III-R criteria for social phobia except the criterion which states that social phobia is not diagnosed when it is secondary to disabling physical pathology, which included visual disorders, Charcot–Marie–Tooth disease, stuttering, polio, muscle twitches, hyperhidrosis, and Bell's palsy. Phenelzine was used successfully in this group, the majority of whom were helped within the dose range of 45–105 mg per day. Such findings suggest that social phobia secondary to medical problems may respond equally well to some of the same treatments that help primary social phobia.

Tranylcypromine (Parnate)

Tranylcypromine was first reported to be effective in social phobia by Versiani, Mundim, Nardi, and Liebowitz (1988). Thirty-two social phobic patients were enrolled in a 1-year open trial of tranylcypromine at doses between 40 and 60 mg per day. Four patients dropped out due to lack of efficacy or side effects, although one of these individuals was able to tolerate the medicine at 40 mg per day for more than 2 weeks, the predetermined minimum treatment period for inclusion in the analysis. Improvement was rated as marked if patients could face all feared situations asymptomatically or with only slight discomfort. Improvement was rated as moderate if anxiety in some but not all phobic situations had improved and there was persistence of some avoidance behavior. Improvement rates were: 62% (18 of 29) showed marked improvement, 17% (5 of 29) showed moderate improvement, and 21% (6 of 29) showed no improvement.

Most common side effects of tranylcypromine were orthostatic dizziness (75%), insomnia (45%), daytime sleepiness (41%), loss of libido (38%), tiredness (21%), nausea (17%), and diarrhea (10%).

Versiani, Nardi, and Mundim (1989) reported a second open trial with tranylcypromine in 81 patients with social phobia. At week 8, the mean dose was 58.2 mg per day ($SD = 6.4$). A statistically significant reduction in score was seen relative to baseline on the CGI Severity measure, which changed from 5.2 ($SD = 0.9$) to 1.5 ($SD = 1.0$). LSAS scores changed from a baseline mean of 90.4 ($SD = 18.7$) to a week 8 score of 28.2 ($SD = 17.9$). The most frequent side effects were loss of libido (59%), orthostatic hypotension (55%), and nausea (18%).

Reversible Inhibitors of Monoamine Oxidase A

There have been some investigations with a new group of MAOIs—reversible inhibitors of monoamine oxidase (RIMAs)—that are selective for the A subtype of the enzyme and whose effects can be rapidly reversed. MAO A selective inhibitors affect the breakdown of norepinephrine and serotonin but permit continued degradation of other substrates, such as dopamine, which are metabolized by both the A and B forms. Tyramine is metabolized by MAO A in the gastrointestinal tract, but the short half-life and reversibility of MAO inhibition by RIMAs makes dietary restrictions, for the most part, unnecessary. Furthermore, other medications containing sympathomimetics, such as phenylephrine and phenylpropanolamine, can be taken safely with MAO A selective inhibitors because of their rapid reversibility by competitive inhibition in the presence of other substrates. Therefore, RIMAs enjoy a considerable advantage of safety and patient acceptability in comparison to the older generation MAOIs. However, their efficacy remains in some question, as indicated by the following reviews of the two major RIMAs, moclobemide (marketed outside the United States as Aurorix or Manerix) and brofaromine.

Moclobemide (Aurorix, Manerix)

In the aforementioned study by Versiani et al. (1992), moclobemide was significantly more effective than was placebo at week 8 on the LSAS, CGI, SAD, and Willoughby Personality Inventory. No other significant differences were found.

At week 8, 5 of 26 moclobemide patients were withdrawn from the study due to nonresponse, and 4 more dropped out at weeks 9 and 10 for other reasons. Therefore, only 17 of the original 26 remained for evaluation at week 16. In this subgroup, moclobemide proved to be efficacious, with 82% of this group continuing to be classified as responders.

Side effects of moclobemide between weeks 1 and 8 were insomnia (19%), sleepiness (15%), dry mouth (11%), headache (11%), constipation (8%), orthostatic hypotension (4%), and loss of libido (4%). All had disappeared or lessened by week 16.

Bisserbe, Lepine, and G. R. P. Group (1994) reported a 12-week open trial with moclobemide in 35 patients who met DSM-III-R criteria for social phobia. Patients were treated with doses ranging from 300 to 600 mg per day. Unfortunately, 18 patients dropped out of the study before completing the full 12 weeks of treatment. Withdrawal was due to side effects in 8 cases, with insomnia being the most frequent (5 cases). Four subjects withdrew due to lack of efficacy, 2 because of depression, and 2 for reasons unrelated to medication. One grand mal seizure occurred, and 1 patient withdrew due to early response.

Patients were rated on the CGI and LSAS. At week 4, 29% (8 of 28) of remaining patients were rated as much or very much improved on the CGI. At week 8, 50% (12 of 24) and at week 12, 94% (17 of 18) were rated as much or very much improved. On the LSAS, patients showed improvement on both the anxiety and avoidance subscales. LSAS scores on the Avoidance subscale changed from a baseline mean of 33 ($SD =$

10.3) to 10.5 (SD = 13.4), and on the Fear subscale changed from a baseline mean of 41.3 (SD = 10.7) to 15 (SD = 14.1).

Three further studies of moclobemide have been completed. A worldwide multicenter trial found moclobemide to be more effective than placebo on several measures, while a U.S. multicenter trial found little difference between treatment groups, although a dose effect was noted. A single-center U.S. study by Schneier and colleagues (F. Schneier, personal communication, December 1994) found a drug response rate of 22% versus a placebo response rate of 10%.

Brofaromine

In a double-blind, 12-week, placebo-controlled study, van Vliet, den Boer, and Westenberg (1992) reported efficacy for the RIMA brofaromine relative to placebo in 30 patients. A 12-week double-blind continuation phase was provided for week 12 responders.

The dose of brofaromine was gradually increased from 50 mg per day to 150 mg per day. Rating scales included the LSAS, SCL-90, and Hamilton Anxiety Scale. Plasma levels of serotonin, 5-hydroxyindoleacetic acid (5-HIAA), melatonin, and homovanillic acid (HVA) were measured. Brofaromine was significantly more effective than was placebo from week 8 onward according to the LSAS and the Hamilton Scale, and at endpoint on the SCL-90 interpersonal sensitivity, obsessive–compulsive, and phobia scales. Eighty percent of brofaromine patients and 14% of placebo patients judged themselves to be responders, although criteria for response were not provided. Using a final Hamilton Anxiety Scale score of less than 10 as criterion for response, the authors found 73% of brofaromine patients and 0% of placebo patients to have been responders.

The most common side effects of the drug were insomnia (73%), weight loss (60%), nausea (53%), anorexia (47%), and increased nervousness (20%). Placebo-related side effects were nausea (21%), weight loss (14%), and anorexia (7%).

Biological measures indicated that brofaromine led to an increase in serotonin and melatonin and a reduction of 5-HIAA and HVA. These findings are consistent with the drug's known action and indicate that the dose was biologically active. However, no information was provided as to whether these biological indices correlated with any of the clinical measures.

One placebo patient and 11 brofaromine patients entered the continuation phase. Further significant improvement occurred on the Hamilton Anxiety Scale.

Humble, Fahlen, Koczkas, and Nilsson (1992) reported on a study in which 77 patients who met DSM-III-R criteria for social phobia were randomized to receive either brofaromine or placebo for 12 weeks. Patients were rated on the CGI, LSAS, and Hamilton Anxiety Scale. Eight patients were withdrawn from the study (1 for lack of efficacy, 6 for side effects, and 1 for other reasons).

Of the 69 patients who completed the 12-week phase, 79.4% of the brofaromine patients were rated much or very much improved on the CGI, compared to 25.6% of the placebo group. On the LSAS, patients receiving brofaromine were significantly improved on both the Anxiety and Avoidance subscales. A statistically significant improvement was also demonstrated on the Hamilton Anxiety Scale in patients receiving brofaromine. Side effects were mild and transient, the most frequent being sleep disturbance. Fahlen and Nilsson (1992) went on to examine the effects of brofaromine and placebo in a sugroup of 63 patients. Within this subgroup, 60% met criteria for avoidant personality disorder before treatment. Notably, the occurrence of avoidant personality disorder was reduced from 62% to 19% in the brofaromine group, compared to a drop of 59% to 44% in the placebo group.

Summary of Studies

Studies that have used MAOIs in the treatment of social phobia are presented in Table 14.1. The results of these studies show that older-generation MAOIs are reasonably effective in reducing symptomatology associated with social phobia. Phenelzine has been the most extensively studied, with three large double-blind placebo-controlled studies showing efficacy in two-thirds or more of the patients who received the drug. There can be little doubt that phenelzine effectively treats most components of social phobia, although side effects and dietary restrictions impose major limitations on widespread use of the drug. Tranylcypromine offers promise, based upon two open studies, but again side effects and dietary restrictions are major limitations. The RIMAs moclobemide and brofaromine have shown promise in the treatment of social phobia. However, all of the positive studies have taken place outside of the United States, and recent work with moclobemide in the United States suggests a much less robust response. The reasons for these discrepancies are unclear. Whether they have to do with ethnocultural factors, sampling differences, or other unknown reasons remains to be established. In the three positive studies, the RIMAs were clearly effective, especially brofaromine. Even with the above qualifications, there may still be a role for RIMAs where they are available because of their greater safety and superior side-effect profile relative to other MAOIs.

TABLE 14.1. Studies of Monoamine Oxidase Inhibitors in Treatment of Social Phobia

Reference	Design	N	Treatments studied and drug dose	Outcome
Bisserbe et al. (1994)	Open trial	35	Moclobemide, 300–600 mg per day	At week 4, 29% (8/28) rated as improved; at week 8, 50% (12/24) improved; at week 12, 94% (17/18) improved.
Gelernter et al. (1991)	Placebo-controlled, and each pill group received self-exposure instructions	65	Alprazolam, 2.1–6.3 mg per day; phenelzine, 30–90 mg per day; cognitive-behavioral therapy (CBT)	On self-ratings, all treatments equally effective, with phenelzine superior on one scale; on physician ratings, phenelzine superior to alprazolam and placebo (CBT not rated); at follow-up, phenelzine and CBT maintained efficacy; alprazolam and placebo associated with relapse.
Humble et al. (1992)	Placebo-controlled	77	Brofaromine, dose not reported	79% of patients on brofaromine were much or very much improved on CGI at week 12, compared at 26% patients on placebo.
Liebowitz et al. (1986)	Open trial	11	Phenelzine, 45–90 mg per day	64% (7/11) of patients markedly improved; 36% (4/11) moderately improved.
Liebowitz et al. (1992)	Placebo-controlled	74	Phenelzine, 45–90 mg per day; atenolol, 50–100 mg per day	64% (16/25) of patients on phenelzine, 30% (7/23) on atenolol, and 23% (6/23) on placebo improved at week 8.
Oberlander et al. (1994)	Open trial	11	Phenelzine, 45–105 mg per day	Improvement in social anxiety symptoms; variable improvement in underlying physical pathology, depending on type.
van Vliet et al. (1992)	Placebo-controlled	30	Brofaromine, 150 mg per day	80% (12/14) of patients on brofaromine improved, and 14% (2/14) on placebo improved.
Versiani et al. (1988)	Open trial	32	Tranylcypromine, 40–60 mg per day	62% (18/29) had marked responses, 17% (5/29) had moderate response, and one patient had no response.
Versiani et al. (1989)	Open trial	81	Tranylcypromine, 40–60 mg per day	CGI Severity at baseline was 5.2 (mean); at week 8, 1.5 (mean); % response not given.
Versiani et al. (1992)	Placebo-controlled	78	Moclobemide, 100–600 mg per day; phenelzine, 15–90 mg per day	At week 8, mean CGI Severity scores were 1.5, 2.4, and 4.1 for phenelzine, moclobemide, and placebo, respectively; response rates not provided; moclobemide and phenelzine both superior to placebo on two main clinician-rated social phobia scales.

343

Moclobemide is now available for use in most countries, but not in the United States. Brofaromine is not available because its manufacturer has withdrawn the drug from worldwide clinical investigation for reasons unrelated to its efficacy in social phobia.

BETA BLOCKERS

Nonclinical Populations

A variety of studies have been conducted using beta blockers in volunteers with performance-related social anxiety. Drugs that have been studied include propranolol (Inderal), nadolol (Corgard), alprenolol, oxprenolol, and pindolol (Visken). These studies have focused on performance anxiety but not necessarily in people meeting diagnostic criteria for social phobia. While some physical symptoms, for example, sweating and palpitations, may be reduced by beta blockers, other symptoms, such as anticipatory anxiety, phobic avoidance, blushing, and cognitive symptoms, are not believed to be significantly ameliorated by these drugs. It is unclear to what extent symptomatic volunteers studied in earlier investigations may have been troubled by this broader symptom complex. As will be discussed later on, more recent controlled studies in patients with social phobia have not shown favorable results for beta blockers. Results of studies in nonclinical performance anxiety populations are displayed in Table 14.2.

Clinical Populations

In 1981, Falloon, Lloyd, and Harpin conducted a study of social skills training (SST) with either propranolol or placebo, administered double-blind. Their study found no difference between SST–propranolol and SST–placebo, but it suffered from a relatively small sample and lack of a drug-only group. More recent studies have evaluated the beta blocker atenolol in treatment-seeking patients with a DSM-III-R diagnosis of social phobia. Atenolol was selected because of its poor ability to penetrate the blood–brain barrier, thereby providing a test of the hypothesis that its benefits may be due to peripheral effects. It might also be less likely to have depression-inducing side effects than do more centrally active beta blockers, such as propranolol.

Gorman, Liebowitz, Fyer, Campeas, and Klein (1985) reported an open trial of atenolol in 10 patients with social phobia. Doses ranged from 50 to 100 mg per day. Five patients exhibited a marked reduction in social phobia symptoms, and four exhibited a moderate reduction, based upon physician and patient assessment.

In the above mentioned double-blind trial of phenelzine, atenolol, and placebo, Liebowitz et al. (1992) found phenelzine to be more effective than was atenolol in relieving symptoms. Unfortunately, the numbers were too small to compare the results of each treatment convincingly in the two social phobia subtypes. One would conclude from this study that the effects of atenolol were modest at best and not significantly different from placebo.

Turner, Beidel, and Jacob (1994) reported a study comparing atenolol at dosages of 25–100 mg per day to flooding and placebo in social phobia, diagnosed according to DSM-III-R criteria. Seventy-two patients were enrolled into this 12-week study. Comorbid diagnoses were present as follows: dysthymia (39%), generalized anxiety disorder (39%), and avoidant personality disorder or obsessive–compulsive personality disorder (35%). Behavior therapy patients were seen for 90 minutes once or twice per week, for a total of 20 sessions. Sessions 1–16 comprised therapist-assisted *in vivo* and imaginal exposure. Sessions 17–20 were therapist-directed, but not accompanied, individualized *in vivo* homework assignments, used to transition patients into assuming responsibility for continued exposure.

Results showed flooding to be consistently superior to atenolol, which was not statistically superior to placebo. On a composite index of improvement, patients who received flooding were moderately or significantly improved in 89% of cases, atenolol patients were improved in 47%, and placebo patients were improved in 44%. This study sample exhibited high comorbidity, but it is unclear to what extent it differs in this respect from most other clinical trials of social phobia, which have generally failed to report comorbid diagnoses.

Summary of Studies

Results of beta blocker studies in nonclinical and clinical samples are presented in Tables 14.2 and 14.3, respectively. Atenolol has been the most studied drug overall, with encouraging results from one open trial. However, two recent double-blind studies, controlled against placebo and other active treatments, have failed to demonstrate convincingly positive effects for atenolol. It is still possible that certain individuals respond well to a beta blocker over the long term, and it is also possible that some individuals may benefit from intermittent use of a beta blocker in specific performance situations. Propranolol is the beta blocker most commonly used in this way.

BENZODIAZEPINES

Alprazolam (Xanax)

To date there have been two open trials with alprazolam (Lydiard, Laraia, Howell, & Ballenger, 1988; Reich & Yates, 1988) and one controlled study (Gelernter et al., 1991) in patients with social phobia.

TABLE 14.2. Studies of Beta Blockers in Nonclinical Performance Populations

Reference	Design	N	Drugs studied and dose	Population	Outcome
Brantigan, & Joseph (1982)	Placebo-controlled crossover of a single dose	29	Propanolol, 40 mg	Musicians	Decreased heart rate, no statistically significant change in performance.
Drew et al. (1983)	Placebo-controlled crossover of a single dose	35	Propanolol, 120 mg	Students taking a test	Improvement in both mental and verbal skills.
Gates et al. (1985)	Placebo-controlled crossover of a single dose	34	Nadolol, 20 mg, 40 mg, and 80 mg	Singers	Decreased heart rate.
Hartley et al. (1983)	Placebo-controlled crossover of a single dose	16	Propanolol, 40 mg	Speakers	Decreased heart rate.
James & Savage (1984)	Placebo-controlled crossover of a single dose	31	Nadolol, 40 mg; diazepam, 2 mg	Musicians	Decreased heart rate with nadolol, no reduction in anxiety with either drug.
James et al. (1983)	Placebo-controlled crossover of a single dose	30	Pindolol, 5 mg	Musicians	Decreased heart rate, subjective improvement in performance.
James et al. (1977)	Placebo-controlled crossover of a single dose	24	Oxprenolol, 40 mg	Musicians	No change in heart rate, reduced overt "nervousness."
Liden & Gottfries (1974)	Placebo-controlled crossover of a single dose	11	Alprenolol, 50–100 mg	Musicians	Subjectively decreased performance anxiety.
Neftel et al. (1982)	Placebo-controlled	22	Atenolol, 100 mg	Musicians	Decreased heart rate.
Siitonen & Janne (1976)	Placebo-controlled crossover of a single dose	17	Oxprenolol, 40 mg	Bowlers	No improvement in bowling scores.

TABLE 14.3. Studies of Beta Blockers in Treatment of Social Phobia

Reference	Design	N	Treatments studied and drug dose	Outcome
Gorman et al. (1985)	Open trial	10	Atenolol, 50–100 mg per day	Five showed marked, four moderate, and one, no improvement.
Falloon et al. (1981)	Placebo-controlled; all patients received social skills training	16	Propranolol, 160–320 mg per day	Both groups improved, but no difference between propanolol and placebo.
Liebowitz et al. (1992)	Placebo-controlled	74	Atenolol, 50–100 mg per day; phenelzine, 45–90 mg per day	At week 8, 30% (7/23) on atenolol, 64% (16/25) on phenelzine, and 23% (6/26) on placebo improved.
Turner et al. (1994)	Placebo-controlled	72	Atenolol, 25–100 mg per day; flooding	At week 8, 47% improvement on atenolol, 44% improvement on placebo, and 89% improvement on flooding.

Lydiard et al. (1988) described four patients treated with alprazolam between 3 and 8 mg per day. All four patients showed a marked reduction in their symptomatology and a resolution of their avoidant behaviors, but no mention was made of treatment duration or speed of recovery.

Reich and Yates (1988) treated 14 patients over 8 weeks. Additional Axis I diagnoses included major depression (n = 6), dysthymia (n = 1), and simple phobia (n = 5). The mean dose of alprazolam at week 8 was 2.9 mg per day (range = 1−7 mg per day), with 11 of 14 patients receiving no more than 3 mg per day. Ten patients were very much improved and 4 were much improved on the CGI, yielding an overall improvement rate of 100%. One week after the drug was discontinued, no significant differences were seen on any rating scale relative to baseline, demonstrating that symptoms had returned. Principal side effects were sedation and mild disinhibition, which responded to dose adjustment.

Gelernter et al. (1991) compared phenelzine, alprazolam, placebo, and CBT as described above. Mean alprazolam dose was 4.2 mg per day (SD = 1.3). This double-blind study found a 38% response rate with alprazolam based on FQ scores and a weakly significant effect for alprazolam relative to placebo on the physician-rated measure of work and social adjustment. Following discontinuation of alprazolam, symptoms had generally returned at 2-month follow-up, implying that the reappearance of anxiety was not merely related to benzodiazepine withdrawal. The incidence of side effects was not reported in this study.

Clonazepam (Klonopin)

Clonazepam has been evaluated in a number of studies. Versiani et al. (1989) treated 40 social phobic patients with clonazepam over an 8-week period. At week 8, the mean dose was 3.8 mg per day (SD = 0.5). Statistically significant lowering of the CGI Severity and LSAS scales were noted at week 8 relative to baseline. Mean CGI scores were 5.0 (SD = 0.6) at baseline and 2.1 (SD = 1.1) at week 8. Baseline LSAS was 81.6 (SD = 16.5), and week 8 LSAS was 31.6 (SD = 21.5). The most common side effects from clonazepam were sleepiness (67%), loss of libido (67%), and memory problems (35%).

Munjack, Baltazar, Bohn, Cabe, and Appleton (1990) studied 23 patients with generalized social phobia who received clonazepam or no treatment for 8 weeks. Twenty-three patients entered this study, of whom 3 dropped out in the initial treatment phase for a variety of reasons. Twenty patients completed treatment, with the two treatment groups being matched for baseline severity of social phobia. Of the 10 clonazepam patients, 3 were very much improved, 3 much improved, 3 minimally improved, and 1 unchanged. On the self-rated CGI, marked improvement occurred in 1 patient, moderate improvement in 8 patients and little improvement in 1 patient. In the 10 patients who were assigned to the no-treatment control, 1 was markedly improved, 1 was mildly improved on the clinician-rated CGI, and 1 patient was improved on the self-rated CGI. Significant treatment effects were observed within the clonazepam group from baseline to week 8 on the LSAS, SAD, and FNE. Principal side effects were sedation (70%), irritability (20%), and incoordination (20%). The following side effects occurred in 10% of subjects (1 instance each): derealization, encopresis, weakness, ataxia, memory impairment, lightheadedness, middle insomnia, and polydipsia.

Ontiveros and Fontaine (1990) treated five social phobic patients with clonazepam. By week 8, one patient was very much improved and four patients were much improved on the CGI. The only side effect was mild drowsiness, seen in two patients. No follow-up data were available following discontinuation of clonazepam, except for one person who remained symptom free over the next year.

Reiter, Pollack, Rosenbaum, and Cohen (1990) treated 11 social phobic patients with clonazepam at a dose range of 0.75 to 3 mg per day (mean = 1.7 mg). Eighty-two percent (9 of 11) showed some degree of improvement, 6 of whom achieved very much improvement, 1 much improvement, and 2 minimal improvement. No data were provided with regard to duration of treatment, side effects, or discontinuation.

Davidson, Ford, Smith, and Potts (1991) reported an open trial of clonazepam in 26 patients with social phobia. Treatment continued for an average of 11.3 months, with a range of 1 to 20 months, and maximum doses varied from 0.5 to 5.0 mg per day, with a mean of 2.1 mg per day. At the time of taper from clonazepam, 42% of patients (11 of 26) were very much improved, 42% (11 of 26) were much improved, and 15% (4 of 26) were minimally or not improved. The most common side effects were sedation/tiredness (27%), memory or concentration problems (15%), coordination problems (12%), sexual impairment (12%), blurred vision (8%), and weight gain (8%). For the 15 patients who experienced adverse reactions, dose reduction attenuated the intensity of these events.

This open long-term study was followed by a 10-week double-blind placebo-controlled evaluation of clonazepam in 75 patients with social phobia (Davidson et al., 1993). A number of different clinician ratings and patient self-ratings were used, including the CGI, LSAS, and Hamilton Depression Scale, as well as the FNE, FQ, and SDS. Response was generally fully evident by week 6, although a number of statistically significant differences were observed as early as week 2. At the end of treatment, 78% of patients had responded to clonazepam versus 20% to placebo, according to the CGI. Drug effects were observed on all of the above-mentioned symptom-rating scales, except for the Hamilton Depression Scale.

Side effects were measured by means of a 35-item self-rated checklist (Davidson et al., 1990), which compared clonazepam to placebo on the basis of "anytime" increase relative to baseline. The following treatment-emergent symptoms occurred more frequently with clonazepam: anorgasmia (44% vs. 6%), unsteadiness (62% vs. 20%), forgetfulness (44% vs. 20%), and impaired concentration (35% vs. 15%).

Bromazepam

Versiani et al. (1989) reported the use of bromazepam, which is not currently available in the United States, for treating patients with social phobia. In an open trial with 10 patients, bromazepam was given for 8 weeks at an average daily dose of 26.4 mg per day (*SD* = 4.9). Statistically significant reductions in scores on the CGI, LSAS, Hamilton Anxiety Scale, and SDS were all seen at week 8 relative to placebo. CGI Severity improved from a baseline mean of 5.0 (*SD* = 0.8) to a final visit mean of 1.3 (*SD* = 0.5). The LSAS was reduced from a baseline mean of 69.3 (*SD* = 20.5) to a final visit mean of 15.8 (*SD* = 9.1). The most frequent side effects were sleepiness (100%) and memory problems (40%).

Summary of Studies

Results of benzodiazepine studies in social phobia are presented in Table 14.4. In two open trials, alprazolam has demonstrated successful reduction of symptoms, having a relatively rapid onset of action within the first 2 weeks. Unfortunately, both open trials of alprazolam produced a high relapse rate once the medication was stopped, as also was found in the placebo-controlled trial by Gelernter et al. (1991). In the Gelernter et al. study, alprazolam had effects that were marginal at best. The initial success of clonazepam in open trials was confirmed by Davidson et al. (1993) in their double-blind study. Bromazepam was effective in one open study by Versiani et al. (1989). The small sample and limited results allow us to draw no more than tentative conclusions as to the drug's effectiveness, and it is presently unavailable in the United States. With regard to benzodiazepines, further studies are clearly indicated: It is our sense that clonazepam is a highly effective compound in this group of patients. Benzodiazepines need to be evaluated over a longer period of maintenance therapy, followed by slow double-blind placebo substitution and taper. It is presently

TABLE 14.4. Studies of Benzodiazepines in Treatment of Social Phobia

Reference	Design	N	Treatments studied and drug dose	Outcome
Davidson et al. (1991)	Open trial	26	Clonazepam, 1–3 mg per day	85% (22/26) of patients improved.
Davidson et al. (1993)	Placebo-controlled	75	Clonazepam, 1–3 mg per day	On clonazepam, 78% (29/37) improved, while only 20% (7/35) on placebo improved.
Gelernter et al. (1991)	Placebo-controlled with each pill group receiving self-exposure instructions	65	Alprazolam, 2.1–6.3 mg per day; phenelzine, 30–90 mg per day; cognitive-behavioral therapy (CBT)	On self-ratings, all treatments equally effective, with phenelzine superior on one scale; on physician ratings, phenelzine superior to alprazolam and placebo (CBT not rated); at follow-up, phenelzine and CBT maintained efficacy; alprazolam and placebo associated with relapse.
Lydiard et al. (1988)	Open trial	4	Alprazolam, 3–8 mg per day	All (4/4) cases improved.
Munjack et al. (1990)	No-treatment control	20	Clonazepam, 1–6 mg per day	On clonazepam, 60% (6/10) improved, while only 10% (1/10) of control group improved.
Ontiveros & Fontaine (1990)	Open trial	5	Clonazepam, 2–4 mg per day	All (5/5) cases improved.
Reich & Yates (1988)	Open trial	14	Alprazolam, 1–7 mg per day	All (14/14) cases were moderately to markedly improved.
Reiter et al. (1990)	Open trial	11	Clonazepam, 0.75–3 mg per day	85% (9/11) of cases improved.
Versiani et al. (1989)	Open trial	10	Clonazepam, mean dose 3.8 mg per day; bromazepam, mean dose 26.4 mg per day	CGI Severity for clonazepam at baseline was 5.0 (mean); at week 8, 2.1 (mean); response rate not given. CGI Severity for bromazepam at baseline was 5.0 (mean); at week 8, 1.3 (mean); response rate not given.

unknown to what extent benzodiazepines can be combined with cognitive-behavioral treatments or whether they potentiate or detract from the effects of CBT.

SELECTIVE SEROTONIN REUPTAKE INHIBITORS

Fluoxetine (Prozac)

Sternbach (1990) described the successful use of fluoxetine (Prozac) in two social phobic patients. In the first patient, lorazepam (Ativan) and amitriptyline (Elavil) had recently been discontinued because of alcohol abuse and side effects. The patient was started on fluoxetine at 20 mg every other day and increasing up to 40 mg per day after 2 weeks. Five weeks into treatment, a marked reduction of symptoms was noted. The second patient had failed to respond to 2 years of psychodynamic and behavioral therapy but showed a 90% reduction in symptoms after being started and maintained on 20 mg per day fluoxetine.

Schneier, Chin, Hollander, and Liebowitz (1992) assessed the response of 12 patients who had been treated with fluoxetine. The starting dose was 20 mg per day in 8 patients, 10 mg per day in 3 patients, and 5 mg per day in 1 patient. The CGI improvement rate was 67% ($n = 8$) much or very much improved. In two patients, prior treatment with propranolol and alprazolam had proven ineffective, and in another case, methylphenidate (Ritalin) was added to reverse the sedation that fluoxetine produced. Duration of improvement ranged from 6 weeks to 5 months. Responders and nonresponders had similar mean daily doses of fluoxetine, 25.8 mg per day and 25.0 mg per day, respectively. The effects of prior drug treatment were briefly examined. In three instances, fluoxetine was as effective as phenelzine had been in the past without as many side effects. In several fluoxetine responders, previous treatment with benzodiazepines, buspirone, or beta blockers had been ineffective.

Black, Uhde, and Tancer (1992) studied 14 patients with generalized social phobia. Fluoxetine was given at doses ranging from 10 to 100 mg per day (mean = 41.4 mg per day). Of these 14 patients, 4 had concurrent panic disorder, and one each had atypical depression, dysthymic disorder, and somatization disorder. Seventy-one percent (10 of 14) showed moderate or marked improvement on fluoxetine on the SPDSC (Liebowitz et al., 1986). Three of 4 patients who were on another anxiolytic medication improved and, within this group, 2 of 3 responders were on benzodiazepines. In these cases, improvement may have been due to fluoxetine-induced increases in serum benzodiazepine levels as opposed to a primary effect of fluoxetine. Three patients who had previously shown a good response to phenelzine were entered into this study, of whom 2 reported fluoxetine to be as effective as phenelzine had been. The third patient, who had previously responded to phenelzine, reported less marked symptom reduction on fluoxetine but was unable to tolerate more than 10 mg per day fluoxetine due to akathisia. With regard to side effects from fluoxetine, 2 patients were not able to tolerate higher doses because of akathisia, 1 was discontinued because of alopecia, 1 patient's dose had to be titrated upward slowly because of diarrhea, and 1 patient's dose had to be titrated slowly because of headaches and nausea.

Van Ameringen, Mancini, and Streiner (1993) reported on 16 patients who received fluoxetine at doses ranging from 20 to 60 mg per day. Most patients also had a comorbid diagnosis of another anxiety or affective disorder, and all suffered from generalized social phobia. The authors rated clinical improvement on the basis of an 11-point CGI, ranging from -5 (severe deterioration) to $+5$ (greatest improvement). A patient was judged to be a responder if he or she exhibited moderate, large, or great improvement. Because of the construction of this scale, it is difficult to compare against the conventional 7-point CGI that has been used in most other trials. Of the 16 patients who entered the study, 3 dropped out early because of side effects. Using their own criteria, the authors classified 10 of the 13 (76.9%) completing patients as responders and 3 (23.1%) as nonresponders. Of the 10 responders, 2 were greatly improved, 6 exhibited large improvement, and 2 showed moderate improvement. Response was seen at 4 weeks in three instances, at 8 weeks in five instances and at 12 weeks in one instance. The mean time until response was approximately 7 weeks. Although social phobia was felt to be the primary diagnosis at the time of study enrollment, the improvement seen in these 10 patients may have been secondary to improvement in their comorbid diagnoses. Against this is the fact that depression ratings and global phobic avoidance did not show a significant difference from baseline to finish, while social phobia scores were lowered.

Fluvoxamine (Luvox)

den Boer, van Vliet, and Westenberg (1994) reported on a placebo-controlled 12-week study using fluvoxamine in 30 patients who met DSM-III-R criteria for social phobia. Dosage started at 50 mg per day for the first week, and gradually increased up to 150 mg per day. Treatment efficacy was measured using the LSAS, SCL-90, Hamilton Anxiety Scale, and STAI. One patient in the fluvoxamine group dropped out due to nausea, and one patient on placebo dropped out due to lack of efficacy. At 12 weeks, fluvoxamine-treated patients showed statistically significant improvement on all scales relative to the placebo group. After the initial 12-week period, patients were given the opportunity to continue on their current medication for a further 12 weeks. Fourteen of the 16 patients on fluvoxamine chose to continue. During this follow-up period, further improvement was seen in general anxiety and on both subscales of the LSAS.

Summary of Studies

The results of these open trials with fluoxetine in social phobia are reviewed in Table 14.5. At the present time, only one double-blind, placebo-controlled study has been reported using fluvoxamine. Most studies of SSRI treatment of social phobia are based on the use of fluoxetine, but ongoing studies are taking place with sertraline (Zoloft) and paroxetine (Paxil). There is no particular reason to expect major differences between the various SSRI drugs. The four open studies of fluoxetine reveal that substantial benefit occurred in 58–100% of patients with social phobia. While the Schneier series (Schneier et al. 1992) suggested that 20 mg per day is adequate for some social phobics, other reports indicate that higher doses may be needed. We do not yet know whether symptom improvement occurs as rapidly with SSRIs as it can with benzodiazepines or phenelzine.

OTHER MEDICATIONS

Buspirone (BuSpar)

Buspirone is a nonbenzodiazepine, azaspirone, anxiolytic with a different side-effect profile from benzodiazepines and no risk of inducing physical dependence.

Munjack et al. (1991) published an open trial of buspirone in 17 social phobic patients. Eleven of the 17 patients completed the 12-week trial, receiving an average dose of 48 mg per day (range 35–60 mg per day). The 6 patients who dropped out included 2 patients who never returned after enrollment, 2 who dropped out due to inability to meet the time commitment to the study, and 2 who had side effects. Of the remaining 11 patients, 6 reported a moderate reduction of symptoms at 4 weeks. At 8 weeks, 4 patients noted marked improvement, 5 noted moderate improvement, and 2 reported minimal improvement. The response rate of those who entered treatment was 53% (9 of 17).

TABLE 14.5. Studies of Selective Serotonin Reuptake Inhibitors in Treatment of Social Phobia

Reference	Design	N	Drugs studied and dose	Outcome
Black et al. (1992)	Open trial	14	Fluoxetine, 10–100 mg per day	71% (10/14) of patients improved.
den Boer et al. (1994)	Placebo-controlled	30	Fluvoxamine, 50–150 mg per day	At week 12, patients on fluvoxamine were significantly more improved on all scales compared to the placebo group.
Schneier et al. (1992)	Open trial	12	Fluoxetine, 20–80 mg per day	58% (7/12) of patients improved.
Sternbach (1990)	Open trial	2	Fluoxetine, 20–40 mg per day	Both (2/2) patients improved.
Van Ameringen et al. (1993)	Open trial	13	Fluoxetine, 20–60 mg per day	77% (10/13) of patients improved.

Schneier et al. (1993) treated 17 social phobic patients with buspirone in an open trial. Forty-seven percent (8 of 17) of patients were judged to be much or very much improved on the CGI at week 12. A post hoc assessment of responders and nonresponders showed that responders received a mean buspirone dose of 56.9 mg per day, compared to a mean dose of 38.3 mg per day for nonresponders. This would suggest that, provided patients can tolerate the drug, there is benefit from raising the dose to higher levels. It is also noted that patients showed maximum improvement by 4 weeks and that after that time no further change was observed.

Clark and Agras (1991) treated 34 social phobic performing musicians with buspirone and placebo, given double-blind, as well as CBT or no psychotherapy, in a 2 × 2 design. Their version of CBT was not identical to the treatment developed by Heimberg et al. (1990). The mean dose of buspirone in this 6-week trial was 32 mg per day (range 15−60 mg per day). The authors found buspirone to be not significantly different from placebo on objective and subjective measures, but CBT was significantly more effective than either buspirone or placebo−no psychotherapy. It is possible that the short duration and relatively low dose of buspirone made this an inadequate test of the drug.

Studies of buspirone in social phobia are summarized in Table 14.6. Overall, while buspirone may offer benefit in social phobia, the results appear to be neither as dramatic nor as consistently found as in other treatments described. The one controlled trial of buspirone failed to show significant improvement relative to placebo. The dose of buspirone needed to reduce fear and avoidance seems to be in the upper range, and this may be a limiting factor on the basis of side effects.

Tricyclic Antidepressants

Imipramine (Tofranil)

Imipramine appears to be less effective than phenelzine in reducing social phobic symptoms and interpersonal sensitivity in depression (Liebowitz et al., 1984; Zitrin, Klein, Woerner, & Ross, 1983). However, Benca, Matuzas, and Al-Sadir (1986) reported two social phobics who showed a rapid resolution of symptoms after 2 to 4 weeks of treatment with imipramine at 250 mg per day. Panic attacks were prominent features in their clinical picture, and they were also characterized by having mitral valve prolapse, rendering these patients rather atypical. Zitrin et al. (1983) found no improvement among patients with social phobia treated with imipramine or placebo.

TABLE 14.6. Studies of Buspirone in Treatment of Social Phobia

Reference	Design	N	Treatments studied and drug dose	Outcome
Clark & Agras (1991)	Partially double-blind 2 × 2 design: drug, placebo; CBT, no CBT	34	Buspirone, 15–60 mg per day	CBT + placebo, 100% improved; CBT + buspirone, 67% improved; buspirone, 57% improved; placebo, 60% improved.
Munjack et al. (1991)	Open trial	17	Buspirone, 35–60 mg per day	82% (9/11) of patients who completed study improved.
Schneier et al. (1993)	Open trial	17	Buspirone, 15–60 mg per day	47% (8/17) of patients improved; at doses of 45 mg per day or greater, 67% (8/12) improved.

Clomipramine (Anafranil)

Clomipramine has been studied by Beaumont (1977) and Pecknold, Mc-
Clure, Appeltauer, Allen, and Wrzesinski (1982). Beaumont found only
modest improvement in a mixed population of social phobic and agoraphobic patients. In the study by Pecknold et al., combined treatment with
clomipramine and L-tryptophan did not produce any greater improvement
than did clomipramine and placebo, thus suggesting that the additional
serotonergic input through L-tryptophan made little difference. However
this should not be construed as negating the possible importance of serotonergic mechanisms in social phobia.

Clonidine (Catapres)

The alpha-adrenergic agonist clonidine (Catapres) appears to be helpful
in patients with panic disorder and generalized anxiety disorder (Hoehn-
Saric, Merchant, Keyser, and Smith, 1981). Goldstein (1987) reported
one social phobic patient with severe blushing who did not respond to
propranolol, phenelzine, or alprazolam, but who responded rapidly and
effectively to clonidine. This drug deserves further study in social
phobia, since blushing is often reported to be a particularly troublesome
symptom.

Bupropion (Wellbutrin)

Emmanuel, Lydiard, and Ballenger (1991) reported beneficial effects of
bupropion (Wellbutrin) in one patient with social phobia. The drug was
given at 300 mg per day. Bupropion is devoid of serotonergic effects and
has a selective catecholaminergic action. One complicating factor in this
particular report was the comorbid occurrence of major depression. Our
personal experience with bupropion in a limited number of patients with
social phobia has not been encouraging.

SUMMARY

A number of studies in the literature now indicate the successful pharmacological treatment of social phobia with a wide range of drug classes. Nine
double-blind, placebo-controlled studies have now been completed. These
studies evaluated 8 drugs (phenelzine $n = 3$, moclobemide $n = 1$, brofaromine $n = 2$, clonazepam $n = 1$, alprazolam $n = 1$, atenolol $n = 2$,

fluvoxamine $n = 1$, buspirone $n = 1$). Positive results occurred in all three phenelzine trials, as well as in the published studies of moclobemide, brofaromine, fluvoxamine, and clonazepam. Alprazolam had, at best, equivocal effects in the only double-blind trial to date. Negative results occurred in both atenolol studies and in the study of buspirone. Other drugs, such as imipramine, clomipramine, fluoxetine, tranylcypromine, bromazepam, bupropion, and clonidine have been reported as benefiting some patients with social phobia, although these conclusions are based upon case reports or open clinical trials in generally small samples.

The MAOIs, especially phenelzine, have been the most extensively studied and appear to be the most efficacious medications in social phobia, possibly along with clonazepam. Disadvantages of the older nonselective, irreversible MAOIs involve the risk of life-threatening side effects, i.e., hypertensive crisis, other troublesome side effects, and the dietary and medication restrictions that must be followed to avoid such an event and that may lead to poor compliance. RIMAs hold out the promise for safer and more acceptable pharmacotherapy in social phobia, as compared to phenelzine and tranylcypromine, although their effectiveness may be somewhat less than the nonselective MAOIs.

Beta blockers have been widely studied and appear to be disappointing in recent controlled trials. However, they do remain a popular standby for intermittent use in advance of public presentations or performances by musicians, students, and so on. It is possible that they are reasonably effective in discrete social phobia or in any person who experiences distressing, sympathetically mediated anxiety symptoms prior to some form of public presentation.

With regard to benzodiazepines, clonazepam has proven effective in one study, and alprazolam of questionable benefit in one study. Whether the two drugs are really different in their effects needs further examination. It is possible that study design and/or sampling factors may explain the discrepancy. Both studies have shown a high relapse rate in symptomatology once medication was discontinued. In the double-blind trial of clonazepam, there was a 71% relapse rate 4 weeks after termination, which included a 2-week drug taper and a 2-week medication-free follow-up period. However, it is our impression that the rate of taper, as well as the time of taper, may be important factors with regard to relapse rates and withdrawal symptoms.

The SSRIs appear to offer potential for symptom relief in social phobia without serious side effects and are much better tolerated than are the older generation MAOIs. They also seem to be more easily tolerated by social phobic patients than by those with panic disorder (Schneier et al., 1992). More placebo-controlled, double-blind studies are needed to demonstrate the benefit of SSRIs.

FUTURE RESEARCH DIRECTIONS
AND CLINICAL CONSIDERATIONS

Over the past 10 years, our knowledge of the pharmacotherapy of social phobia has grown, and it now leads us to consider further important but unstudied areas. Little is known about who is most likely to respond to a particular treatment. The issue of predictors can now be studied, as data have accumulated on a substantial number of patients. With clonazepam, for example, we have demonstrated that patients are less likely to respond well if they have a greater number of comorbid disorders and higher initial severity of symptoms on the LSAS (Davidson, Tupler, & Potts, 1994).

A second question arises from the fact that behavioral inhibition and social avoidance in childhood are often associated with social phobia during adolescence or early adulthood. We can ask, therefore, whether early recourse to pharmacotherapy might help to prevent the development of more pervasive and disabling social phobic states in later life. The long-term repercussions of such intervention at an early point would have significant implications both for individual life satisfaction and more general socioeconomic status.

We must determine for how long pharmacotherapy needs to be given and at what rate discontinuation might be undertaken. Could relapse rates be somewhat less after a period of prolonged, successful pharmacotherapy that has allowed the individual to make a much more successful adjustment to life? Is cognitive behavioral treatment important in this context? So far, the clinical data reviewed in this chapter find a relatively high relapse rate following discontinuation of benzodiazepines and MAOIs within 4 months of initiating treatment. Would this still be the case after 2 years of successful treatment?

Studies examining the combined effects of pharmacotherapy and psychosocial treatments are limited (Clark & Agras, 1991; Falloon et al., 1981). Little is known about the benefits or effects of combining the two treatments, especially in generalized social phobia, which is seen more frequently in clinical settings than is the discrete subtype.

Finally, is there any reason to suggest differential drug effectiveness in the social phobia subtypes? Perhaps beta blockers are more effective in discrete social phobia than in generalized social phobia. On the other hand, when buspirone is effective, perhaps its success is more apparent in generalized social phobia than in discrete social phobia. There is little evidence that buspirone can be used effectively on an as-needed basis, and the same must be said for SSRI and MAOI drugs.

When pharmacotherapy is under consideration, the clinician must always consider the relevance of concomitant medical and psychiatric illnesses, issues of compliance, and how possible side effects are likely to affect the patient. With regard to social phobia, the use of benzodiazepines must be weighed against any history of prior substance abuse. Tricyclic antidepressants are often poorly tolerated by social phobic individuals who are distressed by dry mouth, sweating, or tremor when speaking in front of others. It is also important to consider whether medication needs to be taken on a continual basis or an as-needed basis, and whether or not medication should be prescribed for a short-term or long-term basis. Overall, the goals of pharmacotherapy for social phobia can be summarized as (1) to lessen anticipatory and actual fear of social situations; (2) to reduce physiological symptoms, such as blushing, sweating, and trembling; (3) to decrease avoidance; (4) to reduce maladaptive cognitive distortions; and (5) to treat associated comorbidity. These issues are important in selecting a particular drug, and will be expanded upon in greater detail by Liebowitz and Marshall (Chapter 15, this volume).

REFERENCES

American Psychiatric Association. (1980). *Diagnostic and statistical manual of mental disorders* (3rd ed.). Washington, DC: Author.

American Psychiatric Association. (1987). *Diagnostic and statistical manual of mental disorders* (3rd ed., rev.). Washington, DC: Author.

Beaumont, G. (1977). A large open multicenter trial of clomipramine in the management of phobic disorders. *Journal of International Medical Research, 5*(Suppl. 5), 116–129.

Beck, A. T., Ward, C. H., Mendelson, M., Mock, J., & Erbaugh, J. (1961). An inventory for measuring depression. *Archives of General Psychiatry, 4*, 561–571.

Benca, R., Matuzas, W., & Al-Sadir, J. (1986). Social phobia, MVP, and response to imipramine. *Journal of Clinical Psychopharmacology, 6*, 50–51.

Bisserbe, J. C., Lepine, J. P., & G. R. P. Group. (1994). Moclobemide in social phobia. *Clinical Neuropharmacology, 17*(Suppl. 1), 88–94.

Black, B., Uhde, T. W., & Tancer, M. E. (1992). Fluoxetine for the treatment of social phobia. *Journal of Clinical Psychopharmacology, 12*, 293–295.

Brantigan, C. O., Brantigan, T. A., & Joseph, N. (1982). Effects of beta-blockade and beta-stimulation on stage fright. *American Journal of Medicine, 72*, 88–94.

Clark, D. B., & Agras, W. S. (1991). The assessment and treatment of performance anxiety in musicians. *American Journal of Psychiatry, 148*, 598–605.

Davidson, J. R. T., Ford, S. M., Smith, R. D., & Potts, N. L. S. (1991). Long-term treatment of social phobia with clonazepam. *Journal of Clinical Psychiatry, 52*(11, Suppl.), 16–20.

Davidson, J. R. T., Kudler, H. S., Smith, R. D., Mahorney, S. L., Lipper, S. L., Hammett, E. B., Saunders, W. B., & Cavenar J. O. (1990). Treatment of posttraumatic stress disorder with amitriptyline and placebo. *Archives of General Psychiatry, 4*, 259–269.

Davidson, J. R. T., Potts, N. L. S., Richichi, E., Krishnan, K. R. R., Ford, S. M., Smith, R., & Wilson, W. H. (1993). Treatment of social phobia with clonazepam and placebo. *Journal of Clinical Psychopharmacology, 13*, 423–429.

Davidson, J. R. T., Tupler, L. A., & Potts, N. L. S. (1994) Treatment of social phobia with benzodiazepines. *Journal of Clinical Psychiatry, 55*(6, Suppl.), 28–32.

den Boer, J. A., van Vliet, I. M., & Westenberg, H. G. (1994). Recent advances in the psychopharmacology of social phobia. *Progress in Neuro-Psychopharmacology and Biological Psychiatry, 18,* 625–645.

Derogatis, L. R., Lipman, R. S., & Covi, L. (1973). SCL-90: An outpatient psychiatric rating scale. *Psychopharmacological Bulletin, 9,* 13–28.

Drew, P. J. T., Barnes, J. N., & Evans, S. J. W. (1983). The effect of acute B-adrenoceptor blockade on examination performance. *British Journal of Psychiatry, 19,* 782–786.

Emmanuel, N. P., Lydiard, R. B., & Ballenger, J. C. (1991). Treatment of social phobia with bupropion. *Journal of Clinical Psychopharmacology, 11,* 276–277.

Fahlen, T., & Nilsson, H. L. (1992, May). *Social phobia, personality traits and brofaromine.* Paper presented at the 145th annual meeting of the American Psychiatric Association, Washington DC.

Falloon, I. R., Lloyd, G. G., & Harpin, R. (1981). The treatment of social phobia: Real-life rehearsal with non-professional therapists. *Journal of Nervous and Mental Disease, 169,* 180–184.

Gates, G. A., Saegert, J., Wilson, N., Johnson, L., Shepherd, A., & Hearne, E. M. (1985). Effect of beta-blockade on singing performance. *Annals of Otolology, Rhinology and Laryngology, 94,* 570–574.

Gelernter, C. S., Uhde, T. W., Cimbolic, P., Arnkoff, D. B., Vittone, B. J., Tancer, M. E., & Bartko, J. J. (1991). Cognitive-behavioral and pharmacological treatments of social phobia: A controlled study. *Archives of General Psychiatry, 38,* 938–945.

Goldstein, S. (1987). Treatment of social phobia with clonidine. *Biological Psychiatry, 22,* 369–372.

Gorman, J. M., Liebowitz, M. R., Fyer, A. J., Campeas, R., & Klein, D. F. (1985). Treatment of social phobia with atenolol. *Journal of Clinical Psychopharmacology, 5,* 298–301.

Guy, W. (1976). *ECDEU Assessment Manual for Psychopharmacology* (rev.). Rockville, MD: U.S. Department of Health, Education and Welfare.

Hamilton, M. (1959). The measurement of anxiety states by rating. *British Journal of Medical Psychology, 32,* 50–55.

Hamilton, M. (1960). A rating scale for depression. *Journal of Neurology, Neurosurgery and Psychiatry, 23,* 56–62.

Hartley, L. R., Ungapen, S., Davie, I., & Spencer, D. J. (1983). The effect of beta adrenergic blockade on speaker's performance and memory. *British Journal of Psychiatry, 142,* 512–517.

Heimberg, R. G., Dodge, C. S., Hope, D. A., Kennedy, C. R., Zollo, L. J., & Becker, R. E. (1990). Cognitive behavioral group treatment for social phobia: Comparison with a credible placebo control. *Cognitive Therapy and Research, 14,* 1–23.

Hoehn-Saric, R., Merchant, A. F., Keyser, M. L., & Smith, V. K. (1981). Effects of clonidine on anxiety disorders. *Archives of General Psychiatry, 38,* 1278–1282.

Humble, M., Fahlen, T., Koczkas, C., & Nilsson, H. L. (1992, May). *Social phobia: Efficacy of brofaromine vs. placebo.* Paper presented at the 145th annual meeting of the American Psychiatric Association, Washington DC.

James, I. M., Burgoyne, W., & Savage, I. T. (1983). Effect of pindolol on stress-related disturbances of musical performance: Preliminary communication. *Journal of Royal Society of Medicine, 76,* 194–196.

James, I. M., Griffith, D. N., Pearson, R. M., & Newby, P. (1977). Effects of oxprenolol on stage fright in musicians. *Lancet, 2,* 952–954.

James, I. M., & Savage, I. T. (1984). Beneficial effect of nadolol on anxiety-induced disturbances of performance in musicians: A comparison with diazepam and placebo. *American Heart Journal, 108,* 1150–1155.

Kendall, P. C., & Grove, W. M. (1988). Normative comparisons in therapy outcomes. *Behavioral Assessment, 10,* 147–158.

Liden, S., & Gottfries, C. G. (1974). Beta-blocking agents in the treatment of catecholamine-induced symptoms in musicians. *Lancet, 2,* 529.

Liebowitz, M. R. (1987). Social phobia. *Modern Problems of Pharmacopsychiatry, 22,* 141–173.

Liebowitz, M. R., Fyer, A. J., Gorman, J. M., Campeas, R., & Levin, A. (1986). Phenelzine in social phobia. *Journal of Clinical Psychopharmacology, 6,* 93–98.

Liebowitz, M. R., Quitkin, F. M., Steward, J. W., McGrath, P. J., Harrison, W., Rabkin, J., Tricamo, E., Markowitz, J. S., & Klein, D. F. (1984). Phenelzine versus imipramine in atypical depression: A preliminary report. *Archives of General Psychiatry, 44,* 669–677.

Liebowitz, M. R., Schneier, F. R., Campeas, R., Hollander, E., Hatterer, J., Fyer, A., Gorman, J., Papp, L., Davies, S., Gully, R., & Klein, D. F. (1992). Phenelzine vs atenolol in social phobia: A placebo-controlled comparison. *Archives of General Psychiatry, 49,* 290–300.

Lydiard, R. B., Laraia, M. T., Howell, E. F., & Ballenger, J. C. (1988). Alprazolam in the treatment of social phobia. *Journal of Clinical Psychiatry, 49,* 17–19.

Marks, I. M., & Mathews, A. M. (1979). Brief standard self-rating for phobic patients. *Behaviour Research and Therapy, 17,* 263–267.

Mizes, J. S., & Crawford, J. (1986). Normative values on the Marks and Mathews Fear Questionnaire: A comparison as a function of age and sex. *Journal of Psychopathology and Behavioral Assessment, 8,* 253–262.

Mountjoy, C. Q., Roth, M., Garside, R. F., & Leitch, I. M. (1977). A clinical trial of phenelzine in anxiety, depressive and phobic neurosis. *British Journal of Psychiatry, 131,* 486–492.

Munjack, D. J., Baltazar, P. L., Bohn, P. B., Cabe, D. D., & Appleton, A. A. (1990). Clonazepam in the treatment of social phobia: A pilot study. *Journal of Clinical Psychiatry, 51*(Suppl. 5), 35–40.

Munjack, D. J., Burns, J., Baltazar, P. L., Brown, R., Leonard, M., Nagy, R., Koek, R., Crocker, B., & Schafer, S. (1991). A pilot study of buspirone in the treatment of social phobia. *Journal of Anxiety Disorders, 5,* 87–98.

Neftel, K. A., Adler, R. H., Kappell, L., Rossi, M., Kaser, H. E., Bruggesser, H. H., & Vorkauf, H. (1982). Stage fright in musicians: A model illustrating the effects of beta-blockers. *Psychosomatic Medicine, 44,* 461–469.

Oberlander, E. L., Schneier, F. R., & Liebowitz, M. R. (1994). Physical disability and social phobia. *Journal of Clinical Psychopharmacology, 14,* 136–143.

Ontiveros, A., & Fontaine, R. (1990). Social phobia and clonazepam. *Canadian Journal of Psychiatry, 35,* 439–441.

Pecknold, J. C., McClure, D. J., Appeltauer, L., Allan, T., & Wrzesinski, L. (1982). Does tryptophan potentiate clomipramine in the treatment of agoraphobia and social phobic patients? *British Journal of Psychiatry, 140,* 484–490.

Reich, J. R., & Yates, W. (1988). A pilot study of treatment of social phobia with alprazolam. *American Journal of Psychiatry, 145,* 590–594.

Reiter, S. R., Pollack, M. H., Rosenbaum, J. F., & Cohen, L. S. (1990). Clonazepam for the treatment of social phobia. *Journal of Clinical Psychiatry, 51,* 470–472.

Schneier, F. R., Chin, S. J., Hollander, E., & Liebowitz, M. R. (1992). Fluoxetine in social phobia [Letter to the editor]. *Journal of Clinical Psychopharmacology, 12,* 62–63.

Schneier, F. R., Saoud, J. B., Campeas, R., Falloon, B., Hollander, E., Coplan, J., & Liebowitz, M. R. (1993). Buspirone in social phobia. *Journal of Clinical Psychopharmacology, 13,* 251–256.

Sheehan, D. (1984). *The anxiety disease.* New York: Scribner.

Siitonen, L., & Janne, J. (1976). Effect of beta-blockade during bowling competitions. *Annals of Clinical Research, 8,* 393–398.

Solyom, C., Solyom, L., LaPierre, Y. Pecknold, J., & Morton, L. (1981). Phenelzine and exposure in the treatment of phobias. *Biological Psychiatry, 16,* 239–247.

Solyom, L., Heseltine, G., McClure, D., Solyom, C., Ledwidge, B., & Steinberg, G. (1973). Behavior therapy versus drug therapy in the treatment of phobic neurosis. *Canadian Psychiatric Association Journal, 18,* 25–31.

Spielberger C .D., Gorsuch R. L., & Lushene R. E. (1970). *Manual for the State–Trait Anxiety Inventory.* Palo Alto, CA: Consulting Psychologist Press.

Sternbach, H. (1990). Fluoxetine treatment of social phobia. *Journal of Clinical Psychopharmacology, 10,* 230–231.

Turner, S. M., Biedel, D., & Jacob, R. G. (1994) Social phobia: A comparison of behavior therapy and atenolol. *Journal of Consulting and Clinical Psychology, 62,* 350–358.

Tyrer, P., Candy, J., & Kelly, D. (1973). A study of the clinical effects of phenelzine and placebo in the treatment of phobic anxiety. *Psychopharmacology, 32,* 237–254.

Van Ameringen, M.V., Mancini, C., & Streiner, D.L. (1993). Fluoxetine efficacy in social phobia. *Journal of Clinical Psychiatry, 54,* 27–32.

van Vliet, I. M., den Boer, J. A., & Westenberg, H. G. (1992). The pharmacotherapy of social phobia: Clinical and biochemical effects of brofaromine, a reversible MAO-A inhibitor. *European Neuropsychopharmacology, 2,* 21–29.

Versiani, M., Mundim, F. D., Nardi, A. E., & Liebowitz, M. R. (1988). Tranylcypromine in social phobia. *Journal of Clinical Psychopharmacology, 8,* 279–282.

Versiani, M., Nardi, A. E., & Mundim, F. D. (1989). Fobia social. *Jornal Brasileiro de Psiquiatria, 38,* 251–263.

Versiani, M., Nardi, A. E., Mundim, F. D., Alves, A. B., Liebowitz, M. R., & Amrein, R. (1992). Pharmacotherapy of social phobia: A controlled study with moclobemide and phenelzine. *British Journal of Psychiatry, 161,* 353–360.

Watson, D., & Friend, R. (1969). Measurement of social-evaluative anxiety. *Journal of Consulting and Clinical Psychology, 33,* 448–457.

Willoughby, R. R. (1932). Some properties of the Thurstone Personality Schedule and a suggested revision. *Journal of Social Psychology, 3,* 401–424.

Zitrin, C. M., Klein, D. F., Woerner, M. G., & Ross, D. (1983). Treatment of phobias: A comparison of imipramine and placebo. *Archives of General Psychiatry, 40,* 125–138.

CHAPTER FIFTEEN

Pharmacological Treatments: Clinical Applications

MICHAEL R. LIEBOWITZ
RANDALL D. MARSHALL

In comparison with other anxiety disorders, social phobia has only recently been recognized as amenable to psychopharmacological treatment. There are several reasons for this. The symptoms of social phobia have been viewed as normal personality traits and equivalent to shyness, as manifestations of avoidant personality disorder, or, in very narrow terms, as performance anxiety. Such problems have traditionally been treated exclusively with psychotherapy. However, recent research findings, reviewed by Potts and Davidson (Chapter 14, this volume), now affirm that social phobia is quite responsive to psychopharmacologic treatment and that such treatment can be of enormous clinical benefit. Furthermore, while nonpharmacological treatment approaches are also effective for social phobia, unpublished results from a recent comparative trial by Liebowitz and Heimberg (1995) suggest that pharmacotherapy may work more rapidly and have somewhat more potent acute effects, although cognitive-behavioral treatment gains seem to be more durable at follow-up assessment. Finally, clinical experience suggests that there are patients who do not improve significantly despite having participated in appropriate psychotherapy for social phobia. Therefore, given the prevalence, early onset, chronic course, often extensive impairment, and secondary comorbidity of social phobia, the proper application of pharmacotherapy for this disorder is of the utmost importance.

Two aspects of the clinical pharmacological treatment of social phobia will receive considerable attention in this chapter. The first is the evaluation itself. This includes issues of assessment, differential diagnosis, presentation of a rationale for pharmacotherapy to the patient, and related concerns. The second aspect is the actual treatment, including medication selection and administration, the role of the pharmacotherapist, assessment of progress, and combination with nonpharmacological treatments.

THE PSYCHIATRIC EVALUATION FOR SOCIAL PHOBIA

Assessment of a patient with social phobia for possible pharmacotherapy, as with psychiatric consultations in general, should proceed simultaneously along two paths. The first involves taking a thorough descriptive history of the chief complaint; present illness; past psychiatric symptom and treatment history; medical, social, and family history; and mental status examination (see Greist, Kobak, Jefferson, Katzelnick, & Chene, Chapter 9, this volume). At the same time, the astute clinician establishes an empathic alliance with the patient, coming to understand something of the patient's experience and conveying that understanding so that the patient can agree or express modifications. At the completion of a consultation, one aspires to both an accurate diagnosis and assessment of impairment and an emotional connection with the patient such that he or she feels both understood and enlightened as to the nature of his or her difficulties (Docherty & Feister, 1985). In most cases of social phobia, the patient should feel hopeful by the end of consultation about being helped by appropriate treatment.

One hour for an initial consultation will usually suffice, although a complicated evaluation can require 90 minutes. First, the history of the present illness should be obtained, as it establishes the context and relative importance for all other clinical information. The patient may need to be gently reminded of this initial focus if he or she shifts the emphasis to family, childhood, or past treatment before completing the history of present illness. One might say, for example, "I would like to hear more about _____, but first I need to get a better understanding of what is troubling you now." This is followed in the standard fashion by inquiry into the history of past psychiatric illness and treatment; medical, social, and family histories; and the mental status examination.

The essence of social phobia is the "persistent fear of one or more social or performance situations in which the person is exposed to unfamiliar people or to possible scrutiny by others. The individual fears that he or she will act in a way (or show anxiety symptoms) that will be humiliating or embarrassing" (American Psychiatric Association, 1994, p. 416). This can range from discrete performance anxiety in an individual who is otherwise socially comfortable and has many intimate relationships to severe generalized social phobia in an individual with almost total interpersonal isolation. The patient may often minimize or be unaware of the extent of the interpersonal fear and/or avoidance, so that it is necessary to explore this in detail to obtain a complete clinical picture. Here one must review the range of performance and social situations normally encountered, specifically inquiring about both fear and avoidance (see Greist, Kobak, Jefferson, Katzelnick, & Chene, Chapter 9, this volume, for a description of the Liebowitz Social Anxiety Scale).

Even after a pattern of social avoidance is established, certain other conditions that could contribute to this pattern must be considered, and in some cases excluded, before the diagnosis of social phobia can be made. Paranoid or schizoid features are also associated with avoidance and isolation. Social withdrawal may be symptomatic of major depression, although this tends to be more episodic than in social phobia (Schneier, Spitzer, Gibbon, Fyer, & Liebowitz, 1991; Reich, Noyes, & Yates, 1989). Dysthymia, however, may also manifest itself in some symptoms of social withdrawal. Additionally, many patients with social phobia also meet criteria for dysthymia. Careful clinical judgment is important in establishing the primary problem.

Social phobia can also follow the onset of unexpected panic attacks, although in such cases the patient's primary fear is of having a panic attack and consequently needing medical attention (when help from others would be needed) or suffering public embarrassment because of obvious distress. Patients with generalized social phobia can also meet criteria for avoidant personality disorder, but this does not appear to have any particular implications with regard to pharmacotherapy (Liebowitz et al., 1992). The distinction may in fact be primarily one of severity (Schneier et al., 1991).

Just as social avoidance may be because of panic disorder rather than social phobia, panic attacks may be precipitated by social phobia. We first became interested in social phobia after an encounter with a patient who presented with panic attacks on subways. He was diagnosed with panic disorder and treated with imipramine, to which he did not respond despite adequate doses and blood levels. Further interviews with the patient revealed that he experienced panic only if he sensed another passenger was scrutinizing him, suggesting social phobia. Unlike the typical patient with panic disorder, he was perfectly comfortable on the subway if he had the entire car to himself. Thus, when a patient reports panic attacks, it is necessary to explore the precipitating circumstances and whether the individual is typically more comfortable in the presence of others (suggestive of panic disorder) or alone (suggestive of social phobia).

Certain conditions frequently complicate social phobia, including affective disorders and alcoholism (Kessler et al., 1994; Schneier, Chin, Hollander, & Liebowitz, 1992; Schneier et al., 1989). Both have implications for pharmacotherapy selection (see below).

The fourth edition of the *Diagnostic and Statistical Manual of Mental Disorders* (DSM-IV; American Psychiatric Association, 1994) excludes from the diagnosis of social phobia individuals whose symptoms are secondary to embarrassment caused by another disorder, such as stuttering, or a familial or Parkinsonian tremor. There is, however, no empirical evidence that treatment response would differ from social phobia that fully meets DSM-IV criteria (see below).

At the end of the consultation, the physician is prepared to formulate a diagnostic impression and propose a plan. This may consist of treatment recommendations or further testing and evaluation if deemed necessary (i.e., medical examination, laboratory testing, cognitive testing, or other information-gathering procedures). The latter may include an interview with a significant person in the patient's life, with or without the patient present. This can be particularly helpful in assessing adolescents with social phobia, who often minimize their difficulty. A teenager, for example, may deny having any interest in going to parties, when it seems clear that he or she is too terrified to attend.

RECOMMENDING MEDICATION FOR SOCIAL PHOBIA

Given that many people are anxious about and perhaps avoid performance situations, the question arises as to what level of distress and/or impairment justifies consideration of pharmacotherapy. In general we believe that anyone meeting the DSM-IV severity/impairment criterion is sufficiently ill to justify appropriate medication or psychotherapy—that is, if the avoidant behavior secondary to social phobia interferes with occupational functioning, usual social activities, or relationships with others, or if there is marked distress about having the fear.

Once it is established that the patient is an appropriate candidate for therapy, how should the issue of medication treatment be presented? Many patients have not previously heard the term "social phobia" (although this is becoming less true as the disorder receives increasing media coverage). Most will tend to understand their impairment as extreme shyness, as a long-standing personality trait ("I have always been this way"), or as something to be treated exclusively by psychotherapy.

There are several approaches to conveying the rationale for pharmacotherapy. One strategy is to cite the treatment research literature. The physician may say, "Although it may seem difficult to understand how a medication could be helpful, research studies have shown this to be true." Another strategy is to emphasize the anxiety that drives phobic avoidance and suggest that medication can directly ameliorate that anxiety and, hence, the accompanying interpersonal difficulties. A third strategy, particularly for generalized social phobia, is to identify the construct of interpersonal hypersensitivity, which is an excessive vulnerability to becoming severly dysphoric in the face of any rejection, criticism, or rebuff (Boyce, Parker, Barnett, Cooney, & Smith, 1991; Davidson, Zisook, Giller, & Helms, 1989). There is marked interpersonal hypersensitivity in severe social phobia, which appears to be specifically modified by at least some of the pharmacotherapeutic regimens now utilized for this disorder, such as the monoamine oxidase inhibitors (MAOIs). Helping patients recognize the role that hypersensitivity to rejection may have played in their lives and then suggesting that it can be directly modified often helps to establish a therapeutic alliance and to gain acceptance of pharmacotherapy. These approaches are complementary and available to the clinician depending upon the individual circumstance.

The principal role of the pharmacotherapist is, of course, to select and administer the medication. This requires familiarity with the range of benefits and side effects of the various classes of medications available for social phobia (elaborated below). It also requires more than passing familiarity with the disorder itself, so that efficacy of treatment can be gauged at various stages and informed decisions made about dosage alterations or medication change, augmentation with psychosocial approaches, attempts at tapering the drug, and so forth. It is also essential to the treatment that the pharmacotherapist take a warm, hopeful, supportive stance. The physician can then effectively encourage the patient to enter previously avoided situations once the medications have begun to take effect, and the patient will accurately report both benefits and problems in the treatment.

The special difficulties of these patients in the therapeutic relationship should be kept in mind. There may be strong fears of being judged and critically scrutinized by the physician, consistent with the disorder. If this leads to minimizing reports of anxiety or side effects, the treatment is jeopardized. If the therapy is at risk, it may become necessary to address this issue, with an emphasis on the physician's nonjudgmental and supportive stance. A strong positive alliance, within which the goals and process of treatment are mutually understood, should be actively sought and maintained.

Proper medication selection is crucial, and the pharmacotherapist has a growing list from which to choose. Assuming there is no history of prior medication treatment, the pharmacotherapist and patient can consider the following classes of medicines: *MAOIs*, including both irreversible compounds (phenelzine [Nardil], tranylcypromine [Parnate], or isocarboxazid [Marplan]) and selective reversible compounds (moclobemide [Aurorix] or brofaromine, both unavailable in the United States); high-potency *benzodiazepines*, such as clonazepam (Klonopin) or alprazolam (Xanax); *selective serotonin reuptake inhibitors (SSRIs)*, such as fluoxetine (Prozac), fluvoxamine (Luvox), sertraline (Zoloft), or paroxetine (Paxil); *beta-adrenergic blockers*, such as propranolol (Inderal, others); or *atypical anxiolytics*, such as buspirone (BuSpar).

MEDICATION SELECTION

The first consideration is whether medication might be appropriately prescribed for only occasional use. Although the evidence from clinical studies is lacking, clinical experience suggests that many individuals whose symptoms are limited to occasional events such as public speaking or performance benefit from propranolol taken as needed (*pro re nata*, p.r.n.) (see below).

For patients whose social or performance anxiety occurs more frequently, maintenance regimens are required. Since there is as yet no series of studies comparing the different classes of medications found effective in social phobia, medication selection is somewhat subjective and influenced by the knowledge and prior experience of the physician.

Monoamine Oxidase Inhibitors

Our approach is to consider the standard MAOI phenelzine as the reference medication for social phobia but not necessarily as the first-line treatment for all patients.

As detailed elsewhere in this volume (see Potts & Davidson, Chapter 14, this volume), phenelzine is the most extensively studied pharmacological agent for social phobia, with four double-blind, placebo-controlled trials documenting its efficacy (Liebowitz et al., 1992; Gerlenter et al., 1991; Versiani et al., 1992; Liebowitz & Heimberg, 1995). Across studies, phenelzine benefited about two-thirds of patients. At this point, the evidence also suggests that social phobia responds to phenelzine regardless of severity. Phenelzine does not appear to lose efficacy with continued administration, although there is often substantial loss of gains if it is discontinued, even after 6–9 months of treatment. While the likelihood of discontinuation-induced relapse may be lessened with longer treatment, with adjunctive cognitive-behavioral therapy (these issues are currently the subject of planned investigations), or with treatment at an earlier stage of the illness (adolescence instead of adulthood), at present phenelzine must be considered a treatment rather than a cure for social phobia. These limitations, however, may apply to all medication treatments and would not mitigate against the choice of phenelzine. It is, rather, more relevant to consideration of pharmacological versus psychotherapeutic treatment, since the effects of cognitive-behavioral psychotherapy appear to be more durable.

Although controlled data are lacking, tranylcypromine (another irreversible MAOI) also appears to be helpful for social phobia and can be recommended if phenelzine is poorly tolerated or unavailable.

What particularly makes one pause when considering the administration of phenelzine or tranylcypromine for social phobia are their two major disadvantages: the risk of hypertensive reaction if a low tyramine diet and related precautions are not strictly followed, and the high incidence of side effects.

The reversible selective MAOIs (moclobemide, brofaromine) are safer and better tolerated than are standard MAOIs, since they have a much-reduced risk of both hypertensive reactions and adverse effects. It is not yet established whether their efficacy is comparable to that of the irreversible MAOIs, however. In the one controlled trial demonstrating efficacy for moclobemide (Versiani et al., 1992), the drug was superior to placebo but somewhat less effective than phenelzine. A recent open trial (Bisserbe, Lepine, & G. R. P. Group, 1994) also showed promising results. Several recent placebo-controlled studies suggest only modest efficacy in social phobia. Moclobemide is marketed in Europe for depression by Hoffmann−La Roche, but that company does not intend to pursue marketing of moclobemide in the United States.

There are two controlled trials of brofaromine for social phobia (van Vliet, den Boer, & Westenberg, 1992; Fahlen, Humble, Koczkas, & Nilsson, 1995). However, brofaromine was recently withdrawn from clinical trials by Ciba Geigy, so that it is not currently available for either clinical or investigatory use.

Non-MAOI Medications for Social Phobia

Alternatives to MAOIs include benzodiazepines, SSRIs, and nonbenzodiazepine anxiolytics.

Two high-potency benzodiazepines, clonazepam (Davidson et al., 1993; Munjack, Baltazar, Bohn, Cabe, & Appelson, 1990) and alprazolam (Gelernter et al., 1991), have been tested in controlled studies. In general, there is better empirical support for the effectiveness of clonazepam. The drugs are relatively safe but, like phenelzine, have a high incidence of adverse effects, including drowsiness, ataxia at higher doses, and physical dependence with continued use. Because many persons with social phobia use alcohol to self-medicate, the cross-reactivity of benzodiazepines with alcohol is another concern (Schneier et al., 1989). Current alcoholism is a contraindication to maintenance benzodiazepine treatment, but whether this is the case for past alcoholism as well is more controversial. Our view is that past alcoholism is a relative contraindication to maintenance benzodiazepine therapy because of the risk of reactivating the substance abuse. It is not an absolute contraindication if suitable alternatives are lacking. In summary, these drugs appear to be reasonable alternatives to the standard MAOIs for social phobia.

Of the SSRIs, fluvoxamine and fluoxetine have the best-documented efficacy to date. The first controlled trial of an SSRI showed fluvoxamine to be effective (den Boer, van Vliet, & Westenberg, 1994). Three uncontrolled, open clinical trials suggest efficacy for fluoxetine (Black, Uhde, & Tancer, 1992; Schneier, Chin, et al., 1992; Van Ameringen, Mancini, & Streiner, 1993). The SSRIs as a class are relatively safe and well tolerated by patients and thus may prove to be a reasonable first-line alternative to standard MAOIs. Hepatotoxicity is a potential concern for those individuals with a history of chronic alcoholism, but this is also true for the MAOIs. Further controlled trials of the SSRIs are needed for social phobia.

The nonbenzodiazepine anxiolytic buspirone has been studied in one controlled trial of musicians with predominantly discrete social phobia and performance anxiety (Clark & Agras, 1991). Buspirone at only moderate doses (30 mg per day) was no more effective than placebo and was less effective than cognitive-behavioral therapy. By contrast, one open series found patients who tolerated dosages of 45 mg per day or greater did experience modest benefit (Schneier et al., 1993). The overall response rate was 47% for those treated for 2 weeks or more (Schneier et al., 1993). Further controlled study is also needed for buspirone in social phobia.

The clinical impression has been that tricyclic antidepressants are not helpful in social phobia, although controlled data, for the most part, are lacking. Other reasons for this supposition are that tricyclics are less helpful for atypical depression than are MAOIs and are particularly ineffective in ameliorating chronic interpersonal hypersensitivity (Liebowitz et al., 1984).

PRACTICAL GUIDELINES
FOR MEDICATION TREATMENT

What follows are detailed descriptions of how to prescribe each of the above medications for the treatment of social phobia. We then conclude with a discussion of general issues pertinent to all pharmacological treatments, such as integration of medication and psychotherapy, duration of treatment, and evaluation of progress.

Phenelzine

Phenelzine is the most commonly used and best studied of the MAOIs for social phobia and for anxiety disorders in general. It may also be safer than tranylcypromine, with a lower risk of spontaneous hypertensive reactions—which may rarely occur without any documented dietary indiscretion. Before starting any MAOI, the side effects must be reviewed and the dietary precautions stressed, with a clear discussion of the risks of not following the diet. We often give patients a prescription for nifedipine 10 mg (an antihypertensive calcium channel blocker), to be taken sublingually in the event of a hypertensive reaction.

The usual starting dose of phenelzine is 15 mg per day taken in the morning to reduce interference with sleep. After 3 days, the dosage can be increased to 30 mg per day taken as a single A.M. dose. The dosage for the second week can be increased to 45 mg per day, still as a single A.M. dose, then to 60 mg per day in the 3rd and 4th weeks. Clinical benefit may appear after 4–6 weeks of therapy. If progress is not apparent or seems suboptimal and side effects are not prohibitive, the dosage can be increased to a maximum of 75 mg–90 mg per day.

Patients benefiting from phenelzine seem to report simultaneous decreases in both fear and avoidance of interpersonal and performance situations. Some need to be coaxed into entering previously avoided situations as a way of discovering, or at least evaluating, improvement. A confidence-building, positive experience usually leads naturally to increased self-exposure and further progress.

One occasional side effect of phenelzine that may be less common with other medications for social phobia is disinhibition. Phenelzine may in fact precipitate full-blown mania, in which case it must be immediately discontinued. Antimanic therapy may even become necessary in these cases. Especially for individuals with a history of hypomania (bipolar II) or bipolar disorder, caution must be exercised with close monitoring throughout treatment.

Milder forms of disinhibition, however, respond to lowering of the dosage, as illustrated by the following case.

The patient was a 17-year-old boy with generalized social phobia who had dropped out of high school because of severe anxiety in interacting with classmates and teachers. He also rarely saw friends, went out only at night (to avoid strangers as much as possible), and could not tolerate talking to a cashier in a store. There was also a history of depression and features of mild obsessive–compulsive disorder.

Initially treated with atenolol (Tenormin; cardioselective beta blocker), he felt some improvement in anxieties at school and with strangers. However, he was still frightened to talk to peers or teachers. The atenolol was stopped, his symptoms worsened, and he considered dropping out of school again. After phenelzine was begun, however, there was progessive improvement in anxiety level and socialization as the dose was increased. At a dosage of 75 mg per day, he became disinhibited and developed behavior problems in school: his teachers reported he was "chasing girls" in the hall, slamming doors, shouting, and being generally disruptive. His behavior normalized after phenelzine dosage was lowered to 45 mg per day, on which dose he was able to finish high school and enroll in college.

Clonazepam and Alprazolam

Clonazepam or alprazolam can be initiated at 0.5 mg three times daily (*ter in die*, t.i.d.), although some patients may not tolerate more than 0.25 mg t.i.d. because of drowsiness. Dosage can be gradually increased as needed, up to 4–6 mg per day of alprazolam or 2–4 mg per day of clonazepam. Alprazolam's shorter half-life necessitates frequent dosing, up to four times daily (*quater in die*, q.i.d.). Alprazolam also sometimes has a mood-elevating effect, and therefore may be preferable to clonazepam in patients with comorbid depressive features, since the latter drug can depress mood. On the other hand, clonazepam is easier to taper and discontinue than is alprazolam, since the withdrawal symptoms are generally less uncomfortable. Several weeks are usually needed to withdraw patients from substantial doses of either drug, and discontinuing the last 1 mg can be particularly trying. In our experience, if the difficulty is compounded by the return of symptoms, adding phenelzine may help complete the benzodiazepine taper. Other benzodiazepines may also help with social phobia, but they have not been studied for this indication.

Fluoxetine, Other SSRIs

A recent controlled trial of fluvoxamine supports its efficacy for social phobia. Fluoxetine is the only other SSRI for which published reports are available, and doses higher than 20 mg per day over 6–12 weeks were sometimes required for substantial benefit. Investigations of other SSRIs such as sertraline and paroxetine are under way, with promising initial findings. Social phobia differs from panic disorder in that patients can usually tolerate a starting dose of 20 mg per day of fluoxetine without experiencing hyperstimulation—provided there is no history of unexpected panic attacks.

If further controlled trials confirm these preliminary findings, the SSRIs could become first-line drugs for the treatment of social phobia because of their favorable safety and side-effect profile. Patients may be told, for example, that phenelzine is likely to be helpful, but that an initial trial of an SSRI is worthwhile because it is relatively safer and easier to take over the long-term. This also prepares the patient for a second drug trial if the first is unsuccessful. The physician should explain that this might involve a 2–3-month SSRI trial, to be followed by a taper and a 2–5-week drug-free interval (2 weeks for sertraline and paroxetine, 5 weeks for fluoxetine). Some patients prefer to maximize their chances of improvement as soon as possible and begin with phenelzine.

Moclobemide

Moclobemide can be initiated at 100 mg twice daily (*bis in die*, b.i.d.), and increased by 200 mg total daily dose every 5–7 days. It tends to have far fewer side effects than does phenelzine. The effective dose range, however, is unclear. Versiani et al. (1992) prescribed up to 600 mg per day, and current research in social phobia uses up to 800–900 mg per day. Symptomatic improvement tends to be slow. In Versiani's study, efficacy compared to placebo was not demonstrated after 4 weeks of treatment but did appear by 8 weeks. Further, patients showing benefit after 8 weeks continued to improve between weeks 8 and 16, which was not true for the phenelzine group in that study.

Beta Blockers

Beta blockers are usually prescribed only for occasional use. Although atenolol and propranolol have not proven superior to placebo in controlled investigations of social phobia (Falloon, Lloyd, & Harpin, 1981; Liebowitz et al., 1992; Turner, Beidel, & Jacob, 1994), anecdotal experience suggests that they are effective for specific and circumscribed performance anxiety, especially for signs of sympathetic hyperarousal such as tremor. Their efficacy may be limited to these instances and, hence, would not emerge in a study that included generalized social phobia. This hypothesis is consistent with the large analogue literature (in nonclinical populations) supporting the efficacy of beta blockers for performance anxiety in musicians, pistol shooters, bowlers, and so forth (Liebowitz, Gorman, Fyer, & Klein, 1985).

Propranolol can be taken 45–60 minutes before a performance, and its effects will last about 4 hours. A test dose is always advisable. Patients can take 10–20 mg in a comfortable setting while monitoring their own heart rate. Most healthy individuals (except those very fit athletes with a resting heart rate below 50 beats per minute) tolerate propranolol quite well, especially as the sympathetic arousal of anxiety will partly compensate for the hypotensive side effects.

Performance anxiety can be understood as a positive feedback mechanism in which anxiety and embarrassment induce physical symptoms that compromise performance, in turn causing further anxiety and heightening physical symptoms until the anxiety spins out of control and performance becomes impossible. Propranolol blunts the physical symptoms, such as trembling and tachycardia, in effect interrupting the positive feedback loop. Further gains are probably cognitively mediated. For example, a student with discrete social phobia taking propranolol may experience anticipatory anxiety before a seminar but during the actual presentation will discover that his or her heart is not racing and he or she is not visibly trembling or sweating. This in turn can provide a tremendous feeling of relief, boost confidence, and thereby further improve performance and turn an antici-pated failure into a successful experience. Controlled trials of beta blockers in discrete social phobia are needed.

Buspirone

Buspirone should be initiated at 5 mg 3 times per day or less and can be increased by 5 mg (total daily dose) every three days as tolerated. In Schneier et al.'s (1993) open trial, though the overall response rate was 47%, a more substantial response rate (67%) was observed in the 12 patients who attained a dose of at least 45 mg per day. Some patients may require and tolerate more than 60 mg per day. Both generalized and nongeneralized social phobia appears to respond.

To illustrate: Mr. C was a 40-year-old businessman who had feared speaking at meetings, going to parties, and talking to authority figures for at least 20 years. While not actually highly avoidant, he tolerated these and other social situations with extreme distress. He would experience significant anxiety for days in anticipation of a relatively informal speaking engagement. The anxiety he experienced during public speaking also im-paired his performance.

After 12 weeks of buspirone treatment, his anticipatory, performance, and social anxiety had improved. He still experienced some physical symp-toms of sympathetic arousal during speaking, but these were merely annoying and did not interfere with his performance. He would begin to worry only about an hour in advance of entering a feared situation.

This kind of improvement with mild residual symptoms is typical of buspirone response. The major limitation of treatment is buspirone's ad-verse effects, since high doses appear to be required to achieve benefit.

EVALUATING CLINICAL RESPONSE

To evaluate the outcome of a pharmacological intervention, we look for meaningful improvement in the following areas:

1. Anxiety experienced during a social encounter or performance event and possibly quality of performance and social interaction.
2. Anxiety experienced in anticipation of the feared situation (anticipatory anxiety).
3. Avoidance of social encounters or obligations, relationship opportunities, or performance.
4. Comorbidity related to the social phobia such as secondary depression, demoralization, or alcohol abuse.
5. Overall functional impairment due to the social phobia.

In other words, over the short term, we hope to see symptomatic relief and improved social relatedness and performance. Over the longer term (i.e., 3–6 months), we hope to see increased vocational and/or educational functioning and, especially for individuals with generalized social phobia, improved capacity for more intimate relationships of all kinds— friendships, romantic involvements, relationships with mentor or authority figures, and so forth.

This is exemplified by one young woman in her 20s who had never dated because of severe social anxiety. Soon after successful treatment with phenelzine, she was able to begin chatting with men in her office. Within several months, she was dating, and within a year of beginning treatment, she was involved in her first romantic relationship. Phenelzine treatment seemed to allow her to resume a normal developmental path, with each step requiring time to gain comfort and a sense of mastery.

TREATMENT STRATEGY FOR NONRESPONDERS

After an adequate trial of pharmacotherapy without results, the physician should switch to another class of medications. There are no studies at present predicting differential treatment response, but experienced clinicians have all seen a second medication trial succeed after the first had failed, despite adequate doses and length of treatment, regardless of the medications used.

If a given trial is partially helpful, the practitioner may wish to attempt augmentation before changing medications. Clinically, we have observed that benzodiazepines and beta blockers (p.r.n.) can augment response to an MAOI or SSRI, and many people with social phobia are treated with combination medication regimens. Cognitive-behavioral therapy, either individual or group, can also be combined with medication (see Heimberg & Juster, Chapter 12, this volume). Specially trained therapists can be especially helpful when progress is not optimal and when psychological or personality factors appear to play a significant role in the continued disability. Cognitive-behavioral therapy can also be recommended as an alternative to medication, given its relative safety and durability of benefit in those who respond. Clinically, however, we often observe significant medication response in individuals whose social anxieties and avoidance have not improved after months to years of intensive insight-oriented psychotherapy.

At present we lack the data to guide decisions about which treatment is best for whom. In the absence of data, the individualized treatment algorithm for social phobia, including the initial choice of medication versus psychotherapy, should be made in collaboration by patient and practitioner. Most important, the physician must be aware of the full range of treatments found to be effective for social phobia in order to apply them in an intelligent sequence, especially for hard-to-treat individuals.

MEDICATION MAINTENANCE AND DISCONTINUATION

For patients who respond to medication, and often for patients considering a medication trial, the question arises: "How long should I continue the medicine?" While definitive answers are lacking, studies with MAOIs and benzodiazepines suggest that even after 3–6 months of therapy, there is a high rate of relapse following medication discontinuation. In a recent phenelzine study, responders to 12 weeks of acute treatment were maintained on the effective dose for 6 months and then followed for 6 months without medication (Liebowitz & Heimberg, 1995). Fifty percent of patients relapsed during this follow-up phase.

In presenting the treatment options, the patient can be told that, if medication is helpful, it may need to be continued long term to preserve benefits, with periodic attempts to lower the dose (as a prelude to discontinuation). We are now studying discontinuation after longer treatment trials, as well as whether concomitant cognitive-behavioral therapy will reduce the relapse rate following medication discontinuation.

SPECIAL CASES AND COMORBIDITY

Certain complicated clinical syndromes deserve special mention. One involves social phobia that is comorbid with other anxiety syndromes. In fact, the majority of patients with social phobia also suffer from other Axis I disorders. In the Epidemiologic Catchment Area study, comorbid disorders were diagnosed in 69% of those with social phobia (Schneier,

Johnson, Hornig, Liebowitz, & Weissman, 1992). Controlled studies generally have not examined comorbidity as a factor influencing outcome. Nevertheless, the presence of other diagnoses, such as panic disorder, major depression, obsessive–compulsive disorder, or posttraumatic stress disorder, may have implications for treatment and should be considered in any therapeutic formulation.

In one series of patients with both obsessive–compulsive disorder and social phobia, for example, phenelzine was more effective for both disorders than was fluoxetine (Carrasco, Hollander, Schneier, & Liebowitz, 1992). Usually phenelzine is not considered to be a treatment option for obsessive–compulsive disorder. We have treated such persons whose obsessions and compulsions seemed to be entirely related to interpersonal hypersensitivity and others in whom the obsessions and compulsions appeared to be phenomenologically unrelated to social phobia. Although an SSRI may still be an acceptable first-line treatment, the greater likelihood of an MAOI response should be kept in mind in these instances.

One possible variant of social phobia is paruresis, or the inability to urinate in a public restroom, especially in the presence of others. It is more common in men, perhaps because of the exposure intrinsic to public urinals. Medication regimens effective for other forms of social phobia do not seem to help this problem. Phenelzine in particular may make symptoms worse because of its side-effects (Hatterer et al., 1990).

DSM-IV does not allow the diagnosis of social phobia to be made if the symptoms are secondary to a disorder such as stuttering or tremor (familial or Parkinsonian). However, preliminary evidence suggests that the treatment response of such patients is no different from that of those with "primary" social phobia (Oberlander & Liebowitz, 1993). Pursuing this issue, we have collected a series of eight cases in which patients with social phobic features related to concerns about mild to moderate physical impairments or disfigurements responded well to open clinical trials with phenelzine (Oberlander, Liebowitz, & Schneier, 1994).

Such persons with "secondary" social phobia can be subdivided into those whose social fear/avoidance seems to be excessive for the level of physical disability (implying some component of interpersonal hypersensitivity as well) and those whose social anxiety seems to be a more normative response to marked physical disability or disfigurement (suggesting that interpersonal hypersensitivity may not be a necessary component). However, the fact that many disabled individuals are able to function well socially suggests that problematic social anxiety might be viewed as a symptom regardless of the cognitive content, or referent, of the worry.

We would hypothesize that the former group in particular, because of their interpersonal hypersensitivity, would respond to social phobia treatments. Our impression is that the MAOIs and SSRIs treat social phobia by acting primarily to diminish this trait. At times, the primary medical disability (such as stuttering) may also improve during treatment, since anxiety often plays a role in the symptom (Oberlander & Liebowitz, 1993). We have also observed significant improvement in social anxiety despite actual worsening of the medical disability because of side effects (Oberlander et al., 1994).

While we still have much to learn about the treatment of social phobia, the field has made remarkable advances, considering that before 1985 almost nothing was known about the pharmacotherapy of this condition. This was true despite the fact that social phobia appears to be the third most common psychiatric disorder in the United States, with 12-month prevalence of 8% (Kessler et al., 1994). These new treatments are of enormous clinical importance to individuals who have suffered greatly with severe interpersonal handicaps in the normal pursuit of social, scholastic, and vocational activities. Practitioners can expect to be called on more and more frequently to provide effective medication treatment for patients with social phobia.

REFERENCES

American Psychiatric Association. (1994). *Diagnostic and statistical manual of mental disorders* (4th ed.). Washington, DC: Author.

Bisserbe, J. C., Lepíne, J. P., & G. R. P. Group. (1994). Moclobemide in social phobia: A pilot open study. *Clinical Neuropharmacology, 17* (Suppl. 1), S88–S94.

Black, B., Uhde, T. W., & Tancer, M. E. (1992). Fluoxetine for the treatment of social phobia [Letter to the editor]. *Journal of Clinical Psychopharmacology, 12,* 293–295.

Boyce, P., Parker, G., Barnett, B., Cooney, M., & Smith, F. (1991). Personality as a vulnerability factor to depression. *British Journal of Psychiatry, 159,* 106–114.

Carrasco, J. L., Hollander, E., Schneier, F. R., & Liebowitz, M. R. (1992). Treatment outcome of obsessive–compulsive disorder with comorbid social phobia. *Journal of Clinical Psychiatry, 53,* 387–391.

Clark, D. B., & Agras, W. S. (1991). The assessment and treatment of performance anxiety in musicians. *American Journal of Psychiatry, 148,* 598–605.

Davidson, J. R. T., Potts, N., Richichi, E., Krishnan, R., Ford, S. M., Smith, R., & Wilson, W. H. (1993). Treatment of social phobia with clonazepam and placebo. *Journal of Clinical Psychopharmacology, 13,* 423–428.

Davidson, J. R. T., Zisook, S., Giller, E., & Helms, M. (1989). Symptoms of interpersonal sensitivity in depression. *Comprehensive Psychiatry, 30,* 357–368.

den Boer, J. A., van Vliet, I. M., & Westenberg, H. G. M. (1994). Recent advances in the psychopharmacology of social phobia. *Progress in Neuro-Psychopharmacology and Biological Psychiatry, 18,* 634–636.

Docherty, J. P., & Feister, S. J. (1985). The therapeutic alliance and compliance with psychopharmacology. In R. E. Hales & A. J. Frances (Eds.), *Psychiatry update* (pp. 607–632). Washington, DC: American Psychiatric Association Press.

Fahlen, T., Humble, M., Koczkas, C., & Nilsson, H. L. (1995). [Social phobia: Efficacy of brofaromine versus placebo.] Unpublished data.

Falloon, I. R. H., Lloyd, G. G., & Harpin, R. E. (1981). The treatment of social phobia: Real-life rehearsal with nonprofessional therapists. *Journal of Nervous and Mental Disease, 169,* 180–184.

Gelernter, C. S., Uhde, T. W., Cimboli, P., Arnkoff, D. B., Vittone, B. J., Tancer, M. E., & Bartko, J. J. (1991). Cognitive-behavior and pharmacological treatments of social phobia: A controlled study. *Archives of General Psychiatry, 48,* 938–945.

Hatterer, J. A., Gorman, J. M., Fyer, A. J., Campeas, R. B., Schneier, F. R., Hollander, E., Papp, L. A., & Liebowitz, M. R. (1990). Pharmacotherapy of four men with paruresis. *American Journal of Psychiatry, 147,* 109–111.

Kessler, R. C., McGonagle, K. A., Zhao, S., Nelson, C. B., Hughes, M., Eshleman, S., Wittchen, H., & Kendler, K. S. (1994). Lifetime and 12-month prevalence of DSM-III-R psychiatric disorders in the United States: Results from the National Comorbidity Survey. *Archives of General Psychiatry, 51,* 8–19.

Liebowitz, M. R., Gorman, J. M., Fyer, A. J., & Klein, D. F. (1985). Social phobia: A review of a neglected anxiety disorder. *Archives of General Psychiatry, 42,* 729–736.

Liebowitz, M. R., & Heimberg, R. G. (1995). [A controlled comparison of phenelzine and cognitive behavioral group therapy in social phobia.] Unpublished data.

Liebowitz, M. R., Quitkin, F. M., Steward, J. W., McGrath, P. J., Harrison, W., Rabkin, J., Tricamo, E., Markowitz, J. S., & Klein, D. F. (1984). Phenelzine vs. imipramine in atypical depression: A preliminary report. *Archives of General Psychiatry, 41,* 669–677.

Liebowitz, M. R., Schneier, F., Campeas, R., Hollander, E., Hatterer, J., Fyer, A., Gorman, J., Papp, L., Davies, S., Gully, R., & Klein, D. (1992). Phenelzine vs. atenolol in social phobia: A placebo-controlled comparison. *Archives of General Psychiatry, 49,* 290–300.

Munjack, D. J., Baltazar, P. L., Bohn, P. B., Cabe, D. D., & Appelson, A. A. (1990). Clonazepam in the treatment of social phobia: A pilot study. *Journal of Clinical Psychiatry, 51*(Suppl.), 35–40.

Oberlander, E., & Liebowitz, M. R. (1993). The pharmacology of stuttering: A critique [Letter to the editor]. *American Journal of Psychiatry, 150,* 355.

Oberlander, E., Liebowitz, M. R., & Schneier, F. R. (1994). Physical disability and social phobia. *Journal of Clinical Psychopharmacology, 14,* 136–143.

Reich, J., Noyes, R., Jr., & Yates, W. (1989). Alprazolam treatment of avoidant personality traits in social phobic patients. *Journal of Clinical Psychiatry, 50,* 91–95.

Schneier, F. R., Chin, S. J., Hollander, E., & Liebowitz, M. R. (1992). Fluoxetine in social phobia [Letter to editor]. *Journal Clinical Psychoparmacology, 12,* 62–64.

Schneier, F. R., Johnson, J., Hornig, C. D., Liebowitz, M. R., & Weissman, M. M. (1992). Social phobia: Comorbidity and morbidity in an epidemiologic sample. *Archives of General Psychiatry, 49,* 282–288.

Schneier, F. R., Martin, L. Y., Liebowitz, M. R., Gorman, J. M., Klein, D. F., & Fyer, A. J. (1989). Alcohol abuse and social phobia. *Journal of Anxiety Disorders, 3,* 15–23.

Schneier, F. R., Saoud, J., Campeas, R., Fallon, B., Hollander, E., Coplan, J., Fyer, A. J., & Liebowitz, M. R. (1993). Buspirone in social phobia. *Journal of Clinical Psychopharmacology, 13,* 251–256.

Schneier, F. R., Spitzer, R. L., Gibbon, M., Fyer, A. J., & Liebowitz, M. R. (1991). The relationship of social phobia subtypes and avoidant personality disorder. *Comprehensive Psychiatry, 32,* 496–502.

Turner, S. M., Beidel, D. C., & Jacob, R. G. (1994). Social phobia: A comparison of behavior therapy and atenolol. *Journal of Consulting and Clinical Psychology, 62,* 350–358.

Van Ameringen, M., Mancini, C., & Streiner, D. L. (1993). Fluoxetine efficacy in social phobia. *Journal of Clinical Psychiatry, 54,* 27–32.

van Vliet, I. M., den Boer, J. A., & Westenberg, H. G. M. (1992). Psychopharmacological treatment of social phobia: Clinical and biochemical effects of brofaromine, a selective MAO-A inhibitor. *European Neuropsychopharmacology, 2,* 21–29.

Versiani, M., Nardi, A. E., Mundim, F. D., Alves, A. V., Liebowitz, M. R., & Amrein, R. (1992). Pharmacotherapy of social phobia: A controlled study with moclobemide and phenelzine. *British Journal of Psychiatry, 161,* 353–360.

PART V

Special Populations

CHAPTER SIXTEEN

Children and Adolescents: Assessment and Treatment

ANNE MARIE ALBANO
PATRICIA MARTEN DiBARTOLO
RICHARD G. HEIMBERG
DAVID H. BARLOW

Everyone can recall instances during the early school years when giving an oral report, talking to a "crush," or perfoming in gym class was accompanied by symptoms such as butterflies and blushing. Although the waxing and waning of anxieties and fears during childhood is expected and considered normal (Johnson & Melamed, 1979; King, Hamilton, & Ollendick, 1988), for socially anxious children and teenagers these fears have been found to interfere with development and to hinder mastery and growth (Inderbitzen-Pisaruk, Clark, & Solano, 1992; Kendall et al., 1991; Vernberg, Abwender, Ewell, & Beery, 1992). In this chapter we review the diagnosis, assessment, and treatment of social phobia in children and adolescents. In addition to current prevalence estimates and phenomenological considerations, we review current assessment methodologies for accurate differential diagnosis and treatment planning. Following a review of the relevant treatment literature, we present in detail a promising new group treatment protocol for social phobic adolescents.

PREVALENCE AND CHARACTERISTICS

Prevalence of Social Phobia in Children and Adolescents

Anxiety disorders are the most common category of psychiatric disorders in youth (Bernstein & Borchardt, 1991) and the primary reason for the referral of children and adolescents for mental health services (Beidel, 1991b). Yet there is little information in the literature regarding the prevalence of social phobia in children and adolescents. In two cross-sectional epidemiological studies (Kashani & Orvaschel, 1990; Kashani, Orvaschel, Rosenberg, & Reid, 1989), 21% of children sampled (aged 8, 12, or 17) reported symptoms consistent with diagnosis of an anxiety disorder. Among the individual disorders for these samples, prevalence was 12.9% and 12.4% for separation anxiety disorder and overanxious disorder, respectively, 3.3% for simple phobia, and 1.1% for social phobia. Similar findings were obtained in a longitudinal study conducted in New Zealand (Anderson, Williams, McGee, & Silva, 1987; McGee et al., 1990). In a sample of 792 children evaluated at age 11, the prevalence rates were 3.5% for separation anxiety disorder, 2.9% for overanxious disorder, 2.4% for simple phobia, and 1.0% for social phobia. When the children were reassessed at age 15 (McGee et al., 1990), the overall prevalence rates were 5.9% for overanxious disorder, 2% for separation anxiety disorder, 3.6% for simple phobia, and 1.1% for social phobia. The rates reported for simple and social phobia may be misleading, however, because the most common "simple" fear was the fear of public speaking. By the definition of the revised third edition of the *Diagnostic and Statistical Manual of Mental Disorders* (DSM-III-R; American Psychiatric Association, 1987), fear of public speaking would be considered a social phobia.

Among children referred to an anxiety disorders clinic (Last, Hersen, Kazdin, Finkelstein, & Strauss, 1987), 33% of the sample received a primary diagnosis of separation anxiety disorder, 15% had primary school phobia (described as social in origin), 15% had overanxious disorder, and 15% presented with a major affective disorder. Strauss and Francis (1989) reported that almost 9% of youngsters referred to their anxiety disorders clinic received a diagnosis of social phobia that was unrelated to school refusal. Furthermore, high comorbidity rates were evidenced among childhood anxiety disorders (Last, Strauss, & Francis, 1987). One or more concurrent anxiety disorders were diagnosed in 41% of the children with primary separation anxiety disorder, 63% of the school (social) phobia sample, and 56% of the children with primary overanxious disorder. Strauss, Lease, Kazdin, Dulcan, and Last (1989) reported that their clinic sample of children (ages 5–17) diagnosed with anxiety disorders was uniformly described as socially maladjusted by multiple informants (parents, teachers, self).

At the Center for Stress and Anxiety Disorders of the University at Albany, State University of New York, of the 156 children (ages 7–17) diagnosed with an anxiety disorder, 27 (17.9%) received a principal diagnosis of social phobia. In addition, of the 129 children for whom social phobia was not the principal diagnosis, 25 (19.4%) received a secondary diagnosis of social phobia. Diagnoses were derived from the Anxiety Disorders Interview Schedule for Children and Parents (ADIS-C and ADIS-P; Silverman & Nelles, 1988). Of the children receiving a principal diagnosis of social phobia, 3 were between 7 and 9 years of age, 2 were between 10 and 12 years of age, and 22 were 13 and older. Interestingly, all of these children presented with generalized social phobia, and none were diagnosed with the specific type (e.g., fears of tests or oral presentations). Based on a review of our diagnostic records, it appears that circumscribed fears of one or two social situations are uncommon in children. Such fears appear to generalize to other situations or events and to become part of the phenomenological expression of anxiety characteristic of overanxious disorder or the broad social-evaluative anxiety of generalized social phobia. It remains to be seen whether this finding will hold in the fourth edition of the *Diagnostic and Statistical Manual of Mental Disorders* (DSM-IV; American Psychiatric Association, 1994) for the diagnosis of generalized anxiety disorder in children and adolescents.

Clinical Significance and Persistence of Social Phobia in Children and Adolescents

Several studies have suggested that for many children, fears and anxieties are persistent and cause significant interference in daily functioning (Beidel, 1991b; Strauss, Frame, & Forehand, 1987). The accumulation of some six decades of research has consistently demonstrated the cognitive-developmental progression of children's fears and anxieties (e.g., Graziano, DeGiovanni, & Garcia, 1979; Ollendick, 1983; Ollendick, King, & Frary, 1989). Childhood fears are considered part of normal development. However, the distinction between normal developmental fears and pathological anxiety conditions remains unclear in the literature. Normal developmental fears are expected to be relatively transient and minimally distressing to the child. A fear is considered to be pathological when the magnitude of the anxiety, the intensity of the distress, and the interference in the child's life are such that the child's daily functioning is impaired and the fear does not readily dissipate with time. Operational definitions for these parameters are largely dependent upon individual clinician judgment.

Investigators have well documented age-related increases in social and evaluative fears in late childhood and early adolescence (e.g., Graziano et al., 1979; King, 1993). With increasing ability to understand the complexities of social interaction and to develop negative self-focused attention, the older child becomes capable of fearing negative evaluation from others. Although social anxiety is a common experience among children and adolescents, unremitting anxiety has significant implications for adjustment and development. Investigators have reported that anxious children are identified by their teachers as being less happy than their nonanxious peers (Edelbrock, 1985) and that they are less well liked by peers (Strauss et al., 1987). Moreover, with specific regard to social anxiety in children, research has suggested that such anxiety interferes with the development of adequate social skills and establishment of friendships, resulting in an increase in negative self-evaluation (Rubin, LeMare, & Lollis, 1990). Francis (1990) reports that as a result of avoiding a large variety of social situations, social phobic children evidence pervasive disruption in functioning and constriction of normal activities. Late childhood and early adolescence are especially important times for establishing friendships, peer-group identification, and identity development. During this time, the adolescent begins to test his or her emerging independence and individuality. Experience in dating will influence the adolescent's ability to form long-term relationships (Havighurst, 1972; Johnson & Glass, 1989). Social phobia during this critical period has lasting consequences, as several studies document the onset of social phobia to be in the middle adolescent years with unremitting persistence into adulthood (Öst, 1987; Turner & Beidel, 1989).

Clinical Manifestation of Social Phobia in Youth

In all likelihood, social phobia in children and adolescents is underreported and undertreated because these children are not readily recognized as clinically impaired. Although the relationship between social phobia and behavioral inhibition (BI) is unclear (Rosenbaum, Biederman, Hirshfeld, Bolduc, & Chaloff, 1991), evidence suggests that BI in infants may be associated with the development of social phobia or related anxiety disorders. The reader interested in a review of this literature is referred to Bruch and Cheek (Chapter 8, this volume); however, suffice it to say that about 10% to 15% of Caucasian American children appear to be inhibited as infants and subsequently become overly cautious, quiet, and introverted by school age (Kagan, Reznick, & Snidman, 1988). Only recently has attention turned toward examining this temperamental style as a possible diathesis for later psychopathology.

Shyness is generally accepted in our society, and shy children typically are not a cause of concern or trouble for teachers or parents. Research on shyness reveals that 50–60% of adolescents consider themselves shy and that shy teens are more likely to use alcohol or drugs to feel confident and at ease in social situations (Zimbardo, Pilkonis, & Norwood, 1974; Zimbardo & Radl, 1981). Due to the nature of the disorder, socially anxious children are more likely to endure social situations with distress than to call attention to themselves. In our clinical experience, these children are brought to treatment when the disorder is of sufficient intensity to have interfered with academic progress (such as repeated absences from school) or because the parents report frequent somatic complaints (headaches, stomachaches) or avoidance behaviors that interfere with family and daily activities.

In a study designed specifically to examine the characteristics of social phobia in children, Beidel (1991b) evaluated the clinical presentation of children (mean age = 10.4) with social phobia (n = 18), children with overanxious disorder (n = 11), and normal controls (n = 18). Children were diagnosed via the ADIS-C and ADIS-P, in addition to completing self-report measures and a daily monitoring log and participating in a behavioral test. The social phobic children manifested many of the same characteristics found in adult social phobics. Specifically, they reported significantly lower perceptions of cognitive competence, higher trait anxiety, and higher anxiety during a stressful task than did the overanxious children and normal controls. Moreover, the social phobic children reported a greater number of anxiety-provoking events and greater distress over such events on the daily diary task. When faced with tasks such as giving oral reports or reading aloud, social phobic children demonstrated more behavioral avoidance, crying, and somatic complaints than did the overanxious group. These results were taken as evidence that social phobia in children results in extreme distress and significant interference in daily functioning.

Observations and responses of the social phobic children at our clinic (n = 27) support Beidel's findings. For our sample, thoughts are characterized by negative self-focus and self-deprecation and are accompanied by a range of autonomic symptoms and sensations. Complaints of stomachaches and illness are common, especially among younger children. Behaviorally, younger children may manifest excessive clinging and crying, while the older child is likely to shrink from social contact and avoid being the focus of attention. Table 16.1 presents a summary of social phobic children's responses across the three components of anxiety. Responses represented under the behavioral and physiological categories are characteristic of all phobic children. The social-evaluative fears noted in the cognitive category are principally characteristic of social phobic children.

The children in our sample reported avoiding a wide range of situations, from oral reports and eating in the cafeteria to attending family functions and answering the telephone. At times, refusal to attend school was reported by the children as a means to escape anxiety (Table 16.2).

We have also observed that many social phobic children develop unusual interests for their given age. For example, a number of the children at our clinic pursue solitary hobbies or interests in atypical subjects (e.g., Civil War facts, computer programming, tracking weather reports). We

TABLE 16.1. Behavioral, Physiological, and Cognitive Responses Associated with Social Phobia in Children and Adolescents

Behavioral	Physiological	Cognitive
Crying	Palpitations	Thoughts of
Whining	Nausea	escape
Clinging to parent	Sweating	negative evaluation
Stuttering	Shakiness	failure
Fidgeting	Breathlessness	humilitation
Poor eye contact	Numbing	embarrassment
Mumbling	Headaches	inadequacy
Trembling voice	Increased pulse	self-criticism
Nail biting	Muscle tension	
Avoidance	Butterflies in stomach	
Nervous habits		

Note. Specific examples associated with social phobia were compiled from clinical information gathered from working with these groups.

hypothesize that the absence of more common interests (e.g., videogames, television, teen magazines) may result from limited time spent in social interactions. Consequently, the children are not adequately exposed to these mainstream stimuli and fail to receive adequate social reinforcement from peers. Consistently, they argue that their peers and typical age-related interests are "too immature" as reasons for justifying these alternative pursuits. It is further hypothesized that at some point the atypical interest becomes a means to avoid the usual peer-related activities that trigger social anxiety. It would be interesting to study whether such interests wane with successful treatment of the social phobia.

Differential Diagnosis

As with any anxiety disorder in children and adolescents, social phobia must first be distinguished from an expected degree of heightened self-consciousness and embarrassment that is characteristic of this period of life. Subclinical social anxiety may be expressed through a child's worry about an upcoming oral report, reluctance to enter a novel social situation, such as a new classroom or a party, or a teenager's hesitance in asking for a date. Such anticipatory anxiety is transient and relatively circumscribed. Typically the anxiety dissipates as the child gains experience with the task and through social facilitation by the peer group.

Social phobia may be distinguished from specific (simple) phobias partly on the basis of the focus of the fear. For example, a diagnosis of

TABLE 16.2. Situations That Children and Adolescents with Social Phobia May Fear and/or Avoid

School-related	Other situations
School dances	Parties
Oral presentations	Eating in public
Speaking in class	Dating situations
Walking in the hallways	Using public restrooms
Interacting with peers	Talking with adults
Interacting with teachers, principal, school personnel	Speaking with people in authority (e.g., doctors, store managers)
Taking gym class	Using the telephone
Riding the schoolbus	Attending family functions
Taking tests	Interacting with family members' friends
Writing on the blackboard	Going shopping
Being in the cafeteria	After-school employment
Performing (e.g., in band, chorus, theater)	Meeting new people
Working on group projects	Answering the telephone
Joining clubs, groups, or sports	Starting a conversation
Calling a classmate for homework	Attending sleep-away camp
Returning to school after an absence	
Being teased[a]	
Situations requiring assertiveness[a]	

[a] These situations can commonly occur both in school and in a variety of other situations (e.g., at home, in stores).

specific phobia is made if avoidance of eating in the school cafeteria is motivated by a fear of choking. Social phobia is diagnosed if the child's avoidance is due to the fear of others' evaluations and judgments about such things as how or what the child eats, the child's appearance, or similar personal attributes. The diagnosis of specific phobia is not made if the fear is of embarrassment, humiliation, or evaluation by others.

The diagnosis of overanxious disorder has been dropped from the nomenclature of DSM-IV and subsumed under generalized anxiety disorder (GAD). Children with GAD may have excessive worry and anticipatory anxiety about a number of events or activities that pertain to the quality of their performance in school, athletics, or social events. However, children with GAD experience these worries even when they are not being evaluated by others or the focus of others' attention. The child with GAD may be more likely to endure an evaluative situation with discomfort and complaints than to actively avoid it. Although worry about examinations and school performance may be subsumed under GAD, test anxiety by itself should be diagnosed as a social phobia. These children may display anxious apprehension about upcoming exams, interference in their ability to study or prepare adequately for tests, and heightened arousal resulting in somatic complaints and sleep disturbance. Test phobic children are likely to perform well on homework and during informal discussions about subject material but display marked dysfunction during formal examination situations.

School refusal is a significant potential concomitant behavior of social phobia. However, the motivating conditions for school refusal must be accurately differentiated for appropriate prescriptive treatment planning. For example, children with separation anxiety disorder will often refuse to attend school (or other social situations) for fear of being separated from the primary caretakers. These children are often comfortable socializing in their own home and in outside social settings when accompanied by their parents. Social phobic children display signs of discomfort even when feared social situations occur at home and/or in the presence of their parents.

Selective mutism (formerly elective mutism) is a disorder of childhood characterized by a persistent refusal to speak in selected social situations despite the ability to communicate fluently in spoken language. Children with this disorder typically converse and carry on in a normal speaking voice at home but refuse to speak in school or other social situations where there is an expectation for speaking. Hence, the disorder has the potential to interfere with academic achievement, peer relationships, occupational achievement, and overall social functioning. Black and Uhde (1992) have suggested that selective mutism may, in fact, be a variant of social phobia as opposed to a distinct diagnostic syndrome. Children with selective mutism may evidence excessive shyness, fear of social embarrassment, social isolation and withdrawal, and negativism (American Psychiatric Association, 1994), all of which are characteristics observed in social phobic children. Moreover, investigators have previously identified fear and avoidance of speaking in public or to strangers as among the most common symptoms of social phobics (Uhde, Tancer, Black, & Brown, 1991). Controlled clinical and epidemiological studies of selective mutism and social phobia are warranted in order to determine the relationship between these two disorders. Until then, differential diagnosis will remain a challenge for the clinician. In cases where there is clear evidence of fear and avoidance of social situations and the child refuses to speak in specific situations that require verbal communication, both diagnoses should be assigned.

Avoidance of social interactions is also a presenting feature of major depressive disorder, dysthymia, and thought disorders. In such cases the avoidance is not due to social anxiety, and thus, social phobia should not be diagnosed. In addition, because of the disorder's early and chronic course, children may fail to achieve an expected level of social functioning. Social phobic children may shrink away from contact with others, display little or no eye contact or associated social skills, and prefer solitary activities. However, such deficits are also observed in pervasive developmental disorder (PDD) and, thus, require careful differential diagnosis. The presence of stereotypic behavior, unusual verbal or behavioral fixations, and language anomalies would warrant the consideration of the PDD diagnosis.

ASSESSMENT

A variety of methods pertinent to the assessment of social phobia in children and adolescents will be reviewed. Specifically, the following categories of assessment will be considered: structured interviews, self-report measures, cognitive assessment, self-monitoring, behavioral observation, psychophysiological assessment, and family assessment. Particular attention will be paid to the reliability and validity of each method presented. Additionally, areas that demand future research efforts will be discussed.

Structured Interviews

Recently, leading child anxiety researchers have called for increased use of valid and standardized diagnostic procedures in order for the field to make comparisons of data across settings (e.g., Lann, 1991). There are a number of structured interviews that can be employed to assess psychiatric disorders in children and adolescents (for a review, see Silverman, 1991). Each of these interviews assesses a variety of areas, one of which is the presence of anxiety disorders. Silverman and Nelles (1988) developed the ADIS-C and the ADIS-P in order to provide more thorough coverage of childhood anxiety disorders. Each of these interviews has been revised to be consistent with DSM-IV (e.g., ADIS-C and ADIS-P for DSM-IV; Silverman & Albano, 1995). Although new reliability and validity studies are pending, we have no reason to expect any decrease in the psychometric integrity of these measures.

Each structured interview generally requires that both parent and child are interviewed with complementary versions of the instrument. Additionally, each of these interviews allows evaluators to assign diagnoses based on DSM-III-R criteria. Moreover, all of the structured interviews employed with clinically anxious children cover the same general age range, providing coverage of both children and adolescents.

Despite shared features, structured interviews have been observed to vary widely in their coding and administration (Silverman, 1991). In particular, differences in level of structure demanded by the interview instrument are common. Although all of these assessments require that both child and parent be interviewed, methods regarding order of interview (parent first vs. child first) and integration of interview data in order to determine composite diagnoses often differ.

Unfortunately, due to some of the noted methodological differences among structured interviews, sweeping statements regarding the reliability and validity of these instruments are precluded (Silverman, 1991). Although all structured interviews have demonstrated reliability, differences in methodology for determining interrater reliability often exist (e.g., independent administrations of the interview, videotaping of interview to be observed by a second rater). Moreover, few investigations have allowed researchers to make comparisons of reliability across the childhood anxiety disorders due to small sample sizes. Instead, reliability coefficients are often reported for specific anxious symptoms or the entire class of anxiety disorders rather than for specific diagnostic categories.

At this time, then, there are very few data that would allow a clear delineation of those categories that can be reliably diagnosed. The diagnosis of social phobia in children is no exception. Many studies provide coefficients for phobic disorders without further clarification of reliability for social versus specific phobias. This is probably due to the fact that some of these earlier studies may not have yielded data compatible with the DSM diagnostic system or may have been conducted prior to the publication of the third edition of the *Diagnostic and Statistical Manual of Mental Disorders* (DSM-III; American Psychiatric Association, 1980), in which the diagnosis of social phobia was first established. Nevertheless, there are some more recent studies that provide preliminary evidence of good test–retest and interrater reliability of the diagnosis of social phobia in children (e.g., Beidel, Neal, & Lederer, 1991; Silverman & Eisen, 1992).

Given the limited data on the psychometric soundness of structured interviews, some researchers have cautioned against sole reliance on these measures in clinical work (Ollendick & Francis, 1988). Among the specific criticisms of these interviews were their time-consuming nature, the need for rigorous training of interviewers, and their potential inappropriateness for use with young children. Thus, consideration might be given to the administration of a problem-focused interview to supplement the information obtained from the structured measure (Ollendick & Francis, 1988).

Overall, then, the psychometric properties of structured interviews for the childhood anxiety disorders, including social phobia, have not been fully established. Clearly, further examination of the psychometric properties of the available structured interviews is warranted. Most of the psychometric research completed to date has examined various forms of reliability (e.g., interrater, test–retest). Greater consideration must be given to the validity of the diagnostic categories delineated by these assessments as well. Despite these difficulties, further refinement of structured interviews will allow researchers to make invaluable comparisons across settings.

Self-Report Measures

A number of self-report measures are suited for use with children and adolescents with social phobia. Indeed, a variety of constructs are relevant to the assessment of social phobia, including social skills, self-esteem, general anxiety, and social anxiety and satisfaction. Self-report measures both allow clinical researchers to make comparisons across diagnostic categories and provide a means of tracking treatment progress.

First, there are a few self-report measures that tap general anxiety in children and adolescents and have proven to be both reliable and valid. For example, the State–Trait Anxiety Inventory for Children (STAIC; Spielberger, 1973) is a 40-item scale measuring state and trait anxiety. Children diagnosed with social phobia have been found to have significantly higher STAIC scores than do normal comparison children (Beidel, 1991b). Similarly, the 37-item Revised Children's Manifest Anxiety Scale (RCMAS; Reynolds & Richmond, 1978) is also a measure of chronic anxiety and contains three clinical subscales: physiological, worry/oversensitivity, and concentration. A lie scale also allows an examination of the validity of the child's responses on the measure. This information may be particularly important, given that some anxious children appear to respond to questionnaires in a socially desirable manner (Kendall & Chansky, 1991). Thorough normative data are available for a variety of ages and groups of children for both scales (Reynolds & Paget, 1983; Spielberger, 1973; Strauss, 1988).

In comparison to the instruments available to measure general anxiety in children, relatively little work has been devoted to the development or evaluation of self-report measures that specifically measure social anxiety and avoidance, although a number of such measures have been developed for use with adult social phobics (see McNeil, Ries, & Turk, Chapter 10, this volume, for a review). One exception is an investigation that examined the validity of the Fear of Negative Evaluation (FNE) and the Social Avoidance and Distress (SAD) Scales (Watson & Friend, 1969) with junior high school students (Warren, Good, & Velten, 1984). These scales were originally designed using a college sample and are widely employed to assess social anxiety and avoidance in adults. Preliminary evidence of the concurrent validity of these measures with junior high school students was provided by the significant positive relationship between SAD scores and peer sociometric ratings of social anxiety. Additionally, socially anxious adolescents receiving rational–emotive treatment also evidenced significant reductions in FNE and SAD scores at posttreatment assessment.

The validity of the FNE and SAD with preadolescent populations, however, has not yet been examined. In fact, only two measures specifically addressing childhood social and evaluative anxiety and avoidance have been developed to date. LaGreca and colleagues have provided preliminary evidence of the factor structure, concurrent validity, and internal reliability of their 22-item Social Anxiety Scale for Children—Revised (SASC-R; LaGreca & Stone, 1993; LaGreca, Dandes, Wick, Shaw, & Stone, 1988). This measure consists of three factors similar to those identified in the adult social anxiety literature. In addition to a fear of negative evaluation factor, two social avoidance and distress factors were identified in the SASC-R: Social avoidance of new situations involving unfamiliar peers is tapped by the SAD-New factor, and generalized social avoidance and distress by the SAD-G factor. Confirmatory factor analysis supported this three-factor model for children's social anxiety (LaGreca & Stone, 1993). In addition, adequate reliability and internal consistency were reported for the measure. Future research is warranted to further examine the convergent and discriminant validity of this promising measure.

Recently, Beidel and colleagues presented preliminary psychometric data on a new measure of social anxiety in children, the Social Phobia and Anxiety Inventory for Children (SPAI-C; Beidel, Turner, & Morris, 1995). The SPAI-C is a 26-item measure suitable for children and adolescents (ages 8 and up). Factor analysis revealed the instrument taps three primary factors: assertiveness/general conversation, traditional social encounters, and public performance. The authors report 2-week and 10-month test–retest reliabilities of .85 and .63, respectively (Morris, Beidel, & Turner, 1993), and the measure differentiates socially anxious from non-anxious children (Beidel et al., 1995). Research is underway examining the SPAI-C's ability to discriminate among samples of anxiety-disordered youth.

Another construct potentially relevant to social anxiety in children is self-esteem, particularly perceived competence in social functioning. Indeed, strong self-esteem in this and other domains may serve to protect children from the development of psychopathological states (e.g., depression; cf. Cole, 1991). Harter's 28-item Self-Perception Profile for Children (SPPC; Harter, 1982, 1985) consists of four subscales, measuring cognitive, physical, social, and general self-worth. The factorial structure of the instrument was found to be stable across age ranges (3rd through 9th graders). One study found that social self-competence as measured by the SPPC was positively related to more popular peer sociometric status. Moreover, anxious children reported feeling less socially competent than did groups of clinic control (e.g., externalizing) and nonreferred children using the SPPC (Strauss et al., 1989). Additionally, children with social phobia also evidenced lower scores on the cognitive subscale of the SPPC in comparison to children with overanxious disorder and nonanxious children (Beidel, 1991b). This measure also has parallel teacher and parent rating forms that have adequate reliability and validity (Harter, 1985).

A final construct that appears to be relevant to the assessment of social phobia in children is social skills. As noted by Heimberg and Juster (see Chapter 12, this volume), poor social behavior is not necessarily related to a deficit in social skills. Social skill, broadly defined, is a hypothetical construct (related to behavioral capacity) that serves as one of many hypotheses to account for poor social behavior. Investigations examining the relationship of social skills deficits to social phobia in children and adolescents are just underway (e.g., Albano, Leung, & Barlow, 1994). Until this relationship is elucidated, we recommend the assessment of social skills as a means to guide treatment planning and goal setting for children and adolescents. The 62-item Matson Evaluation of Social Skills with Youngsters (MESSY; Matson, Rotatori & Helsel, 1983) is one useful measure to tap this construct. The MESSY consists of five factors: overconfident, impulsive/recalcitrant, jealousy/withdrawal, inappropriate assertiveness, and appropriate social skill. All items included in the final version of the scale evidenced adequate test–retest reliability. Anxious children have been found to exhibit social skills deficits as measured by the MESSY in comparison to nonreferred children, most particularly shyness and social withdrawal (Strauss et al., 1989). This measure also has a parallel teacher form.

The Teenage Inventory of Social Skills (TISS; Inderbitzen & Foster, 1992) was developed to identify adolescents with poor social skills and to guide the selection of target behaviors for intervention. The TISS consists of 40 items, 20 items assessing positive social behaviors and 20 assessing negative social behaviors. Two-week, test–retest reliabilities for the positive and negative behavior scales were .90 and .72, respectively, and internal consistencies were .88 for both scales. In addition, evidence for adequate convergent and discriminant validity were reported. While the TISS appears to be a promising measure of social competence, investigations with social phobic adolescents are lacking. Further research with clinical populations are necessary to evaluate the scale's utility as a measure of clinical outcome.

Cognitive Assessment

Cognitive assessment has been an area of increased interest in recent years (Arnkoff & Glass, 1989; D. A. Clark, 1988; Parks & Hollon, 1988). However, relatively little consideration has been given to the measurement of cognitive functioning among anxious children (Francis, 1988; Kendall & Ronan, 1990a; Ollendick & Francis, 1988). Indeed, virtually none of the little work that has been done includes diagnosed samples of anxious children (Francis, 1988). Cognitive assessment of anxious children can be considered to be a complex undertaking, given the dynamic nature of cognitive development and the nature of the thoughts or cognitive processes that are being assessed (i.e., state-dependent and fleeting thoughts that these children typically attempt to avoid; D. M. Clark, 1986; Last, 1988).

Despite these problems, a few measures targeting cognitive variables have recently been developed for use with anxious children. Kendall and Ronan's (1990b) Children's Anxious Self-Statement Questionnaire (CASSQ) is a global measure of the content of anxious children's thoughts. Subjects are asked to endorse the frequency of a number of cognitions during the previous week using a 1 (not at all) to 5 (all the time) rating system. This measure consists of two subscales: negative self-evaluation and positive self-concept and expectations. Preliminary data regarding the reliability and validity of the CASSQ appear promising (Kendall et al., 1991; Ronan, Rowe, & Kendall, 1988). As might be expected, anxious children generally score higher on the negative self-evaluation scale than on the positive scale. The CASSQ also differentiates clinically anxious from nonanxious children (Ronan et al., 1988). Nevertheless, it did not differentiate anxious children from children who were referred to an anxiety clinic but did not meet the criteria for an anxiety disorder (i.e., avoidant disorder, overanxious disorder, separation anxiety disorder), suggesting that it may measure global levels of distress. As noted with other children's self-report measures, further empirical validation of the CASSQ as applied to social phobic children and adolescents is warranted. In comparison to this more global measure, the 40-item Children's Cognitive Assessment Questionnaire (CCAQ), created and revised by Zatz and Chassin (1983, 1985), was developed to assess cognitions following exposure to an anxiety-provoking situation (i.e., test-taking). The CCAQ requires children to reflect upon the thoughts they experienced during the test and then to respond to each listed statement in a yes–no format (e.g., "I am bright enough to do this"; "I really feel stupid"; "I wish I were playing with my friends"). The instrument consists of five subscales, including coping, on- and off-task thoughts, and positive and negative evaluations. With samples of test anxious children, the CCAQ evidenced adequate internal and test–retest reliability (Zatz & Chassin, 1983). Moreover, high test anxious children reported significantly more debilitating cognitions (i.e., off-task thoughts, negative self-evaluative thoughts) than did either moderate or low test anxious subjects during both simulated and naturalistic test-taking situations (Zatz & Chassin, 1983, 1985).

Fox, Houston, and Pittner (1983) employed a think-aloud procedure, as described by Meichenbaum (1977), in order to compare the cognitions of high and low trait anxious children prior to a stressful situation (i.e., a test). This procedure required the children to verbalize their thoughts, which were audiotaped for 2 minutes. The think-aloud procedure was found to be feasible for the assessment of anxious children's cognitions.

Generally, all subjects were able to follow instructions with little difficulty. Adequate interrater reliability was found for the six scales employed to score the think-aloud transcripts (i.e., preoccupation, analytic attitude, avoidant thinking, derogation of other, positive situation-relevant, justification of positive attitude). High trait anxious children responded to an impending anxiety-provoking task with more preoccupation (e.g., "I'm just worried . . . about what we're going to do here and if I understand it"), derogation of other (e.g., "I wish my Mom wouldn't have made me do this"), and justification of a positive attitude (e.g., "I shouldn't worry about that").

Kendall and Chansky (1991) recently reported on the responses of anxious and nonanxious children to a thought-listing assessment following participation in a stressful task (i.e., a 5-minute videotaped improvised speech about themselves). Responses were coded into four categories: neutral, positive, negative, and coping/strategic (cf. Prins, 1986). A number of findings from this preliminary study are of note. First, an overwhelming number of children in both groups reported only positive thoughts or only negative thoughts. In addition, children responding with positive thoughts tended to respond with only a single thought, whereas individuals responding with negative thoughts tended to report multiple thoughts. On the basis of these findings, Kendall and Chansky (1991) suggest that endorsement methods of cognitive assessment may be superior to thought-listing approaches with children, given the "one-track" nature of cognitions reported.

One striking finding from the cognitive assessment literature is that negative cognitions are more strongly related to task performance than are positive cognitions (Zatz & Chassin, 1985). However, a seemingly contradictory finding is that coping self-statements are also frequently reported by anxious children during various cognitive assessments and have been consistently associated with increased anxiety as well as with task interference (Fox & Houston, 1981; Fox et al., 1983; Houston, Fox, & Forbes, 1984; Kendall & Chansky, 1991; Prins, 1986; Zatz & Chassin, 1985). It is assumed, then, that the recurrent use of coping cognitions may debilitate performance of anxious children by distracting them from the actual task at hand. Furthermore, given the noted association of negative thinking to performance, some authors have emphasized the importance of directly targeting the disruption of such thoughts, rather than increasing the number of coping statements, as a primary means of intervention (Kendall & Chansky, 1991).

To date, however, we have little understanding of adaptive cognitive responses of children to stressful situations. Research in the adult literature has found that the cognitions of nondistressed individuals are characterized by a ratio of approximately 1.6:1.0 for positive to negative thoughts (Kendall, Howard, & Hays, 1989; Schwartz & Garamoni, 1986), but no normative data are available for children. Additionally, we have only preliminary evidence regarding the relationship between cognition and other response systems in anxious children (e.g., behavioral performance, subjective anxiety, somatic symptoms). Further examination of the impact of various categories of cognition on these response systems is crucial to our understanding of anxiety.

Self-Monitoring

Self-monitoring of problematic or anxiety-provoking situations is a common component of behavioral assessment and treatment (Bornstein, Hamilton, & Bornstein, 1988). To date, little systematic work has been completed examining the utility of self-monitoring in the assessment of childhood anxiety disorders. One recent investigation has examined the reliability and validity of self-monitoring data collected from test anxious and normal control children (Beidel et al., 1991). This study is particularly relevant to social phobia, since a subset of test anxious children have been found to be concerned with social evaluation in a variety of settings (cf. Beidel & Turner, 1988). In fact, 34% of this sample met DSM-III-R diagnostic criteria for social phobia (Beidel et al., 1991), and test anxiety is listed as an example of social phobia in DSM-IV.

Data from this preliminary study of self-monitoring with anxious children illustrate that children will generally comply with the monitoring task and can provide reliable data (Beidel et al., 1991). Furthermore, anxious children reported significantly more distress and negative and avoidance behaviors than did non-test anxious children, providing evidence of the validity of self-monitoring.

Another interesting investigation that directly compared social phobic and overanxious children on a number of assessment measures, including daily diary data, provides evidence of the utility of self-monitoring with social phobic children (Beidel, 1991b). The social phobic children reported significant levels of daily distress and interference, including more frequent occurrence of negative events and greater distress in reaction to such events (e.g., crying, behavioral avoidance). Children with overanxious disorder did not differ from normal control children in their reported frequency of negative events or emotional distress in such situations. As would be expected, social phobic children reported anxiety in response to social-evaluative situations, such as reading aloud and writing on the blackboard in class.

Behavioral Observation

One cornerstone of behavioral assessment is behavioral observation (Barrios & Hartmann, 1988; Foster, Bell-Dolan, & Burge, 1988). Nonetheless, few standardized measures of behavioral indicators of anxiety in children have been developed. One exception is the Preschool Observation Scale of Anxiety (POSA) constructed by Glennon and Weisz (1978). Raters note the presence of 30 operationally defined behavioral signs of anxiety, such as crying, nail-biting, whining/whimpering, physical complaints, and verbal expressions of fear or worry, using a time-sampling methodology.

The POSA was found to possess good interrater reliability. The validity of the POSA was examined through a comparison of POSA scores to teacher and parent ratings of child anxiety as well as a comparison of the POSA scores to the responses of each child to an experimental manipulation of his or her anxiety state (i.e., attending a testing session with and without the mother present). POSA scores were positively related to others' ratings of the child's general levels of anxiety. Additionally, higher POSA scores were noted for all children during the testing session when their mother was not present. Although this scale has been developed and generally validated using a preschool sample, it may prove to be clinically useful with older samples as well (Ollendick, 1983).

One widely employed measure of behavioral observation is the behavioral avoidance task (BAT), wherein clients are exposed to anxiety-provoking situations and measures of approach and related behaviors are taken (Kendall et al., 1991; Ollendick & Francis, 1988). These tasks often provide rich clinical information regarding a client's responses of coping and avoidance. Unfortunately, they often suffer from a lack of standardization, precluding comparisons across studies. Furthermore, the psychometric properties of this form of assessment have yet to be explored.

Psychophysiological Assessment

Recently, Beidel and colleagues have published a number of investigations of the utility and reliability of psychophysiological assessment with anxious children (Beidel, 1988, 1991a, 1991b; Turner, Beidel, & Epstein, 1991). Although these assessments have just begun to receive attention in the clinical literature, data from developmental psychology indicate that physical responses to stressful situations (e.g., heart rate) may signal the presence of an anxious temperament in a subset of children (Beidel, 1989).

For a variety of groups of socially anxious children, including those with test anxiety or other forms of social phobia, socially relevant tasks, such as reading aloud, have been associated with increased heart rate (Beidel, 1988, 1991b). Interestingly, no baseline differences in physiological arousal were noted between socially anxious and normal control children during these assessments. In contrast to nonanxious children, however, clinical subjects appear to exhibit continually elevated heart rate throughout the task without any evidence of habituation (Beidel, 1988, 1991b; Turner et al., 1991).

Preliminary data regarding the test–retest reliability of various autonomic indicators of arousal in anxious children have been reported (Beidel, 1991a). This investigation examined the physiological reactivity of test anxious and nonanxious children to social-evalutive situations using a BAT format (i.e., a vocabulary test and oral reading task). Assessments were conducted two weeks apart, and both heart rate and blood pressure evidenced stability over time in response to participation in these tasks. Interestingly, test anxious subjects appeared to evidence comparable heightened physiological arousal from time 1 to 2, whereas nonanxious children displayed small decreases in their physiological reactivity.

Family Assessment

The interaction among child and family variables in the etiology and maintenance of anxiety in children and adolescents is an area that has been sorely understudied (Kendall et al., 1991; Mash & Terdal, 1988). Family evaluation has been an extremely fruitful area of research in the study of externalizing disorders (cf. Dadds, 1987; Patterson, 1982; Wahler, 1976; Wahler & Dumas, 1986), yet empirical assessment studies are practically nonexistent for anxious children and their families. It is surprising to find that so little work has been undertaken in this area, given that such research may provide important information for the assessment and treatment of anxious children. For example, global measures of the family milieu examining the nature of the general family environment, as well as problematic issues within the parent–child relationship, might yield interesting findings. Instruments such as the Issues Checklist (IC; Prinz, Foster, Kent, & O'Leary, 1979), Conflict Behavior Questionnaire (Prinz et al., 1979), and the Family Environment Scale (Moos, 1986) could assess descriptive characteristics of families of anxious children as well as suggest areas that might benefit from intervention or further empirical examination.

Fortunately, some very recent work has begun to focus on molecular examinations of the interactions between anxious children and their parents in order to explicate more clearly those factors within the family that may be associated with childhood anxiety (Dadds, Heard, & Rapee, 1992). This work is part of an ongoing treatment outcome study of childhood anxiety disorders that specifically examines the effect of parental involvement in treatment. Areas of particular interest within these family assessments include the family's information-processing style when presented with an ambiguous situation as well as the means by which the family manages such situations. Using the Family Anxiety Coding Schedule

(Dadds, Heard, & Rapee, 1994), these specific interactions will be examined and analyzed. Such data will provide invaluable information regarding the complex interactions of child and family characteristics in the maintenance of childhood anxiety.

Conclusions

Researchers have just begun to explore methods for comprehensive assessment of anxiety in children. Relatively little work has been undertaken examining the utility of assessment techniques with various diagnostic categories, including social phobia. Clearly, examinations of diagnostic differences are crucial to our understanding of the nature of childhood anxiety disorders. For example, there are few data to indicate that diagnostic categories differ on many of the aforementioned self-report measures, such as the STAIC or RCMAS (cf. Beidel, 1991b). Similarly, there is some evidence that anxiety-disordered children are not differentiated from children with externalizing disorders on some of these instruments (cf. Strauss et al., 1989). Continued consideration of self-report instruments that would tap specific key features of each diagnostic category is essential. In this regard, the SASC-R and SPAI-C are particularly promising. Moreover, given the relevance of constructs such as self-competence and social skills to the diagnosis of social phobia, future assessments should empirically examine the interrelationships of these constructs in a multimethod fashion (cf. Strauss et al., 1989). In this way, related strengths and deficits associated with social anxiety can then be examined and targeted during treatment.

Future work would greatly benefit from assessments that explore the interrelationship of cognitions, behaviors, and physiological responses associated with social anxiety. There have been few studies that have assessed the cognitions of anxious children. The convergence of findings from multiple cognitive assessment measures needs to be addressed using samples of anxious children, since it has been reported in the adult literature that different cognitive assessment methods appear to yield different results, perhaps by tapping different dimensions of cognitive activity (Clark, 1988; Kendall & Hollon, 1981). Further evidence of the reliability and validity of these assessments with anxiety-disordered children, particularly at various developmental levels, is warranted. In order to allow for comparisons across studies, it is imperative that scoring of cognitive assessments (e.g., thought listings) be standardized in the future (Kendall & Chansky, 1991). In addition, cognitive characteristics found to be associated with particular diagnostic categories (e.g., social phobia, overanxious disorder) need to be explicated (Kendall & Chansky, 1991; Last, 1988). Last, one area of study that has greatly contributed to our understanding of the cognitive experience of anxious adults has been the examination of information-processing biases in the face of threatening stimuli (MacLeod & Mathews, 1991; see Elting & Hope, Chapter 11, this volume). Similar work may contribute to our understanding of childhood anxiety as well.

Clearly, the area of behavioral assessment of childhood anxiety demands further empirical attention. Specifically, standardized measures of behavioral indicators of anxiety, such as the POSA, are necessary in order to make comparisons of data. In addition, valid and reliable behavioral observations are required in order to allow a greater understanding of the interrelationship of these responses to other systems (e.g., cognitions). Future work needs to be directed toward a more thorough understanding of the psychophysiological correlates of anxiety in anxious children, including those with social phobia. Some stimulating initial data have been provided that merit further attention. To date, the studies that have been conducted have used BATs in order to examine the differential effects of potentially anxiety-provoking situations on autonomic response. Additionally, comprehensive and multimodal assessments that examine the interrelationship between social anxiety and other related constructs (e.g., family characteristics, social skills, self-competence) are clearly warranted. For each assessment method, normative data must be gathered and consideration given to developmental differences that may affect the administration of and/or data collected from these methods. The work completed to date provides a promising beginning to these future endeavors.

TREATMENT

Pharmacotherapy

Although a number of pharmacological agents have been found useful in the treatment of adults with social phobia (see Potts & Davidson, Chapter 14, this volume), the literature on the pharmacological treatment of children with this anxiety disorder is practically nonexistent. In fact, few placebo-controlled trials have been conducted examining the efficacy of pharmacological treatment of any anxiety disorder in children and adolescents. Briefly, we review the limited literature examining the pharmacological treatment of avoidant disorder and selective mutism in children.

Simeon and Ferguson (1987) report on a single-blind uncontrolled trial of alprazolam in a group of children with avoidant and overanxious disorders. Results indicated a decrease in both child- and parent-rated anxiety symptoms for both diagnostic groups, while cognitive functioning also improved with treatment. In a controlled study of 30 children with avoidant disorder and overanxious disorder, minor improvement was noted for the avoidant disorder group, although no overall differences were found between alprazolam and placebo (Simeon et al., 1992). Thus far, the use of benzodiazepines in the treatment of childhood anxiety is largely based upon physician preference and not on controlled outcomes. Kutcher, Reiter, Gardner, and Klein (1992) caution that adverse effects and paradoxical reactions occasionally noted in benzodiazepine treatment of adults have not been adequately investigated in children.

There are two single-case studies of medication treatment of selective mutism in children. Golwyn and Weinstock (1990) report on the use of phenelzine in the treatment of a 7-year-old girl with a 2-year history of mutism. The authors describe the child as shy, unable to take oral exams, and "frozen" with fear when asked to speak. However, the patient did not avoid school or social functions and easily separated from her parents. Previous trials of behavior therapy and amantadine (200 mg per day) were unsuccessful. Phenelzine was titrated to a dose of 52.5 mg per day by 12 weeks, at which time she began conversing with others at her day-care center. At the start of school (week 16), she freely conversed with teachers, peers, and her doctors. Phenelzine was tapered and withdrawn by week 24, with gains maintained 5 months later.

Black and Uhde (1992) describe the treatment of a 12-year-old female who had never spoken in school. The patient avoided many social situations, including parties, using public bathrooms, being the focus of others' attention, and any interactions with strangers. She spoke on the telephone to only a few friends, but never in person. The patient had an unsuccessful trial of outpatient "psychotherapy" at age 5, and a similar unsuccessful trial of behavioral therapy at age 11. The authors initially prescribed desipramine but it was discontinued due to lack of efficacy. Following 4 weeks of fluoxetine (20 mg per day), the patient began a new school year speaking freely with adults and peers. Moreover, she gave oral reports, conversed freely with classmates, and attended social activities such as parties without distress. Gains were maintained at 7 months; however, the patient maintained a rigid passive–aggressive manner. She continued to refuse to speak with her treating physicians or to openly acknowledge that she was taking medication.

As previously discussed, questions regarding the appropriate nosological classification for the syndrome of selective mutism warrant serious consideration. The two case studies described above illustrate the phenomenological similarities of selective mutism and social phobia. There is a striking absence of systematic, placebo-controlled studies of medications for either disorder in children and adolescents. Yet, given the shared characteristics of the disorders, these case reports point toward the potential efficacy of pharmacotherapy as applied to selectively mute and social pho-

bic youth. Controlled trials have demonstrated the effectiveness of phenelzine, clonazepam and other compounds in the treatment of social phobic
adults (Potts & Davidson, Chapter 14, this volume; Liebowitz et al., 1992).
Similar pharmacological trials for social phobia in children and adolescents
should be rigorously pursued.

Psychosocial Treatment

It is relatively recently that attention has been turned toward the treatment
of childhood anxiety, and in doing so, clinicians have drawn upon the
adult literature in guiding treatment development. In an exhaustive and
comprehensive review of the treatment literature, Barrios and O'Dell
(1989) reviewed the literature on the behavioral treatments of children's
fears and anxieties. More recently, two reviews have focused specifically
on simple and social phobia (Beidel & Morris, 1993; King, 1993). The
most striking finding of these reviews was the lack of any systematic,
controlled, and methodologically sound treatment study of social phobia
in children or adolescents. Overall, studies to date have failed to utilize
standardized diagnostic, treatment, and outcome assessment methods.
However, given the recent advances in the assessment of social phobia in
children, the treatment literature provides a rich basis for the development
of effective therapeutic interventions.

Researchers have investigated the efficacy of a broad range of treatments for shyness, public speaking, and social-evaluative anxiety in youth,
including systematic desensitization and related procedures (e.g., Kondas,
1967; Wolpe, 1958, 1961), prolonged exposure (Kandel, Ayllon, & Rosenbaum, 1977), modeling (Evers & Schwarz, 1973; Matson, 1981), contingency management (Clement & Milne, 1967), and self-management training (Fox & Houston, 1981). A thorough analysis of this literature is beyond
the scope of this chapter. Rather, we will review several studies that have
examined the efficacy of treatments involving behavioral exposure and
skills training for social anxiety in youth. Readers interested in a more
thorough discussion should consult the aforementioned reviews (Barrios
& O'Dell, 1989; Beidel & Morris, 1993; King, 1993).

In the adult treatment literature, combined cognitive and exposure
treatments have been the most frequently investigated psychosocial intervention for social phobia (Hope & Heimberg, 1993; see Heimberg & Juster,
Chapter 12, this volume). Although no definitive conclusions may be
drawn as to whether adding cognitive therapy to exposure bolsters therapeutic effectiveness, the data suggest that cognitive interventions may be
an important component of the psychosocial treatment of adult social
phobics (Hope & Heimberg, 1993). These data support the contention that

social phobics' fear of negative evaluation is a cognitive construct and, thus, requires a direct cognitive intervention (Butler, 1989; Hope & Heimberg, 1993). Similarly, investigators who have examined the treatment of shyness and social-evaluative anxiety in youth identify both behavioral and social problem-solving skills as requiring direct intervention (e.g., Christoff et al., 1985). Although there are no controlled studies on the treatment of social phobia in youth (as defined in DSM-III-R or DSM-IV), several studies examined the treatment of nonclinical problems such as test anxiety and shyness in children.

Several investigators have demonstrated the effectiveness of cognitive restructuring techniques in the treatment of evaluation anxiety in children (e.g., Cavallaro & Meyers, 1986; Fox & Houston, 1981; Stevens & Pihl, 1983). The focus of treatment of test anxious children has been on modifying maladaptive self-statements that may interfere with task-oriented problem-solving behaviors. For example, Cavallaro and Meyers (1986) compared the effectiveness of relaxation training plus study skills (RSS) and relaxation training plus cognitive restructuring (RCR) to a no-contact control condition in reducing test anxiety in a sample of 67 11th-grade girls. Subjects randomly assigned to the treatment groups received six sessions of RSS or RCR over 4 weeks. RCR was effective in reducing subjects' test anxiety, but RSS training was not. The addition of the cognitive restructuring component resulted in greater anxiety reduction for students with good study habits than for those with poor study habits. Although controlled investigations of the effectiveness of these procedures with clinical samples have not been conducted, preliminary evidence suggests that cognitive restructuring techniques may be effective for specific forms of social anxiety in youth.

Franco, Christoff, Crimmins, and Kelly (1983) reported on the effectiveness of combined conversational skills training and behavioral practice in the treatment of an extremely shy 14-year-old boy. The subject was described as having chronic shyness and deficient relationships with peers, as having no friends his own age, and as being prone to isolating himself from relatives and neighbors. A multiple baseline across behaviors was employed, targeting four conversational behaviors: conversational questions, speech acknowledgements/reinforcers, eye contact, and affective warmth. The subject received 30 half-hour sessions over a 15-week period of skills training involving education, modeling, and corrective feedback. Additionally, following each session, the subject engaged in a 10-minute conversation with a novel partner. There was marked improvement when treatment successively targeted each behavior. In addition, these results were supported by global ratings of the subject's social skill by peer judges, conversational partners, his teachers, and the subject himself.

Although the study was uncontrolled and limited by the absence of standardized diagnostic and behavioral measures, Franco et al. (1983)

provide an exceptional early treatment model for the application of behavioral exposure combined with specific skills training for shy adolescents. Extending this paradigm, Christoff et al. (1985) treated six shy adolescents in an eight-session behavioral group. Subjects first received four sessions of social problem-solving skills training, followed by four sessions of conversational skills training. Conversational skills were modeled by therapists and then rehearsed by subjects. Extended and unstructured conversations between pairs of adolescents were utilized to practice and refine skills. Between-session homework to practice each target skill was then assigned. This group intervention was successful in increasing the frequency of daily social interactions and resulted in more positive reports of social interaction skill and more positive patterns of self-evaluation for the group. In addition, global ratings of ease of conversing with others and social interactions were taken from the subjects, their parents, and teachers, and these ratings supported the external validity of the intervention. Gains were maintained at 5-month follow-up.

Christoff et al. (1985) conceptualize effective social functioning as an integration of specific behavioral social skills (e.g., initiate conversations, assertiveness) and social problem-solving skills (e.g., planning practical ways to meet others). It is likely that shyness and/or social phobia interfere with the development of these skills or arrest the refinement of these skills in children and adolescents by limiting access to situations in which they may practice. Although social phobia was not the specific target of the Franco et al. (1983) and Christoff et al. studies, shyness may be viewed as a variant of social anxiety. Consequently, the use of extended, unstructured conversations between adolescent subjects provided an ecologically valid condition for practicing social skills and gaining experience with peer interactions.

Cognitive-Behavioral Group Treatment for Adolescent Social Phobia

In the remainder of this chapter we describe a newly developed treatment protocol for social phobic adolescents that is currently being evaluated in a controlled clinical trial. The cognitive-behavioral group treatment protocol for social phobic adolescents (CBGT-A; Albano, Marten, & Holt, 1991; Marten, Albano, & Holt, 1991) integrates the procedures used in our successful treatment for adult social phobia (Heimberg et al., 1990; Hope & Heimberg, 1993) with the skill-building elements necessary for effective social functioning as outlined by Christoff and colleagues. Thus, CBGT-A addresses the specific cognitive-developmental needs of this age group. In all of our child and adolescent treatment programs, we emphasize that children are not little adults, and hence, in modifying methods developed on adult patients, we cannot merely simplify the vocabulary and expect success. Treatment of the social phobic child or adolescent must take into account the patient's social milieu, cognitive-developmental level, and behavioral skill levels. The protocol allows for all skill levels to be addressed while focusing on specified individual target behaviors through the use of individualized fear and avoidance hierarchies. Patients' individual goals are identified and specific behavioral targets are addressed within the group format. Hierarchies are developed in an individual pretreatment assessment session with the therapists. A completed hierarchy will have 10 situations rated for fear and avoidance by the patient on a 0–8 scale (see example in Table 16.3). Items are derived by having the patient brainstorm situations that cause significant anxiety and by using situations identified earlier in both the child and parent diagnostic interviews. Prior to each session, the adolescents rate each hierarchy item for fear and avoidance, providing an ongoing measure of change.

The overall goals of the CBGT-A program are to teach adolescents to master their social phobias and concomitant avoidance of social situations by learning to control excessive anxiety and cope with normal, expected levels of anxiety. Specific skills that can decrease the distress and/or interference that result from social anxiety are taught and reviewed in group. Additionally, treatment focuses on having group members face personally relevant social situations in a structured and graduated manner during both within- and between-session exposures to difficult situations. These exposures are hypothesized to hold several key implications for the success-

TABLE 16.3. Individual Fear and Avoidance Hierarchy

Item	Fear rating[a]	Avoidance rating[a]
1. Asking a clerk for something in a store	8	7
2. Being asked a question in class	6	4
3. Giving an oral presentation	8	3
4. Talking to kids I don't know	7	4
5. Introducing myself to new people	7	5
6. Writing on the blackboard in class	5	5
7. Paying a cashier	4	5
8. Talking to a grownup (e.g., teacher)	5	4
9. Calling up a classmate for homework	7	5
10. Going to parties with people I don't know well	7	6

Note. Patient was a 14-year-old, Caucasian female, who participated in the CBGT-A program.
[a] Ratings from 0–8: 0 = no anxiety, do not avoid at all; 4 = definitely anxious, sometimes avoid situation; 8 = very severe/continuous anxiety and panic, invariably avoid the situation.

ful treatment of social phobic adolescents. First, behavioral exposures provide a means for the patient to directly confront stimuli that trigger their anxiety and avoidance. Thus, exposures are maintained for an extended period in order to effect habituation to the feared stimuli. Next, exposures provide an opportunity for the patient to apply his or her coping skills, rather than escape the anxiety or merely endure the situation with distress. Skills may then be tested, practiced, and mastered by the patient. But perhaps the most significant contribution of behavioral exposure is that the patient gains concrete evidence to disconfirm his or her maladaptive beliefs about the feared social situation. Up until this point, the adolescents' fears have been fueled by untested assumptions that have been treated as facts.

The CBGT-A protocol is divided into two eight-session phases: (1) psychoeducation and skills training, and (2) behavioral exposure. Sessions are 1.5 hours in length and conducted by a team of cotherapists. Groups are conducted with four to six participants. Table 16.4 presents a summary of specific session plans.

During the psychoeducation and skill-building phase, therapists present basic information about the treatment program and treatment rationale and educational material about the nature of social anxiety. As treatment progresses, various skill-building modules are introduced and reviewed, including modules for social skills, problem-solving skills, assertiveness, and cognitive restructuring. Modeling, behavioral shaping, and role-play techniques are utilized by the therapists to illustrate the coping strategies introduced during this phase.

Each session contains a scheduled snack time midway through the meeting. Our assessment of these youngsters revealed that the overwhelming majority avoid eating in public, and thus, the snack time provided a naturalistic activity for the initial modeling and shaping of prosocial behaviors. During the skill-building phase, the desensitization of eating in public and the shaping of delivering oral presentations are the focus of snack time. Group process activities and behavioral "mini-exposures" are targeted during the second phase of treatment.

Phase two (behavioral exposure) is concentrated on simulated within-session and *in vivo* exposures to each adolescent's feared social situations. Each group member works through his or her individual hierarchy of feared social situations and is "double exposed" by participating as a role-player in the exposures of other group members. During these exposures, observable behavioral goals are identified, along with anxiogenic automatic thoughts and rational coping responses. An example of an exposure plan is illustrated in Table 16.5.

In this example, the target patient and therapists chose the hierarchy item "calling up a classmate for homework" for the simulated exposure.

TABLE 16.4. Outline of CBGT-A Protocol

Individual pretreatment assessment
Devise patient's individual fear and avoidance hierarchy

Session 1 (parents attend)
Discuss ground rules for group
Obtain patients' and parents' description of social situations that cause anxiety
Introduce group to the cognitive-behavioral model of social anxiety
Snack time practice: therapists share information about themselves; informal mingling
Present overview of treatment and rationale
Review workbooks and monitoring technology
Assign homework: self-monitoring, treatment goals

Session 2 (parents attend)
Review self-monitoring
Describe three-component model of anxiety
Dissect a social situation into the three components
Snack time practice: therapists describe surviving a socially embarrassing moment
Elicit and discuss expectations for treatment
Discuss examining individual responses within the three components; encourage "detective work"
Assign homework: self-monitoring, life goals

Session 3
Review: self-monitoring, goals, model of anxiety
Labeling distortions: introduction to automatic thoughts (ATs)
Therapists role-play ATs
Snack time practice: relaxation and guided imagery
Rational responses: countering anxiogenic thoughts
Review of session
Assign homework: self-monitoring, workbook AT forms

Session 4
Review: self-monitoring, AT forms, cognitive counters
Introduce four steps of cognitive restructuring
Therapists role-play cognitive restructuring
Snack time practice: therapist deals with a problem
Steps to problem solving
Review of session
Assign homework: self-monitoring, workbook forms, cognitive restructuring, and problem solving

Session 5
Review: self-monitoring, workbook forms, cognitive restructuring, and problem-solving skills
Therapists model social skills versus "unskilled"
Social skills training I: identifying social skills and five steps to improve weaknesses
Snack time practice: shaping oral reading skills; each member reads aloud a paragraph provided by
   the therapists
Social skills training II: introduction to assertiveness training
Review of session
Assign homework: self-monitoring, social skills workbook forms, assertiveness monitoring, prepare a
   paragraph on a hobby or pastime to read aloud

Session 6
Review: self-monitoring, workbook forms, social skills
Social skills training III: review of skill-building steps and focus on perspective taking
Group role-play: conversing in the cafeteria
Snack time practice: reading prepared paragraphs
Social skills IV: assertiveness training continues
Review of session
Assign homework: self-monitoring, assertiveness workbook forms, assertiveness skill practice

(Table continues on next page.)

TABLE 16.4. (*Continued*)

Session 7
Review: self-monitoring, workbook forms, social skills
Review of skills learned to date: cognitive restructuring, problem solving, social skills
Treatment rationale: simulated exposures
Evaluating expectations: "How much better should I be by now?"
Snack time practice: group interaction exercise
Parents: how to access support and be understood
Assign homework: self-monitoring, review of skills

Session 8 (parents attend)
Review: self-monitoring homework
Review of expectations: "What should have changed by now?"
Treatment rationale: simulated and between-session exposures
Snack time: informal socializing
Role-play: perspective taking; parents and teens switch roles and deal with a social situation
Enlisting support: parents and teens are engaged in discussion on how to help "coach" the teen through
   the exposure phase
Assign homework: self-monitoring

Sessions 9–14
Review: self-monitoring and exposure homework
Simulated exposure #1
Snack time practice: specific mini-exposures to situations such as accepting compliments, giving critical
   feedback to a friend, etc.
Simulated exposure #2
Assign homework: individual hierarchy items are assigned for between-session exposures

Session 15 (parents attend)
Review: self-monitoring and exposure homework
Exposures: each group member is targeted in a simulated exposure that all parents observe
Snack time: informal socializing
Expectations and future plans: focus on maintaining treatment gains
Assign homework: as outlined in sessions 9–14

Session 16
Review: self-monitoring and exposure homework
Final exposures
Snack time: termination pizza party
Processing of termination and relapse prevention

Therapists assisted the patient in identifying specific behavioral goals, and as this phase of treatment progressed, the other group members also provided input in identifying goals, automatic thoughts, and rationale responses. During each 10-minute exposure, anxiety ratings (0–100 Subjective Units of Distress scale [SUDs]) were taken every minute from the subject, followed by the reciting of the chosen rational response. A therapist kept a record of the patient's behavior, noting the occurrence of a behavioral target such as asking a question about schoolmates. Upon completion, therapists reviewed the exposure with the patient, processing and addressing mastery of the exposure or any encountered difficulties. A chart was drawn for the patient illustrating the curve of her SUDs ratings, allowing her to visually inspect the habituation of her anxiety.

TABLE 16.5. Simulated Exposure Example

Hierarchy situation: Calling up a classmate for homework

Behavioral goals
1. Introduce self.
2. Ask for missed homework in social studies and algebra class.
3. Ask two additional questions about schoolmates and/or activities.

Automatic thoughts
"She'll think I'm stupid."
"I've never called her before, why should she talk to me?"
"I won't know what to say."

Rational responses
"It's okay to be nervous; I'm not used to calling people."
"I've seen her in school and she's always been nice to me."
"I've rehearsed this in my mind, and know how to talk to people."
"Even if she can't talk right now, it could be for all kinds of reasons and not because of me."

In situations where SUDs ratings remain elevated, the patient is encouraged to identify impediments to habituation (e.g., generating automatic thoughts without a countering response) and receives feedback from the group about his or her performance. Often, the adolescents are unaware that subjective anxiety does not necessarily hinder overt behavior. Thus, the exposure provides an opportunity to demonstrate that in spite of subjective feelings of anxiety, overt behavior may continue without any obvious impairment. In addition, therapists assist group members to recognize and accept normal levels of anxiety, such as the experience of sweaty palms and butterflies that may accompany giving an oral report or asking someone for a date. Group members are encouraged to allow this anxiety to occur, while maintaining focus on their task and coping skills. Because the sensations and accompanying awareness of anxiety has become the adolescent's first signal to escape and avoid, tolerance of normal levels of anxiety must be gradually reinforced and developed. At the end of each session, the adolescents are assigned personally relevant between-session *in vivo* exposures from their individual hierarchies and are encouraged to apply anxiety management skills in naturally occurring anxiety-provoking situations.

In addition to continued exposures, the final two sessions focus on termination and relapse prevention. Skills are reviewed and coping plans discussed in regards to anticipated upcoming events (e.g., proms, starting high school or college). The adolescents are encouraged to continue conducting their own exposures to such events. In addition, "relief" is identified as a marker for social anxiety. It is explained to the participants that if a person feels relieved when a social situation is cancelled or postponed, this should prompt an examination of the thoughts about entering the situation. The identification of any anxious thoughts (e.g., "Whew, I really wouldn't know what to say"; "There may not be anyone there I know") then becomes the cue that social anxiety is creeping in and the situation must be confronted. The adolescents are instructed to then devise a coping and exposure plan and to enter the situation repeatedly until they master their anxiety.

Parent Participation

Research on the treatment of adult anxiety disorders has demonstrated that the inclusion of a family member may significantly enhance the effects of treatment and may also address the severe interpersonal problems that sometimes accompany the anxiety disorders (Barlow, Mavissakalian, & Hay, 1981; Barlow, O'Brien, & Last, 1984; Cerny, Barlow, Craske, & Himadi, 1987). The involvment of parents in the treatment of childhood anxiety disorders has been the exception (Barlow & Seidner, 1983), rather than the rule, with parents typically seen separately for instruction in contingency management procedures (see Barrios & O'Dell, 1989, and Braswell, 1991). In the treatment of adolescent social phobia, we have opted to include parents in some sessions because the adolescent functions within the family system, with their primary support coming from family members.

Parents are actively involved in selected CBGT-A sessions. In the first two sessions, parents attend along with their child in order to receive education about the nature and maintenance of social phobia and to develop realistic and appropriate expectations for their child's behavior and treatment. At session 8, parents again attend so that we may directly address the feelings and behavioral reactions of the adolescents and their parent(s) regarding family interactions influenced by the adolescent's social phobia. Perspective taking (accomplished through role reversals) and effective communication strategies are targeted in this session. In addition, we address the parents' expectations for their child after having attended the first half of the program. Parents and adolescents are then given a description of the second phase of treatment.

At session 15, parents again attend the group and watch exposures in progress. In this session (usually lasting 2 hours), each adolescent engages in a 10-minute exposure, followed by a processing of the experience by the adolescents and their parents. Termination and relapse prevention are addressed. We encourage families to discuss anxiety-provoking situations and brainstorm coping and exposure plans for entering and managing them. Finally, parents are given specific feedback on their roles as "coaches" for the adolescent in applying their skills after termination. Although the inclusion of parents in the active treatment program makes intuitive sense, we are currently conducting a controlled clinical trial evaluating the impact of the parental involvement on the overall effectiveness of CBGT-A.

Preliminary Effectiveness and Future Directions

Empirical data examining the effectiveness of CBGT-A are forthcoming; however an early pilot investigation provided strong support for the protocol. In Albano, Marten, Holt, Heimberg, and Barlow (in press), we present data on five adolescents who completed the CBGT-A treatment protocol with parent participation. The sample consisted of three males and two females (ages 13–16) who, on the basis of the ADIS-C and ADIS-P interviews, were diagnosed with social phobia, generalized type. All five adolescents presented with comorbid conditions, mainly overanxious disorder and mood disorders. Independent evaluations, completed at 3 months posttreatment, revealed that social phobia had decreased to subclinical levels for all but one adolescent. At 1-year follow-up, four subjects were completely free of any mental disorder, and social phobia had remitted to subclinical levels in the remaining subject. Despite continued physiological arousal during the standardized BAT tasks (elevated heart rate), the subjects reported a substantial decrement in subjective anxiety. Moreover, the mean number of negative cognitions decreased while neutral thoughts increased during the BAT. The results suggest that subjects' interpretation of heightened physiological arousal and the task at hand changed from an anxiogenic, negative self-focus to a nonanxious and nonthreatening interpretation.

These results are encouraging and have prompted a systematic examination of the protocol. In addition to examining the relative effectiveness of the protocol and involvement of parents, questions regarding the indirect impact of this prescriptive cognitive-behavioral intervention on comorbid conditions are being addressed. Moreover, it remains to be seen whether severe behavioral dysfunction, such as that evidenced in school refusal resulting from social anxiety, can be adequately treated within the context of this protocol.

SUMMARY AND CONCLUSIONS

The purpose of this chapter was to examine our current understanding of social phobia in children and adolescents. Social phobia is a disruptive and debilitating condition for children and adolescents. Research has documented the chronicity of social phobia, yet only recently has attention turned toward examining its full impact on the developing child. Numerous studies have documented disruption of peer relations, self-concept, and academic and occupational functioning, and that such disruption continues well into adulthood. Longitudinal research on behavioral inhibition suggests that it may be a significant diathesis for further psychopathology. Clearly, attention must be turned toward the elucidation of those factors that may foster the emergence of social phobia. Parent pathology, family environment, behavioral inhibition, and social–environmental variables must all be examined for their potential role in the development and maintenance of this serious disorder. We are now beginning to develop adequate assessment methodologies for social phobic children and adolescents. Continued advances in the development of psychometrically sound diagnostic and assessment instruments will help us to a greater understanding of the nature of social phobia in youth. Furthermore, we have begun to develop effective treatments for social phobia in youth. It is clear that both pharmacological and psychosocial treatments warrant serious study. Overall, there is a serious need for prospective, longitudinal studies in which standardized assessment methods are used to examine social phobia and its impact. Advances in the understanding of the etiology of this disorder and early detection and intervention of social phobic children and adolescents may prevent a lifetime of anxiety and distress.

REFERENCES

Albano, A. M., Leung, A. L., & Barlow, D. H. (1994, November). *Assessment and remediation of social skills deficits in social phobic adolescents: A preliminary study.* Paper presented at the annual meeting of the Association for Advancement of Behavior Therapy, San Diego, CA.

Albano, A. M., Marten, P. A., & Holt, C. S. (1991). *Therapist's manual for cognitive-behavioral group therapy for adolescent social phobia.* Unpublished manuscript, State University of New York, Albany.

Albano, A. M., Marten, P. A., Holt, C. S., Heimberg, R. G., & Barlow, D. H. (in press). Cognitive-behavioral group treatment for adolescent social phobia: A preliminary study. *Journal of Nervous and Mental Disease.*

American Psychiatric Association. (1980). *Diagnostic and statistical manual of mental disorders* (3rd ed.). Washington, DC: Author.

American Psychiatric Association. (1987). *Diagnostic and statistical manual of mental disorders* (3rd ed., rev.). Washington, DC: Author.

American Psychiatric Association. (1994). *Diagnostic and statistical manual of mental disorders* (4th ed.). Washington, DC: Author.

Anderson, J. C., Williams, S., McGee, R., & Silva, P. A. (1987). DSM-III disorders in preadolescent children. *Archives of General Psychiatry, 44,* 69–76.

Arnkoff, D. B., & Glass, C. R. (1989). Cognitive assessment in social anxiety and social phobia. *Clinical Psychology Review, 9,* 61–74.

Barlow, D. H., Mavissakalian, M., & Hay, L. R. (1981). Couples treatment of agoraphobia: Changes in marital satisfaction. *Behaviour Research and Therapy, 19,* 245–255.

Barlow, D. H., O'Brien, G. T., & Last, C. G. (1984). Couples treatment of agoraphobia. *Behavior Therapy, 15,* 41–58.

Barlow, D. H., & Seidner, A. L. (1983). Treatment of adolescent agoraphobics: Effects on parent–adolescent relations. *Behaviour Research and Therapy, 21,* 519–526.

Barrios, B. A., & Hartmann, D. P. (1988). Fears and anxieties. In E. J. Mash & L. G. Terdal (Eds.), *Behavioral assessment of childhood disorders* (2nd ed., pp. 196–262). New York: Guilford Press.

Barrios, B. A., & O'Dell, S. L. (1989). Fears and anxieties. In E. J. Mash & R. A. Barkley (Eds.), *Treatment of childhood disorders* (pp. 167–221). New York: Guilford Press.

Beidel, D. C. (1988). Psychophysiological assessment of anxious emotional states in children. *Journal of Abnormal Psychology, 97,* 80–82.

Beidel, D. C. (1989). Assessing anxious emotion: A review of psychophysiological assessment in children. *Clinical Psychology Review, 9,* 717–736.

Beidel, D. C. (1991a). Determining the reliability of psychophysiological assessment in childhood anxiety. *Journal of Anxiety Disorders, 5,* 139–150.

Beidel, D. C. (1991b). Social phobia and overanxious disorder in school-age children. *Journal of the American Academy of Child and Adolescent Psychiatry, 30,* 545–552.

Beidel, D. C., & Morris, T. L. (1993). Avoidant disorder of childhood and social phobia. *Child and Adolescent Psychiatric Clinics of North America, 2,* 623–638.

Beidel, D. C., Neal, A. M., & Lederer, A. S. (1991). The feasibility and validity of a daily diary for the assessment of anxiety in children. *Behavior Therapy, 22,* 505–517.

Beidel, D. C., & Turner, S. M. (1988). Comorbidity of test anxiety and other anxiety disorders in children. *Journal of Abnormal Child Psychology, 16,* 275–287.

Beidel, D. C., Turner, S. M., & Morris, T. L. (1995). A new inventory to assess childhood social phobia: The Social Phobia and Anxiety Inventory for Children. *Psychological Assessment, 7,* 73–79.

Bernstein, G. A., & Borchardt, C. M. (1991). Anxiety disorders of childhood and adolescence: A critical review. *Journal of the American Academy of Child and Adolescent Psychiatry, 30,* 519–532.

Black, B., & Uhde, T. W. (1992). Elective mutism as a variant of social phobia. *Journal of the American Academy of Child and Adolescent Psychiatry, 31,* 1090–1094.

Bornstein, P. H., Hamilton, S. B., & Bornstein, M. T. (1988). Self-monitoring procedures. In A. R. Ciminero, K. S. Calhoun, & H. E. Adams (Eds.), *Handbook of behavioral assessment* (pp. 176–221). New York: Wiley.

Braswell, L. (1991). Involving parents in cognitive-behavioral therapy with children and adolescents. In P. C. Kendall (Ed.), *Child and adolescent therapy: Cognitive-behavioral procedures* (pp. 316–351). New York: Guilford Press.

Butler, G. (1989). Issues in the application of cognitive and behavioral strategies to the treatment of social phobia. *Clinical Psychology Review, 9,* 91–186.

Cavallaro, D. M., & Meyers, J. (1986). Effects of study habits on cognitive restructuring and study skills training in the treatment of test anxiety with adolescent females. *Techniques: A Journal for Remedial Education and Counseling, 2,* 145–155.

Cerny, J. A., Barlow, D. H., Craske, M. G., & Himadi, W. G. (1987). Couples treatment of agoraphobia: A two-year follow-up. *Behavior Therapy, 18,* 401–415.

Christoff, K. A., Scott, W. O. N., Kelley, M. L., Schlundt, D., Baer, G., & Kelly, J. A. (1985). Social skills and social problem-solving training for shy young adolescents. *Behavior Therapy, 16,* 468–477.

Clark, D. A. (1988). The validity of measures of cognition: A review of the literature. *Cognitive Therapy and Research, 12,* 1–20.

Clark, D. M. (1986). Cognitive therapy for anxiety. *Behavioural Psychotherapy, 14,* 283–294.

Clement, P. W., & Milne, D. C. (1967). Group play therapy and tangible reinforcers used to modify the behaviour of 8-year-old boys. *Behaviour Research and Therapy, 5,* 301–312.

Cole, D. A. (1991). Preliminary support for a competency-based model of depression in children. *Journal of Abnormal Psychology, 100,* 181–190.

Dadds, M. R. (1987). Families and the origins of child behavior problems. *Family Process, 26,* 341–357.

Dadds, M. R., Heard, P. M., & Rapee, R. M. (1992). The role of family intervention in the treatment of child anxiety disorders: Some preliminary findings. *Behaviour Change, 9,* 171–177.

Dadds, M. R., Heard, P. M., & Rapee, R. M. (1994). Behavioral observation. In T. H. Ollendick, N. J. King, & W. Yule (Eds.), *International handbook of phobic and anxiety disorders in children* (pp. 349–364). Boston: Allyn & Bacon.

Edelbrock, C. (1985, June). *Teachers' perceptions of childhood anxiety and school adjustment.* Paper presented at the Conference on Anxiety Disorders in Children: Implications for School Adjustment, Cape Cod, MA.

Evers, W. L., & Schwarz, J. C. (1973). Modifying social withdrawal in preschoolers: The effects of filmed modeling and teacher praise. *Journal of Abnormal Child Psychology, 1,* 248–256.

Foster, S. L., Bell-Dolan, D. J., & Burge, D. A. (1988). Behavioral observation. In A. S. Bellack & M. Hersen (Eds.), *Behavioral assessment: A practical handbook* (3rd ed., pp. 119–160). New York: Pergamon Press.

Fox, J. E., & Houston, B. K. (1981). Efficacy of self-instructional training for reducing children's anxiety in an evaluative situation. *Behaviour Research and Therapy, 19,* 509–515.

Fox, J. E., Houston, B. K., & Pittner, M. S. (1983). Trait anxiety and children's cognitive behaviors in an evaluative situation. *Cognitive Therapy and Research, 7,* 149–154.

Francis, G. (1988). Assessing cognition in anxious children. *Behavior Modification, 12,* 267–280.

Francis, G. (1990). Social phobia in childhood. In C. G. Last & M. Hersen (Eds.), *Handbook of child and adult psychopathology: A longitudinal perspective* (pp. 163–168). New York: Pergamon Press.

Franco, D. P., Christoff, K. A., Crimmins, D. B., & Kelly, J. A. (1983). Social skills training for an extremely shy young adolescent: An empirical case study. *Behavior Therapy, 14,* 568–575.

Glennon, B., & Weisz, J. R. (1978). An observational approach to the assessment of anxiety in young children. *Journal of Consulting and Clinical Psychology, 46,* 1246–1257.

Golwyn, D. H., & Weinstock, R. C. (1990). Phenelzine treatment of elective mutism: A case report. *Journal of Clinical Psychiatry, 51,* 384–385.

Graziano, A. M., DeGiovanni, I. S., & Garcia, K. A. (1979). Behavioral treatment of children's fears: A review. *Psychological Bulletin, 86,* 804–830.

Harter, S. (1982). The Perceived Competence Scale for Children. *Child Development, 53,* 87–97.

Harter, S. (1985). *Manual for the Self-Perception Profile for Children.* Denver, CO: University of Denver.

Havighurst, R. J. (1972). *Developmental tasks and education.* New York: McKay.

Heimberg, R. G., Dodge, C. S., Hope, D. A., Kennedy, C. R., Zollo, L. J., & Becker, R. E. (1990). Cognitive behavioral group treatment for social phobia: Comparison with a credible placebo control. *Cognitive Therapy and Research, 14,* 1–23.

Hope, D. A., & Heimberg, R. G. (1993). Social phobia and social anxiety. In D. H. Barlow (Ed.), *Clinical handbook of psychological disorders: A step-by-step treatment manual* (pp. 99–136). New York: Guilford Press.

Houston, B. K., Fox, J. E., & Forbes, L. (1984). Trait anxiety and children's state anxiety, cognitive behaviors, and performance under stress. *Cognitive Therapy and Research, 8,* 631–641.

Inderbitzen, H., & Foster, S. L. (1992). The Teenage Inventory of Social Skills: Development, reliability, and validity. *Psychological Assessment, 4,* 451–459.

Inderbitzen-Pisaruk, H., Clark, M. L., & Solano, C. H. (1992). Correlates of loneliness in midadolescence. *Journal of Youth and Adolescence, 21,* 151–167.

Johnson, R. L., & Glass, C. R. (1989). Heterosocial anxiety and direction of attention in high school boys. *Cognitive Therapy and Research, 13,* 509–526.

Johnson, S. B., & Melamed, B. G. (1979). The assessment and treatment of children's fears. In B. B. Lahey & A. E. Kazdin (Eds.), *Advances in clinical child psychology* (Vol. 2, pp. 107–139). New York: Plenum Press.

Kagan, J., Reznick, J. S., & Snidman, N. (1988). Biological bases of childhood shyness. *Science, 240,* 167–171.

Kandel, H. J., Ayllon, T., & Rosenbaum, M. S. (1977). Flooding or systematic exposure in the treatment of extreme social withdrawal in children. *Journal of Behavior Therapy and Experimental Psychiatry, 8,* 75–81.

Kashani, J. H., & Orvaschel, H. (1990). A community study of anxiety in children and adolescents. *American Journal of Psychiatry, 147,* 313–318.

Kashani, J. H., Orvaschel, H., Rosenberg, T. K., & Reid, J. C. (1989). Psychopathology in a community sample of children and adolescents: A developmental perspective. *Journal of the American Academy of Child and Adolescent Psychiatry, 28,* 701–706.

Kendall, P. C., & Chansky, T. E. (1991). Considering cognition in anxiety-disordered children. *Journal of Anxiety Disorders, 5,* 167–185.

Kendall, P. C., Chansky, T. E., Freidman, M., Kim, R., Kortlander, E., Sessa, F. M., & Siqueland, L. (1991). Treating anxiety disorders in children and adolescents. In P. C. Kendall (Ed.), *Child and adolescent therapy: Cognitive-behavioral procedures* (pp. 131–164). New York: Guilford Press.

Kendall, P. C., & Hollon, S. D. (1981). Assessing self-referent speech: Methods in the measurement of self-statements. In P.C. Kendall & S.D. Hollon (Eds.), *Assessment strategies for cognitive-behavioral interventions* (pp. 85–118). New York: Academic Press.

Kendall, P. C., Howard, B. L., & Hays, R. C. (1989). Self-referent speech and psychopathology: The balance of positive and negative thinking. *Cognitive Therapy and Research, 13,* 583–598.

Kendall, P. C., & Ronan, K. R. (1990a). Assessment of children's anxieties, fears, and phobias: Cognitive-behavioral models and methods. In C. R. Reynolds & R. W. Kamphaus (Eds.), *Handbook of psychological and educational assessment of children: Personality, behavior, and context* (pp. 223–244). New York: Guilford Press.

Kendall, P. C., & Ronan, K. R. (1990b). *Children's Anxious Self-Statement Questionnaire (CASSQ).* Unpublished manuscript, Temple University, Department of Psychology, Philadelphia.

King, N. J. (1993). Simple and social phobias. In T. H. Ollendick & R. J. Prinz (Eds.), *Advances in clinical child psychology* (Vol. 15, pp. 305–341). New York: Plenum Press.

King, N. J., Hamilton, D. I., & Ollendick, T. H. (1988). *Children's phobias: A behavioural perspective.* Chichester, UK: Wiley.

Kondas, O. (1967). Reduction of examination anxiety and "stage-fright" by group desensitization and relaxation. *Behaviour Research and Therapy, 5,* 275–281.

Kutcher, S. P., Reiter, S., Gardner, D. M., & Klein, R. G. (1992). The pharmacotherapy of anxiety disorders in children and adolescents. *Psychiatric Clinics of North America, 15,* 41–67.

LaGreca, A. M., Dandes, S. K., Wick, P., Shaw, K., & Stone, W. L. (1988). Development of the Social Anxiety Scale for Children: Reliability and concurrent validity. *Journal of Clinical Child Psychology, 17,* 84–91.

LaGreca, A. M., & Stone, W. L. (1993). Social Anxiety Scale for Children—Revised: Factor structure and concurrent validity. *Journal of Clinical Child Psychology, 22,* 17–27.

Lann, I. S. (1991). Introduction. *Journal of Anxiety Disorders, 5,* 101–103.

Last, C. G. (1988). Introduction. *Behavior Modification, 12,* 163–164.

Last, C. G., Hersen, M., Kazdin, A. E., Finkelstein, R., & Strauss, C. C. (1987). Comparison of DSM-III separation anxiety and overanxious disorders: Demographic characteristics and patterns of comorbidity. *Journal of the American Academy of Child and Adolescent Psychiatry, 26,* 527–531.

Last, C. G., Strauss, C. C., & Frances, G. (1987). Comorbidity among childhood anxiety disorders. *Journal of Nervous and Mental Disease, 175,* 726–730.

Liebowitz, M. R., Schneier, F., Campeas, R., Hollander, E., Hatterer, J., Fyer, A., Gorman, J., Papp, L., Davies, S., Gully, R., & Klein, D. F. (1992). Phenelzine vs. atenolol in social phobia: A placebo-controlled comparison. *Archives of General Psychiatry, 49,* 1–6.

MacLeod, C., & Mathews, A. M. (1991). Cognitive-experimental approaches to the emotional disorders. In P. R. Martin (Ed.), *Handbook of behavior therapy and psychological science: An integrative approach* (pp. 116–150). New York: Pergamon Press.

Marten, P. A., Albano, A. M., & Holt, C. S. (1991). *Therapist's manual for cognitive-behavioral group treatment for adolescent social phobia with parent participation.* Unpublished manuscript, State University of New York, Albany.

Mash, E. J., & Terdal, L. G. (1988). Behavioral assessment of child and family disturbance. In E. J. Mash & L. G. Terdal (Eds.), *Behavioral assessment of childhood disorders* (2nd ed., pp. 3–65). New York: Guilford Press.

Matson, J. L. (1981). Assessment and treatment of clinical fears in mentally retarded children. *Journal of Applied Behavior Analysis, 14,* 287–294.

Matson, J. L., Rotatori, A. F., & Helsel, W. J. (1983). Development of a rating scale to measure social skills in children: The Matson Evaluation of Social Skills with Youngsters (MESSY). *Behaviour Research and Therapy, 21,* 335–340.

McGee, R., Fehan, M., Williams, S., Partridge, F., Silva, P. A., & Kelly, J. (1990). DSM-III disorders in a large sample of adolescents. *Journal of the American Academy of Child and Adolescent Psychiatry, 29,* 611–619.

Meichenbaum, D. (1977). *Cognitive-behavior modification: An integrative approach.* New York: Plenum Press.

Moos, R. H. (1986). *Family Environment Scale manual.* Palo Alto, CA: Consulting Psychologists Press.

Morris, T. L., Beidel, D. C., & Turner, S. M. (1993, August). *A new self-report measure of child social phobia: The SPAI-C.* Paper presented at the annual meeting of the American Psychological Association, Toronto, Canada.

Ollendick, T. H. (1983). Anxiety-based disorders. In M. Hersen (Ed.), *Outpatient behavior therapy: A clinical guide* (pp. 273–305). New York: Grune & Stratton.

Ollendick, T. H. & Francis, G. (1988). Behavioral assessment and treatment of childhood phobias. *Behavior Modification, 12,* 165–204.

Ollendick, T. H., King, N. J., & Frary, R. B. (1989). Fears in children and adolescents. Reliability and generalizability across gender, age and nationality. *Behaviour Research and Therapy, 27,* 19–26.

Öst, L.-G. (1987). Age of onset in different phobias. *Journal of Abnormal Psychology, 96,* 223–229.

Parks, C. W., & Hollon, S. D. (1988). Cognitive assessment. In A. S. Bellack & M. Hersen (Eds.), *Behavioral assessment: A practical handbook* (3rd ed., pp. 161–212). New York: Pergamon Press.

Patterson, G. R. (1982). *Coercive family process.* Eugene, OR: Castalia Press.

Prins, P. J. (1986). Children's self-speech and self-regulation during a fear-provoking behavioral test. *Behaviour Research and Therapy, 24,* 181–191.

Prinz, R. J., Foster, S., Kent, R. N., & O'Leary, K. D. (1979). Multivariate assessment of conflict in distressed and nondistressed mother-adolescent dyads. *Journal of Applied Behavior Analysis, 12,* 691–700.

Reynolds, C. R., & Paget, N. D. (1983). National normative and reliability data for the Revised Children's Anxiety Scale. *School Psychology Review, 12,* 324–336.

Reynolds, C. R., & Richmond, B. O., (1978). What I Think and Feel: A revised measure of children's manifest anxiety. *Journal of Abnormal Child Psychology, 6,* 271–280.

Ronan, K. R., Rowe, P., & Kendall, P. C. (1988, November). *Children's Anxious Self-Statement Questionnaire (CASSQ): Development and validation.* Paper presented at the annual meeting of the Association for Advancement of Behavior Therapy, New York.

Rosenbaum, J. R., Biederman, J., Hirshfeld, D. R., Bolduc, E. A., & Chaloff, J. (1991). Behavioral inhibition in children: A possible precursor to panic disorder or social phobia. *Journal of Clinical Psychiatry, 52*, 5–9.

Rubin, K. H., LeMare, L. J., & Lollis, S. (1990). Social withdrawal in childhood: Developmental pathways to peer rejection. In S. R. Asher & J. D. Coie (Eds.), *Peer rejection in childhood* (pp. 217–249). Cambridge, UK: Cambridge University Press.

Schwartz, R. M., & Garamoni, G. L. (1986). A structural model of positive and negative states of mind: Asymmetry in the internal dialogue. In P. C. Kendall (Ed.), *Advances in cognitive-behavioral research and therapy* (Vol. 5, pp. 1–62). New York: Academic Press.

Silverman, W. K. (1991). Diagnostic reliability of anxiety disorders in children using structured interviews. *Journal of Anxiety Disorders, 5*, 105–124.

Silverman, W. K., & Albano, A. M. (1995). *The Anxiety Disorders Interview Schedule for Children and Parents—DSM-IV Version.* New York: Graywind.

Silverman, W. K., & Eisen, A. R. (1992). Age differences in the reliability of parent and child report of child anxious symptomatology using a structured interview. *Journal of the American Academy of Child and Adolescent Psychiatry, 31*, 117–124.

Silverman, W. K., & Nelles, W. B. (1988). The Anxiety Disorders Interview Schedule for Children. *Journal of the American Academy of Child and Adolescent Psychiatry, 27*, 772–778.

Simeon, J. G., & Ferguson, H. B. (1987). Alprazolam effects in children with anxiety disorders. *Canadian Journal of Psychiatry, 32*, 570–574.

Simeon, J. G., Ferguson, H. B., Knott, V., Roberts, N., Gauthier, B., Dubois, C., & Wiggins, D. (1992). Clinical, cognitive, and neurophysiological effects of alprazolam in children and adolescents with overanxious disorder and avoidant disorders. *Journal of the American Academy of Child and Adolescent Psychiatry, 31*, 29–33.

Spielberger, C. (1973). *Manual for the State–Trait Inventory for Children.* Palo Alto, CA: Consulting Psychologists Press.

Stevens, R., and Pihl, R. O. (1983). Learning to cope with school: A study of the effects of a coping skill training program with test-vulnerable 7th-grade students. *Cognitive Therapy and Research, 7*, 155–158.

Strauss, C. C. (1988). Behavioral assessment and treatment of overanxious disorder in children and adolescents. *Behavior Modification, 12*, 234–251.

Strauss, C. C., Frame, C. L., & Forehand, R. (1987). Psychosocial impairment associated with anxiety in children. *Journal of Clinical Child Psychology, 16*, 235–239.

Strauss, C. C., & Francis, G. (1989). Phobic disorders. In C. G. Last & M. Hersen (Eds.), *Handbook of child psychiatric diagnosis* (pp. 170–190). New York: Wiley.

Strauss, C. C., Lease, C. A., Kazdin, A. E., Dulcan, M. K., & Last, C. G. (1989). Multimethod assessment of the social competence of children with anxiety disorders. *Journal of Clinical Child Psychology, 18*, 184–189.

Turner, S. M., & Beidel, D. C. (1989). Social phobia: Clinical syndrome, diagnosis, and comorbidity. *Clinical Psychology Review, 9*, 3–18.

Turner, S. M., Beidel, D. C., & Epstein, L. H. (1991). Vulnerability and risk for anxiety disorders. *Journal of Anxiety Disorders, 5,* 151–166.

Uhde, T. W., Tancer, M. E., Black, B., & Brown, T. M. (1991). Phenomenology and neurobiology of social phobia: Comparison with panic disorder. *Journal of Clinical Psychiatry, 52,* 31–40.

Vernberg, E. M., Abwender, D. A., Ewell, K. K., & Beery, S. H. (1992). Social anxiety and peer relationships in early adolescence: A prospective analysis. *Journal of Clinical Child Psychology, 21,* 189–196.

Wahler, R. G. (1976). Deviant child behavior within the family: Developmental speculations and behavior change strategies. In H. Leitenberg (Ed.), *Handbook of behavior modification and behavior therapy* (pp. 516–543). Englewood Cliffs, NJ: Prentice-Hall.

Wahler, R. G., & Dumas, J. E. (1986). Maintenance factors in coercive mother–child interactions: The compliance and predictability hypotheses. *Journal of Applied Behavior Analysis, 19,* 13–22.

Warren, R., Good, G., & Velten, E. (1984). Measurement of social-evaluative anxiety in junior high school students. *Adolescence, 19,* 643–648.

Watson, D., & Friend, R. (1969). Measurement of social-evaluative anxiety. *Journal of Consulting and Clinical Psychology, 33,* 448–457.

Wolpe, J. (1958). *Psychotherapy by reciprocal inhibition.* Stanford, CA: Stanford University Press.

Wolpe, J. (1961). The systematic desensitization treatment of neuroses. *Journal of Nervous and Mental Disease, 132,* 189–203.

Zatz, S., & Chassin, L. (1983). Cognitions of test-anxious children. *Journal of Consulting and Clinical Psychology, 51,* 526–534.

Zatz, S., & Chassin, L. (1985). Cognitions of test-anxious children under naturalistic test-taking conditions. *Journal of Consulting and Clinical Psychology, 53,* 393–401.

Zimbardo, P. G., Pilkonis, P. A., & Norwood, R. M. (1974). *The silent prison of shyness* (ONR Tech. Rep. No. Z-17). Stanford: Stanford University.

Zimbardo, P. G., & Radl, S. (1981). *The shy child.* New York: McGraw-Hill.

Index

Adolescents, 163–178, 406–418
  assessment, 395–406
  cognitive-behavioral group treatment,
    410–417
  peer relationships, 174, 175
  shyness development, 163–178
  social phobia prevalence/
    characteristics, 387–395
  treatment, 406–418
Age at onset, 12, 31, 53, 54
Age at presentation, 54, 55
Agoraphobia, 12, 13, 25
Alcohol abuse, comorbidity, 16, 57, 58
Alprazolam (Xanax)
  cognitive-behavioral treatment
    comparison, 292, 293
  literature review, 345, 348, 351
  phenelzine comparison, 337
  practical guidelines, 375
Ambiguous Events Questionnaire, 81
Anafranil (clomipramine), 358
Animal fears, development, 135, 136
Anticipatory anxiety, 74, 75
Antithyroid antibodies, 124, 126
Anxiety Disorders Interview
  Schedule—Revised, 191–193
Anxiety management training, 289, 290
Applied relaxation (see Relaxation
  strategies)
Approach–avoidance tendencies, 147, 148
Assortative mating, 31
Atenolol, 344, 345
  exposure treatment comparison, 291,
    292, 303
  literature review, 344–347
  phenelzine comparison, 115, 335, 336,
    345

Attentional processes, 242–246
  assessment, 242–245
  social phobia allocation of, 52, 70–73,
    82–84, 326
Attributional Style Questionnaire, 238,
  239
Attributions, 106, 107, 238, 239
Atypical depression, comorbidity, 14
Audience Anxiousness Scale, 206, 212
Audiotape-aided thought recall, 249
Aurorix (see Moclobemide)
Automatic thoughts (see Negative
  thoughts)
Autonomic factors, 119, 220–223
Avoidance behavior, assessment, 219
Avoidance conditioning, 147, 148
Avoidant personality disorder
  cognitive-behavioral treatment
    outcome, 297
  cognitive intervention application,
    326–331
  and generalized social phobia, 14, 15
  social phobia relationship, 45

B

Behavioral assessment, 214–219, 402
Behavioral Assessment Test strategies,
  215, 218, 219
Behavioral avoidance task, 403
Behavioral inhibition
  animal research, 145–147
  and conditioning, 145–148
  family studies, 121, 122
  genetic origins, animals, 145, 146
  longitudinal study, 166, 167
  physiological reactivity, 165

427

Behavioral inhibition (*continued*)
  as predispositional factor, 146–148,
    390
Behavioral observations, 214, 215, 402,
    403
Behavioral pharmacology, 114–120
Behavioral techniques (*see* Exposure
    techniques)
Benzodiazepines
  literature review, 345, 348–352, 359
  practical guidelines, 375
  selection of, 372
Beta blockers, 344–347
  in clinical populations, 344, 345
  literature review, 344, 345
  in nonclinical populations, 344
  practical guidelines, 376, 377
Birth cohort effects, 31
Blood pressure, 220–222, 404
Blushing, 12, 47, 220
Brain imaging, 221
Brief Social Phobia Scale, 194–196
Brofaromine, 115, 341, 342, 372
Bromazepam, 350
Bullying, shy children, 174
Bupropion (Wellbutrin)
  dopaminergic activity, 127
  literature review, 358
  and neurobiology, 115
Buspirone (BuSpar)
  cognitive-behavioral treatment
    combination, 293, 294, 304
  cognitive-behavioral treatment
    comparison, 303
  literature review, 354, 356, 357
  practical guidelines, 377
  selection of, 373

C

Caffeine challenge paradigm, 118, 119
Cardiovascular indices, 220–223, 403,
    404
Career functioning, 59
Caseness threshold, 8–10
Catapres (clonidine), 115, 358
Category decision tasks, 245, 246
Challenge paradigms, 117–120
Child-rearing attitudes, 170, 171
Children, 163–178, 387–418
  assessment, 395–406

clinical presentation, 390–392
  differential diagnosis, 392–395
  peer relationships, 174, 175
  pharmacotherapy, 406–408
  psychophysiology, 403, 404
  psychosocial treatment, 408–410
  shyness development, 163–178
  social phobia continuity, 7, 389, 390
  social phobia prevalence/
    characteristics, 387–395
  temperament, 164, 165
Children's Anxious Self-Statement
    Questionnaire, 400
Children's Cognitive Assessment
    Questionnaire, 400
Christchurch/New Zealand study, 22, 23,
    29
Clinical interview, 185–199
  children/adolescents, 395, 396
  technique, 186–189
Clomipramine (Anafranil), 358
Clonazepam (Klonopin)
  literature review, 348–351
  and neurobiology, 115, 116
  practical guidelines, 375
  selection of, 372
Clonidine (Catapres), 115, 358
  challenge, 125, 126
Cognitive-behavioral group therapy
  adolescents, 410–417
    parent participation, 416, 417
  avoidant personality disorder outcome,
    297
  description of, 286
  exposure treatment comparison, 288,
    289
  long-term outcome, 295, 296
  pharmacological treatment comparison,
    292, 293, 303
  state of mind ratio assessment, 250,
    286, 287
  supportive therapy comparison, 286
Cognitive-behavioral treatments,
    261–333
  clinical applications, 310–331
  literature review, 261–305
  long-term outcome, 294–296, 304
  matching of, 285, 296, 297, 304, 305
  outcome predictors, 296, 297
  pharmacological treatment
    combination, 293, 294, 303, 304

pharmacological treatment comparison,
  291–293, 303
research summary, 298–305
Cognitive processes, 69–70, 232–252
  assessment of, 232–252
  case examples, 77–80, 320–323
  model of, 69–90, 232, 233, 318–323
  and negative beliefs, 71–73
  research review, 77, 81–86
  and self-focused attention, 70–73
  treatment implications, 86–90,
    318–323
Cognitive restructuring, 285, 286
  in adolescents, 409
  exposure treatment combination,
    288–291, 301
  research summary, 301, 302
Cognitive therapy, 283–287
  exposure treatment combination,
    287–291, 323–326
  literature review, 283–287
  pharmacological treatment
    comparison, 291–294
  primary aims, 320
  research summary, 301–307
Cohort effects, 31
Colony-intruder test, 149, 150, 152
Comorbidity, 11–16
  diagnostic issues, 11–16
  and pharmacological treatment,
    379–381
  substance abuse, 57, 58
Composite International Diagnostic
  Interview, 28
Computer-administered rating scales,
  196, 197
Conditioned fear, 134–156
  and behavioral inhibition, 145–148
  generalization, 140
  immunization, 139, 140, 154, 155
  individual differences, 147, 148
  inflation effect, 140
  models, 134–151
  observational effects, 137–139
  preparedness theory, 141–145
  social defeat effects on, 152, 153
  temperamental variables, 145–148
  and trauma, 136, 137
Conflict Behavior Questionnaire, 404
Controllability perceptions (*see*
  Uncontrollability perceptions)

Conversation skills
  behavioral assessment test strategy,
    218, 219
  role-play assessment, 217
  training of, adolescents, 409, 410
Cortisol levels, 125, 126
Cultural studies, 7, 8, 22, 23, 25–27

D

Daily logs, 215, 216
Dating Behavior Assessment Test, 217
Dating relationships, 217, 235, 236
Depression
  comorbidity, 14, 58
  differential diagnosis, 13, 14
  self-schemata, 76
Developmental perspective
  negative beliefs, 76, 77
  shyness, 163–178
  social phobia onset, 54
Dexamethasone suppression test, 125, 126
Diagnostic Interview Schedule, 21–27
Diary assessment, 215, 216
Differential diagnosis, 11–16
Discontinuation of medication, 379
Discrete social phobia (*see* Nongeneralized
  social phobia)
Disinhibition, and phenelzine, 374
Dominance, social
  inescapable shock effects on, 152
  observational conditioning, 138
  and preparedness, 142–144
  social fear origin, 135, 138
Dopamine levels, and extraversion, 126,
    127
Dopaminergic system, 125–127
Dot-probe paradigm, 83, 84, 244, 245
Drug therapy (*see* Pharmacological
  treatments)
DSM-I/DSM-II, 4
DSM-III/DSM-III-R, 4, 5
DSM-IV
  social phobia criteria, 5–9
  social phobia subtyping, 7
Dysfunctional beliefs
  assessment, 236, 237
  case formulation, 320–323
  categories of, 75–77
  and cognitive model, 320–323
  in depression versus social phobia, 76

Dysfunctional beliefs (*continued*)
  development of, 76, 77
  video feedback effects, 88
Dysmorphism, 102, 103

E

Early-developing shyness, 165–168,
  175, 176
East Asia studies, 22, 23, 25–27, 29
Edmonton/Canada study, 22, 23
Educational level, 32
Educational–Supportive Group
  Psychotherapy, 286, 287
Elective mutism (*see* Selective mutism)
Electrodermal activity, 221, 222
Endorsement methods, 250, 251
Epidemiologic Catchment Area study, 12,
  22, 23, 25
Epidemiology, 21–36, 387–389
Epinephrine challenge, 118
Escape behavior, 219
Ethological models, 134–156
Evolutionary perspective, 135, 141–145
Expectancies, assessment, 235, 236
Exposure techniques, 280–282
  in adolescents, 408, 409, 412–417
  as "challenge" paradigm, 120
  clinical application, 316–318
  cognitive model implications, 89, 319,
    320
  cognitive treatment combination,
    287–291, 301, 302, 318
    clinical application, 323–326
  limitations in social phobia, 300, 319
  literature review, 280–282
  long-term outcome, 294–296, 300
  pharmacological treatment
    comparison, 291–299
  research summary, 300, 301
Extraversion, dopamine levels, 126, 127

F

Facial expressions, 82–84, 153
Family Anxiety Coding Schedule, 404,
  405
Family environment
  childhood anxiety, assessment, 404, 405
  shyness antecedent, 168–172
  social phobia mediation, 56

Family Environment Scale, 404
Family studies, 32–36, 120–122
  behaviorally inhibited children, 121,
    122
  generalized versus nongeneralized
    social phobia, 34, 35
  shyness, 164
  social phobia rates, 32–36, 121
Fear of femininity, 173
Fear of negative evaluation
  cognitive model, 70–73
  as core social phobia feature, 45, 51
  development of, 54
  treatment outcome predictor, 297
Fear of Negative Evaluation Scale, 51,
  201–212
  in adolescents, 397
  clinical change sensitivity, 247, 248
  factor analysis, 248
  psychometrics, 206, 210–212, 247
  in social phobia assessment, 211, 212,
    247, 248
Fear Questionnaire, 190, 207, 213, 214
Fear Survey Schedule, 214
Fears, 42–46
Fenfluramine challenge, 125
Florence/Italy study, 22, 23, 29
Fluoxetine (Prozac)
  in elective mutism, 116, 407
  literature review, 352, 353, 355
  and neurobiology, 115–117
  practical guidelines, 375, 376
  selection of, 373
Fluvoxamine (Luvox), 353, 354, 373
Friendships, and shyness, 174, 175

G

Gender differences
  shyness, 172, 173
  social phobia prevalence, 29, 30, 55, 56
  in treatment seeking, 55, 56
Gender roles, and shyness, 172, 173
Generalized anxiety disorder
  in children, 393
  diagnosis, 13, 16, 17
  familial transmission, 34, 35
Generalized social phobia
  avoidant personality disorder overlap,
    14, 15
  childhood prevalence, 389

child-rearing influences on, 171, 172
and cognitive-behavioral treatment,
outcome, 297
diagnostic issues, 5–7
dysfunctional beliefs development, 77
heart rate reactivity, 44, 222
versus nongeneralized social phobia,
symptoms, 44, 45
phenelzine response, 336
versus public speaking phobia, heart
rate, 222
traumatic conditioning, 136, 137
Genetics, 32–36, 120–122
Group-administered exposure, 282
Group therapy (*see* Cognitive-behavioral
group therapy)
Growth hormone, clonidine challenge,
125, 126

H

Heart rate, 220–222
children, 403, 404
in orthostatic challenge paradigm, 119
in psychophysiological assessment,
220–222
reactivity, 44
social phobics' estimation of, 82
treatment outcome measure, 222
Help seeking, 55, 56
Heritability index, 35
Heterosexual Adequacy Test, 217
Heterosocial Skill Observational Rating
System, 218
Heterosocial skills, 217–219, 235, 236
Hypothalamic–pituitary–adrenal axis,
124–126
Hypothalamic–pituitary–thyroid axis,
123, 124
Hypothyroidism, 124

I

Imipramine
literature review, 356
and neurobiology, 115–117
Immunization to conditioned fear, 139,
140, 154, 155
Impression motivation (*see* Self-
presentation model)
In vivo exposure (*see* Exposure techniques)

Inderal (*see* Propranolol)
Inescapable shock studies, 148–150,
152, 153
Inflated fear effect, 140
Interaction Anxiousness Scale, 206, 212
Internal–External Locus of Control
Scale, 237
Interpersonal hypersensivity, 370
Interviewing (*see* Clinical interview)
Intimate self-disclosure, 173
Introversion, avoidance conditioning,
147, 148
"Inverted-U anxiety effects," 49
Irrational Beliefs Test, 236, 237
Issues Checklist, 404

K

Klonopin (*see* Clonazepam)

L

Lactate infusions, 118
Late-developing shyness, 165–168, 175, 176
Learned helplessness, 151, 152
Lehrer–Woolfolk Anxiety Symptom
Questionnaire, 214
Levenson Locus of Control Scale, 237, 238
Levodopa challenge, 125
Lexical decision tasks, 245, 246
Liebowitz Social Anxiety Scale, 43, 193,
194, 196
Lifetime prevalence, 21–28
Locus of Control Scale, 237, 238
Loneliness, shyness correlation, 59
Luvox (fluvoxamine), 353, 354, 373

M

Maintenance pharmacotherapy, 379
Manerix (*see* Moclobemide)
Marital status, 30, 31, 58
Matched treatments (*see* Treatment
matching)
Maternal characteristics, 56, 169–172
Matson Evaluation of Social Skills with
Youngsters, 399
McCroskey's Shyness Scale, 213
Medical illness (*see* Secondary social phobia)
Memory biases, 52, 246, 247
MMPI-2, 214

Moclobemide (Aurorix, Manerix)
  literature review, 340, 341
  phenelzine comparison, 337, 338
  practical guidelines, 376
  selection of, 372
Monoamine oxidase inhibitors, 334–344
    (*see also* Phenelzine)
  literature review, 334–344, 359
  neurobiological aspects, 114–117, 127
  practical guidelines, 373–375
  selection of, 371, 372
Motoric assessment, 214–219
Musicians, 346, 356, 373

N

Nardil (*see* Phenelzine)
National Comorbidity Survey, 27, 28
Negative thoughts
  in children, 401, 402
  cognitive model, 50, 51, 71–73,
    320–323
  psychopathology correlation, 249, 250
  and safety behaviors, 73
  and self-schemata, 76, 77, 81, 82
  shyness versus social phobia, 72
  in state of mind ratio, 249, 250
Nongeneralized social phobia
  child-rearing influences on, 171, 172
  and cognitive-behavioral treatment
    outcome, 297
  diagnosis, 16, 17
  dysfunctional beliefs development, 77
  versus generalized social phobia,
    symptoms, 44
  heart rate reactivity, 44
  phenelzine response, 336
  traumatic conditioning, 136, 137
Noradrenergic system, 125, 126
Norepinephrine levels, 119

O

Observational conditioning, 137–139
Obsessive–compulsive disorder, 380
Occupational functioning, 59

P

Panic attacks, 13
Panic disorder with agoraphobia, 12, 13,
    25

Paradoxical strategies, 325
Parental characteristics, 56, 168–172
Parkinson's disease, 127
Parnate (tranylcypromine), 115, 339, 371
Paruresis, 380
Peer relations, and shyness, 174, 175
Perception of uncontrollability (*see*
    Uncontrollability perceptions)
Performance fears
  beta blockers in, 376, 377
  versus social interaction fears, 43
Personal Report of Communication, 213
Personal Report of Confidence as a
    Speaker, 207, 212, 213
Pharmacological treatments
  in children/adolescents, 406–408
  clinical applications, 366–381
  cognitive-behavioral treatment
    combination, 293, 294, 303, 304
  cognitive-behavioral treatment
    comparison, 291–293, 303
  and comorbidity, 379–381
  literature review, 334–361
  maintenance and discontinuation, 379
  and neurobiology, 114–117
  nonresponder strategies, 378, 379
  practical guidelines, 373–378
  rationale, 369, 370
  selection of, 371–373
  and social phobia evaluation, 367–369
Phenelzine (Nardil), 335–339
  cognitive-behavioral treatment
    comparison, 292, 293, 303
  disinhibition side effect, 374
  dosage, 374
  literature review, 335–339
  neurobiological aspects, 114–117
  practical guidelines, 373–375
  in secondary social phobia, 338, 339
  selection of, 371, 372
  in selective mutism, 407
  side effects, 338, 371, 372, 374
Photoplethysmography, 220
Physical attractiveness, 102, 176, 177
Physical impairments/disfigurements,
    380, 381
Physiological assessment, 219–223
Positive thoughts, 249, 250
Postevent processing, 74, 75, 85, 86
"Power of nonnegative thinking," 249
Preattentive processing, 144, 244, 245
Predator fears, 137, 138

Preparedness factors, 141–145
Prevalence, 21–32, 387–389
Probability–Cost Questionnaire, 236
Problem-solving skills training, 284
Propranolol (Inderal)
 in clinical populations, 344–347
 cognitive-behavioral treatment
  combination, 293, 294
 in nonclinical populations, 344
 practical guidelines, 376, 377
Prozac (*see* Fluoxetine)
Psychophysiological assessment,
 219–223, 403, 404
Public self-consciousness, 51, 52, 176, 177
Public speaking anxiety
 behavioral assessment test strategy,
  218, 219
 heart rate, 44, 222
 inverted-U effects, 49
 psychophysiological assessment, 221,
  222
 role-play assessment, 218
Puerto Rico/United States study, 22, 23
Pulse rate, 221, 222 (*see also* Heart rate)

Q

Questionnaire strategy, 247, 248

R

Rational Behavior Inventory, 236, 237
Rational–emotive therapy
 and exposure, 302
 long-term outcome, 295
 relative effectiveness, 284
 treatment matching, 296
Rational self-talk, 289
Rejection hypersensitivity, 370
Relaxation strategies
 literature review, 279, 280, 284, 285
 research summary, 299, 300
 treatment matching, 296, 297
REM latency, 123
Respiratory measures, 221
Reversible monoamine oxidase A
 inhibitors, 339–342, 359, 372, 376
Revised Children's Manifest Anxiety
 Scale, 397, 405
Role-plays, 214, 216–218
 social skill assessment, 216–218
 and thought recall, 249

S

Safety behaviors, 73, 84
 and cognitive model, 320–323
 intervention, 87, 325
 outcome link, 73
 research review, 84
Saudi Arabia study, 7, 8
Schedule for Affective Disorders and
 Schizophrenia, 191, 192
Schizophrenia spectrum disorders, 15
School refusal, 388
Secondary social phobia
 diagnosis, 11
 phenelzine treatment, 338, 339, 380, 381
Selective mutism
 drug studies, 115, 116
 pharmacotherapy, 407
 social phobia relationship, 394
Selective serotonin reuptake inhibitors (*see*
 Serotonin reuptake inhibitors)
Self-Consciousness Scale, 213
Self-control desensitization, 283, 299
Self-discrepancy theory, 239–241
Self-efficacy expectations, 104
Self-Efficacy Questionnaire for Social
 Skills, 235, 236
Self-esteem
 assessment in children/adolescents, 398
 shyness relationship, 175–177
 and trait social anxiety, 101
Self-focused attention
 cognitive model, 51, 70–73
 modification of, 326
 research review, 82–84
 treatment techniques, 87, 88, 326
Self-instructional training, 284, 285, 317
Self-monitoring methods, 215, 216, 402
Self-Perception Profile for Children, 398
Self-presentation model, 94–108
 interpersonal behavior implications,
  105–107
 and state social anxiety, 98–100
 theoretical aspects, 95–98
 and trait social anxiety, 101–105
 treatment implications, 107, 108
Self-Rating Scale, 176, 177
Self-report
 available instruments, 204–214
 in children and adolescents, 397–399
Self-schemata, 75–77
 assessment, 239–241

Self-schemata (*continued*)
  categories of, 75–77
  cognitive intervention, 327–331
Selves Questionnaire, 240, 241
Semistructured clinical interviews,
  190–199
Seoul/South Korea study, 22, 23, 26, 29
Separation stress, monkeys, 155
Serotonergic system, 125, 126
Serotonin reuptake inhibitors
  in elective mutism, 116
  literature review, 352–355, 359
  neurobiological aspects, 115–117
  practical guidelines, 375, 376
  selection of, 373
Sex roles, and shyness, 172, 173
Sexual dysfunction, 146, 147
Shame, 27, 171, 172
Shyness (*see also* Behavioral inhibition)
  developmental factors, 163–178, 390
  early versus late development of,
    165–168
  family environmental antecedents,
    168–172
  gender differences, 172, 173
  longitudinal study, 166–168
  and peer relations, 174, 175
  prevalence, 10, 11
  self-esteem relationship, 175–177
  and sex roles, 172, 173
  social cognition, 72
  social phobia relationship, 10, 11, 41, 42
  socialization processes, 172–175
  subtypes, 43, 44
  temperamental factors, 164, 165, 390
  typology, 165, 166
Simulated Social Interaction Text, 216,
  217
Situation Questionnaire, 213
Situational Expectancies Inventory, 235,
  236
Skin conductance responses, 221, 222
Sleep physiology, 122, 123
Snake fears, 137, 138, 141, 142
Sociability, and shyness, 59
Social Anxiety Scale for Children—
  Revised, 398, 405
Social Avoidance and Distress Scale, 206,
  210–212, 397
Social defeat effects, 150–154
Social dominance (*see* Dominance, social)

Social Effectiveness Therapy, 282
Social Interaction Anxiety Scale, 205–208
Social Interaction Self-Statement Test,
  250, 251
Social Interaction Test, 217
Social Phobia and Anxiety Inventory,
  206–210
Social Phobia and Anxiety Inventory for
  Children, 398, 405
Social Phobia Scale, 205–208
Social phobia subtypes, 43–45
  and cognitive-behavioral treatment
    outcome, 297, 304
  descriptive issues, 43–45
  diagnosis, 16, 17
  quantitative interpretation, 45
Social rejection, 174, 175
Social Reticence Scale, 213
Social skills
  assessment in children/adolescents, 399
  performance deficits in, 299
  role-play tests, 216–218
  social anxiety effects on, 48–50
Social skills training, 262–279
  adolescents, 408–410, 412
  clinical application, 316
  and cognitive restructuring, 278
  exposure comparison, 278
  literature review, 262–279, 298, 299
  long-term outcome, 295
  and propranolol, 279, 304
  research summary, 298, 299
  systematic desensitization comparison,
    262, 276, 277
  treatment matching, 296, 297
Socioeconomic status, 32
Sodium lactate infusions, 118
Specific social phobia (*see* Nongeneralized
  social phobia)
Stanford Shyness Survey, 213
State of mind ratio, 249, 250, 286, 287
State social anxiety, 98–100
State–Trait Anxiety Inventory for
  Children, 397, 405
Stress immunization, 139, 140, 154, 155
Stroop task, 242–244
Structured Clinical Interview for
  DSM-III-R, 191, 192
Structured clinical interviews, 190, 191,
  203, 204, 395, 396
Stuttering, 380, 381

Subliminal conditioning, 144
Submissive behaviors
  conditioning, 138, 142–144
  function of, 107
  preparedness theory, 142–144
  social defeat effect, animals, 150–154
  and uncontrollability perceptions,
    148–150
Substance abuse, comorbidity, 57, 58
Subtyping (*see* Social phobia subtypes)
Suicidal ideation, 58
Suicide attempts, 58
Switzerland study, 28
Symptom Checklist-90-R, 214
Symptom Rating Scales, 193–197
Systematic desensitization
  research summary, 299
  social skills training comparison, 262,
    276, 277
Systematic rational restructuring, 283, 299

T

T₃/T₄ levels, 124, 126
Taijin kyofu-sho, 8, 26, 27
Taipei/Taiwan study, 22, 23, 25
Taped Situation Test, 217
Teenage Inventory of Social Skills, 399
Temperament (*see also* Behavioral
    inhibition)
  and conditioning, 145–148
  family studies, 164
  shyness predisposition, 164, 165, 390
Test anxiety
  in children, 393, 394
  cognitive restructuring, 409
  social phobia relationship, 11, 47
  and test performance, 47
Therapist-assisted guided exposure, 290
Think-aloud procedure, 400, 401
Thought listing, 248, 249, 401
Three-response-systems approach, 202
Thyroid function abnormalities, 123, 124
Thyrotropin-releasing hormone infusion,
    124, 126
Thyroxine levels, 124, 126
Timed Behavioral Checklist, 218
Timidity, 145–147, 150–154

Tofranil (*see* Imipramine)
Trait social anxiety, 101–105
Tranylcypromine (Parnate), 115, 339, 371
Traumatic conditioning, 136, 137
Treatment matching
  clinical value of, 317, 318
  cognitive-behavioral treatments, 285,
    304
  and outcome, 296, 297, 304, 305
  and self-presentation model, 107, 108
Treatment nonresponse, 378, 379
TRH stimulation test, 124, 126
Tricyclic antidepressants, 356, 358, 373
Triiodothyronine levels, 124, 126
Twin studies, 32, 35, 120, 121, 164

U

Unconditional beliefs, 76, 77
Uncontrollability perceptions
  animal studies, 148–150
  and fear conditioning, 148–150
  immunization, 154, 155
  social anxiety role, 148–155
  social defeat parallel, 150–154
  and social dominance change, 152
  in social phobics, 155, 156
  stress-induced analgesia relationship,
    153
  submissiveness increases, 148–150

V

Vicarious conditioning, 137–139
Video feedback, 88, 249
Visual dot-probe paradigm, 83, 84, 244,
    245

W

Wellbutrin (*see* Bupropion)
Willoughby Personality Schedule, 214
Winnipeg/Canada study, 28
Work functioning, 59

X

Xanax (*see* Alprazolam)